101 746 881 8

SHEFFIELD HALLAM UNIVERSITY
LEARNING CENTRE
COLLEGIATE CRESCENT CAMPUS
SHEFFIELD S10 2BP

C ... ITION

DIAGNOSTIC
RADIOLOGY

Multiple Choice Questions

ONE WEEK LOAN

Sheffield Hallam University
Learning and Information Services
Withdrawn From Stock

Commissioning Editor: Michael J. Houston
Project Development Manager: Louise Cook
Project Manager: The Partnership Publishing Solutions
Designer: Sarah Russell

Grainger & Allison's

FOURTH EDITION

DIAGNOSTIC RADIOLOGY
Multiple Choice Questions

Compiled by

Adam W.M. Mitchell MB BS, FRCS, FRCR
Consultant Radiologist, Charing Cross Hospital
Honorary Senior Lecturer, Imperial College
School of Medicine
London, UK

John F. Cockburn MB BCh, MRCP, FRCR, FFRRCSI
Consultant Radiologist
Norfolk and Norwich University Hospital
Norwich, UK

Adrian Lim MB BS, FRCR
Radiology Fellow
Department of Imaging Sciences
Faculty of Medicine
Imperial College School of Medicine
Hammersmith Hospital
London, UK

Edited by

Ronald G. Grainger MB ChB (Hon), MD, FRCP,
DMRD, RFCR, FACR (Hon), FRACR (Hon)
Emeritus Professor of Diagnostic Radiology
University of Sheffield
Honorary Consultant Radiologist
Royal Hallamshire Hospital
and Northern General Hospital
Sheffield, UK

David J. Allison BSc, MD, FRCR, FRCP
Formerly Professor of Imaging
Imperial College School of Medicine
Hammersmith Hospital
London, UK

Andreas Adam MB BS(Hons), FRCP, FRCR, FRCS
Professor of Interventional Radiology
United Medical and Dental Schools of Guy's
and St Thomas' Hospitals
London, UK

Adrian K. Dixon MD, FRCR, FRCP, FMedSci
Professor of Radiology
Addenbrooke's Hospital
University of Cambridge
Cambridge, UK

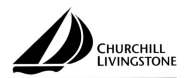

CHURCHILL
LIVINGSTONE

EDINBURGH   LONDON   NEW YORK   OXFORD   PHILADELPHIA   ST LOUIS   SYDNEY   TORONTO   2004

CHURCHILL LIVINGSTONE
An imprint of Elsevier Limited

© 2004, Elsevier Limited. All rights reserved.

The right of Adam WM Mitchell, John C Cookson and Adrian Lim to be identified as authors of this work has been asserted by them in accordance with the Copyright, Designs and Patents Act 1988

No part of this publication may be reproduced, stored in a retrieval system, or transmitted in any form or by any means, electronic, mechanical, photocopying, recording or otherwise, without either the prior permission of the publishers or a licence permitting restricted copying in the United Kingdom issued by the Copyright Licensing Agency, 90 Tottenham Court Road, London W1T 4LP. Permissions may be sought directly from Elsevier's Health Sciences Rights Department in Philadelphia, USA: phone: (+1) 215 238 7869, fax: (+1) 215 238 2239, e-mail: healthpermissions@elsevier.com. You may also complete your request on-line via the Elsevier homepage (http://www.elsevier.com), by selecting 'Customer Support' and then 'Obtaining Permissions'.

First published 2004

ISBN 044307254X

British Library Cataloguing in Publication Data
A catalogue record for this book is available from the British Library

Library of Congress Cataloging in Publication Data
A catalog record for this book is available from the Library of Congress

Notice
Medical knowledge is constantly changing. Standard safety precautions must be followed, but as new research and clinical experience broaden our knowledge, changes in treatment and drug therapy may become necessary or appropriate. Readers are advised to check the most current product information provided by the manufacturer of each drug to be administered to verify the recommended dose, the method and duration of administration, and contraindications. It is the responsibility of the practitioner, relying on experience and knowledge of the patient, to determine dosages and the best treatment for each individual patient. Neither the Publisher nor the authors nor editors assume any liability for any injury and/or damage to persons or property arising from this publication.

The Publisher

The publisher's policy is to use paper manufactured from sustainable forests

Printed in China

Contents

Foreword

Multiple choice questions (MCQs) continue to be of increasing importance as a means of checking the knowledge base of examination candidates. With 'competence' coming under increasing public scrutiny, the fact that a candidate has reached a certain standard in an MCQ provides one objective measure that he or she knows their subject. In addition, an MCQ test is a useful reminder to more senior practitioners that they may have forgotten some aspects of their trade since they qualified!

The authors are to be congratulated in producing these fresh looking questions based on the contents of the fourth edition of Grainger & Allison's *Diagnostic Radiology*. The setting of good, clear and un-ambiguous MCQs is an art form of its own. The range of knowledge tested impressed all of those involved in checking these questions. Perhaps the most stimulating feature was the way the questions and answers prompted a re-read of appropriate sections of the textbook. Especially in areas where the scores were poor!

Some people, unfortunately, find MCQs more difficult than others, even when they seem to have mastered the literature. Practice, practice and more practice is the only real answer. This book, prepared by a group of very enthusiastic radiologists, provides every opportunity.

RG Grainger
DJ Allison
A Adam
AK Dixon

Editorial advice on using this MCQ book

This MCQ book is carefully based on the fourth edition of Grainger & Allison's *Diagnostic Radiology*. All of the answers to these MCQs are supplied in the parent book, and every question and answer is cross-referenced from the MCQ book to the chapter and page of the Grainger and Allison fourth edition. The MCQ book can of course also be used by those persons preferring other parent texts or monographs on specific body systems. Whatever the preferred parent book, the reader should carefully study the appropriate chapter(s) or body systems before attempting the relevant questions in this book.

Many varied format and marking systems are used by different Examination Boards.

ALWAYS CAREFULLY READ THE INSTRUCTIONS OF YOUR EXAMINATION BOARD AT LEAST TWICE BEFORE ATTEMPTING THE ANSWERS.

This book uses the current format (1997) of the Royal College of Radiologists (UK) – 2 papers of 2 hours, each containing 60 randomized questions on imaging and related clinicopathological aspects.

There is a common stem with 5 related questions, each of which should be answered **True** or **False**. Each correct answer gains a point and each incorrect answer loses a point. A **'don't know'** or **no answer** neither gains nor loses a point. **All** of the 5 questions may be True or False, permitting the score for each stem to range from +5 to –5.

Our advice to the readers is to develop their own strategy and timing for answering MCQs by extensive practice on many MCQ papers and books. During the actual examination use the strategy and system that you prefer and with which you are most at ease.
We suggest you practise the following approach:

A. Draw three columns for your answers

Column 1	*Column 2*	*Column 3*
I know this answer	I think I know the answer I'm having an educated guess	I don't have a clue

B. Whilst practising, always place your answer to each question in one of these columns. Always mark your confident answers first, but never leave out an answer to any question.

C. At the end of the simulated practice examinations, add up your answers in each column and work out your percentage accuracy in each group. Only then can you reach a decision on whether you are good guesser or not.

Many authorities advise that if you consistently answer about 80% of the questions and about 80% of your answers are correct, it may well be advisable not to attempt the pure guesswork answers in column 3, as that approach may lose you valuable points.

Most examination Boards advise that the examinee enters his/her choice of True or False answers into the question booklet in the first instance, before transferring them into the definitive answer sheet. Ensure that there is ample time within the allocated examination time to permit this essential transfer of your data to the answer book. Don't rush this transfer as your examination performance depends on it.

Repeated practice on as many MCQs as you can obtain will much improve your performance. Don't panic, be methodical, keep to the allotted time and don't cheat in your practice tests. Enjoy this learning process and good luck in your examinations.

Acknowledgements

Many thanks to Michelle Balmer and Sheryl Banks who helped with typing of the MCQs (**AL**).

With thanks to Dr. Deborah Browne for her love, wisdom and managerial prowess (**JC**).

To Cathy, Elsa and Max (**AM**).

1 Imaging techniques and modalities

Q 1.1 Regarding radioactivity and radioactive substances

A. Nuclides with the same mass number (A) but different atomic number (Z) are referred to as isotopes.

B. Isotopes have the same chemical and, therefore, biological behaviour.

C. Gamma rays and X-rays differ only by the way they are produced.

D. One milliSievert (1 mSv) is equivalent to 1 milliCoulomb per kilogram ($mCKg^{-1}$).

E. The half-life of metastable technetium-99m (^{99m}Tc) is approximately 6 hours.

Q 1.2 Regarding radioactive decay

A. Alpha decay results in the mass number (A) decreasing by two and the atomic number (Z) decreasing by 1.

B. Beta decay occurs when radionuclides with excess protons decay.

C. Beta particles are readily detected outside the body using a dosimeter.

D. When a positron combines with an electron two photons are produced.

E. The rate of decay of an isotope slows down with time.

(Answers overleaf)

A 1.2 Regarding radioactivity and radioactive substances

A. False Nuclides have the same atomic number but different mass numbers.
Ch. 6 Radionuclide Imaging: General Principles, p. 138.

B. True The atomic number is the number of protons (and hence orbiting electrons). The chemical properties of a substance depend on the number of orbiting electrons, and, as isotopes share this number, their chemical properties are the same.
Ch. 6 Radionuclide Imaging: General Principles, p. 138.

C. True They are both forms of electromagnetic radiation. If this originates in the nucleus the product is gamma radiation. If it originates from transformations involving orbital electrons, X-radiation is the result.
Ch. 6 Radionuclide Imaging: General Principles, p. 138.

D. False The Sievert (Sv) is the unit of dose equivalent otherwise expressed in Joules per kg. The unit of exposure is coulomb per Kg previously known as a roentgen.
Ch. 6 Table 6.1, p. 138.

E. True
Ch. 6 Table 6.2, p. 139.

A 1.2 Regarding radioactive decay

A. False Release of an alpha particle results in the mass number decreasing by four and the atomic number by two.
Ch. 6 Radionuclide Imaging: General Principles, p. 139.

B. False Radionuclides with excess neutrons decay by beta emission as expressed by the formula: $^A_ZX = \,^A_{Z+1}Y + \,^0_{-1}e$ + neutrino where $^0_{-1}e$ represents an electron.
Ch. 6 Radionuclide Imaging: General Principles, p. 139.

C. False These high-speed electrons have a short range in tissue and are difficult to detect outside the body.
Ch. 6 Radionuclide Imaging: General Principles, p. 140.

D. True This annihilation reaction is the principle of positron emission tomography.
Ch. 6 Radionuclide Imaging: General Principles, p. 140.

E. False The rate of decay is constant for each radionuclide. The amount of radioactivity reduces with time.
Ch. 6 Radionuclide Imaging: General Principles, p. 140.

Q **1.3**   Concerning imaging in nuclear medicine

A. Pure sodium iodide crystals are the best light emitters for use in gamma cameras.

B. In a gamma camera there are approximately 70 photomultiplier tubes.

C. The collimator in the gamma camera acts as a lens to focus the gamma rays onto the crystal.

D. In a PET scanner mechanical collimation is used to achieve tomographic images.

E. Dedicated PET cameras use sodium iodide crystals as detectors.

Q **1.4**   Regarding radiopharmaceuticals

A. ^{99m}Tc DMSA is retained in the renal cortex.

B. ^{99m}Tc – pertechnetate is used to assess salivary duct patency.

C. ^{99m}Tc – pertechnetate is used to localize Meckel's diverticulum containing gastric mucosa.

D. ^{99m}Tc-labelled red cells are used to detect the site of occult GI blood loss.

E. ^{111}In-pentatreotide acts as a somatostatin analogue that binds to somatostatin receptor positive neuroendocrine tumours.

(Answers overleaf)

A **1.3** Concerning imaging in nuclear medicine

A. False The amount of light emitted from a sodium iodide crystal is increased if a small amount of thallium is added during the growing of the crystal.
Ch. 6 Radionuclide Imaging: General Principles, p. 142.

B. True From the relative sizes of signals from each of these tubes it is possible to decode the X and Y co-ordinates of the photon's interaction with the NaI crystal.
Ch. 6 Radionuclide Imaging: General Principles, p. 142.

C. False X-rays and gamma rays cannot be focused. The function of the parallel hole collimator is to allow through only those rays that are perpendicular to the face of the crystal.
Ch. 6 Radionuclide Imaging: General Principles, p. 142.

D. False Mechanical collimation is not needed because the detector circuitry registers an event only when two co-incidental photons strike the detector pair at almost exactly the same time.
Ch. 6 Radionuclide Imaging: General Principles, p. 144.

E. False The crystal is made from bismuth germanate (BGO). This is the optimal material for detecting 511 keV gamma rays running at high count rates.
Ch. 6 Radionuclide Imaging: General Principles, p. 142.

A **1.4** Regarding radiopharmaceuticals

A. True This is the basis of the DMSA scan that images the number of functioning cortical nephrons.
Ch. 6 Radionuclide Imaging: General Principles, p. 146.

B. True There is active uptake and excretion by the salivary glands.
Ch. 6 Radionuclide Imaging: General Principles, p. 146.

C. True There is active uptake by gastric mucosa.
Ch. 6 Radionuclide Imaging: General Principles, p. 146.

D. True There is extravasation into bowel lumen allowing the pool of signal to be detected.
Ch. 6 Radionuclide Imaging: General Principles, p. 146.

E. True

Ch. 6 Radionuclide Imaging: General Principles, p. 146.

Q **1.5** Regarding the properties of radiopharmaceuticals

A. Pure gamma-ray emitters are preferable for imaging purposes.
B. Allergic reaction to the injection of radiopharmaceutical is less common than with iodinated contrast media.
C. Right heart failure is a potential side effect of ventilation-perfusion scanning.
D. ^{131}Iodine emits gamma rays that are useful in controlling thyrotoxicosis.
E. Urinary excretion of ^{99m}Tc-cyanocobalamin is measured as a test of vitamin B_{12} absorption.

Q **1.6** Factors leading to increased risk of vascular complications from arteriography include

A. Cushing's syndrome.
B. Ehlers-Danlos syndrome Type IV.
C. Systemic hypertension.
D. Wedged catheter position in a vessel.
E. Factor 3 deficiency.

(Answers overleaf)

A **1.5** Regarding the properties of radiopharmaceuticals

A. True Particle emission, Auger electrons and characteristic X-radiation add to patient dose without contributing to the image.
Ch. 6 Radionuclide Imaging: General Principles, p. 146.

B. True In a recent 5-year study of over 750 000 radiopharmaceutical injections no adverse reactions requiring hospitalization were recorded.
Ch. 6 Radionuclide Imaging: General Principles, p. 147.

C. True A sudden increase in pulmonary vascular resistance due to capillary blockage by macroaggregated albumin can exacerbate right heart failure.
Ch. 6 Radionuclide Imaging: General Principles, p. 147.

D. False It emits beta particles that deliver the ablative radiation dose locally in thyroid tissue.
Ch. 6 Radionuclide Imaging: General Principles, p. 147.

E. False ^{57}Cobalt has a longer half-life that is necessary for the Schilling test and is used to label the cyanocobalamin.
Ch. 6 Radionuclide Imaging: General Principles, p. 147.

A **1.6** Factors leading to increased risk of vascular complications from arteriography include

A. True Increased vessel fragility in this condition makes bruising more likely and more extensive.
Ch. 7 Principles, Techniques and Complications of Angiography, p. 150.

B. True Aneurysm formation at the puncture site and at internal sites of even minor catheter-related trauma are complications of angiography in this condition.
Ch. 7 Principles, Techniques and Complications of Angiography, p. 150.

C. True On withdrawal of the catheter, compression above the arterial systolic pressure is required to effect haemostasis. Systemic hypertension, particularly in the obese patient makes bleeding at the puncture site more likely.
Ch. 7 Principles, Techniques and Complications of Angiography, p. 150.

D. True This position predisposes to intimal tears and vessel occlusion, as well as in-situ thrombosis due to stasis. During embolization procedures with particles, wedged catheters predispose to the delivery of embolic material retrogradely towards non-target organs.
Ch. 7 Principles, Techniques and Complications of Angiography, p. 150.

E. False This has not been shown to lead to increased risk of complications of angiography.
Ch. 7 Principles, Techniques and Complications of Angiography, p. 150.

Q **1.7** Regarding angiographic technique

A. During the initial arterial puncture, if there is resistance to passage of the guidewire through the needle, firm forward pressure should be applied.

B. The brachial artery lies lateral to the biceps tendon in the antecubital fossa.

C. During 'axillary' artery puncture, it is the brachial artery that should be punctured.

D. A 5 Fr sheath is recommended for radial arterial puncture.

E. During percutaneous injection of thrombin into a femoral artery pseudoaneurysm, the patient should be anticoagulated to minimize the effects of distal embolization.

Q **1.8** Regarding dual energy X-ray absorptiometry (DXA)

A. For every reduction of one standard deviation in bone mineral density the fracture risk doubles.

B. Osteopenia is defined as a bone mineral density greater than one standard deviation below the age and sex-matched control.

C. Osteoporosis is defined as a bone mineral density greater than 2.5 standard deviations below the young adult mean.

D. In the normal skeleton there is a progressive increase in bone mineral density caudally down the spine.

E. Patients on steroid therapy are likely to fracture at a higher bone mineral density than the ordinary osteoporotic population.

(Answers overleaf)

A **1.7** Regarding angiographic technique

A. False Firm pressure has no place in the manipulation of a guidewire through a needle.
Ch. 7 Principles, Techniques and Complications of Angiography, p. 152.

B. False It lies medial to the biceps tendon in the antecubital fossa.
Ch. 7 Principles, Techniques and Complications of Angiography, p. 153.

C. True The most proximal portion of the brachial artery is cannulated.
Ch. 7 Principles, Techniques and Complications of Angiography, p. 153.

D. False 4 Fr or 3 Fr micropuncture systems are used to minimize the risk of arterial injury and occlusion. Furthermore, many operators routinely administer vasodilators to reduce spasm in the radial artery.
Ch. 7 Principles, Techniques and Complications of Angiography, p. 153.

E. False Femoral arterial pseudoaneurysms arise after inadequate compression of a puncture site. The neck of the lesion is often tiny and well-suited to the injection of 500 or 1000 units of thrombin. Anticoagulation is not required as distal embolization is rare. Compression of a pseudoaneurysm is an alternative technique using an ultrasound probe to identify and then compress the aneurysm neck. It is painful and time consuming, however.
Ch. 7 Principles, Techniques and Complications of Angiography, p. 177.

A **1.8** Regarding dual energy X-ray absorptiometry (DXA)

A. True
Ch. 8 Dual Energy X-ray Absorptiometry, p. 185.

B. False Greater than one standard deviation below the young adult mean.
Ch. 8 Dual Energy X-ray Absorptiometry, p. 188.

C. True
Ch. 8 Dual Energy X-ray Absorptiometry, p. 188.

D. True
Ch. 8 Dual Energy X-ray Absorptiometry, p. 189.

E. True A bone mineral density greater than 1.5 standard deviations less than the young adult mean is an indication for mineral preserving treatment in this group.
Ch. 8 Dual Energy X-ray Absorptiometry, p. 188.

Q **1.9**   **Causes of errors in DXA measurements include**

    A. Aortic calcification.
    B. Paget's disease.
    C. X-ray contrast media.
    D. Vertebral compression fractures.
    E. Anorexia nervosa.

Q **1.10**   **Concerning ultrasound**

    A. The wavelength of the diagnostic insonant ultrasound beam is roughly between 1 and 0.1 mm.
    B. Ultrasound travels more quickly in fat than in watery soft tissue.
    C. Flow reversal in the carotid bulb indicates significant stenosis.
    D. Flow reversal during diastole in the external carotid artery indicates a significant narrowing.
    E. Increased hepatic vein pulsatility is a sign of diffuse liver disease.

(Answers overleaf)

A **1.9** **Causes of errors in DXA measurements include**

A. True May cause a falsely elevated reading.
Ch. 8 Dual Energy X-ray Absorptiometry, p. 192.

B. True May cause an elevated reading masking osteoporosis in unaffected bone.
Ch. 8 Dual Energy X-ray Absorptiometry, p. 192.

C. True Especially barium retained in bowel.
Ch. 8 Table 8.3, p. 192.

D. True When associated with sclerosis there is an elevated bone mineral density.
Ch. 8 Table 8.3, p. 192.

E. True In excessively thin patients, bone edges may be difficult to ascertain. These edges are critical to measurements. Padding with rice bags around the hips may be necessary to simulate soft tissue and allowing accurate estimation of bone edges.
Ch. 8 Dual Energy X-ray Absorptiometry, p. 193.

A **1.10** **Concerning ultrasound**

A. True Velocity = Frequency × wavelength. Wavelength = Velocity divided by frequency. Ultrasound velocity in tissue is 1540 metres per second (1 540 000 mms). The frequency of diagnostic probes varies from around 2 MHz (2 000 000 cycles per second) to 20 MHz. Dividing velocity by frequency yields figures of approximately between 1 and 0.1 mm.
Ch. 3A Ultrasound: General Principles, p. 44.

B. False Approximately 20% more slowly. This makes the depth of echoes arising deep to large fatty regions appear further from the probe than they actually are. An important effect of different velocities at fat/soft tissue interfaces is defocusing and dispersing of the ultrasound beam causing degraded images.
Ch. 3A Ultrasound: General Principles, p. 51.

C. False There is a region on the posterolateral wall of the carotid bulb where flow velocity is normally slow or reversed. This is known as the boundary layer separation zone.
Ch. 3B Vascular Ultrasound, p. 68.

D. False Continuous flow during diastole occurs in a damped waveform beyond a stenosis. Flow reversal may be a normal phenomenon in diastole in this artery due to high peripheral resistance in the external carotid circulation.
Ch. 3B Vascular Ultrasound, p. 68.

E. False Forward flow in the hepatic veins is modulated by cardiac pulsations giving it a complex biphasic appearance. A less pulsatile (damped) hepatic venous trace, however, occurs in diffuse liver disease.
Ch. 3B Vascular Ultrasound, p. 75.

Q **1.11** **Increased through-transmission of ultrasound occurs in the following**

  A. Fibroadenoma.
  B. Hydatid cyst.
  C. Lymphomatous deposits.
  D. Pus.
  E. Haemangioma.

Q **1.12** **Regarding spiral computed tomography (CT)**

  A. Slip rings are required to prevent tangling of cables joining the gantry to the rotating tube-detector assembly.
  B. Spiral CT images are fractionally more sharp than conventional (non-helical) CT images.
  C. Ceramic detectors are now obsolete.
  D. Pitch describes the relationship between the amount of table feed per rotation and the collimator width.
  E. Increasing the pitch lowers the radiation dose.

(Answers overleaf)

A **1.11** **Increased through-transmission of ultrasound occurs in the following**

A. True This tumour in the breast typically has marked 'bright up' beyond it accentuated by dark bands from the edge shadows of its wall.
Ch. 3A Ultrasound: General Principles, p. 53.

B. True Although acoustic shadowing may occur from a calcified cyst wall, through transmission is a feature of non-calcified cysts.
Ch. 3A Ultrasound: General Principles, p. 53.

C. True
Ch. 3A Ultrasound: General Principles, p. 53.

D. True Depending on its fluid content – generally the more fluid, the more through-transmission.
Ch. 3A Ultrasound: General Principles, p. 53.

E. True
Ch. 3A Ultrasound: General Principles, p. 53.

A **1.12** **Regarding spiral computed tomography**

A. True Non-helical systems had to stop and unwind these cables before proceeding with the next slice.
Ch. 4 Whole Body Computed Tomography: Recent Developments, p. 82.

B. False They are slightly less sharp because the slice profile is bell-shaped rather than the sharper rectangular profile of non-helical CT slice profiles.
Ch. 4 Whole Body Computed Tomography: Recent Developments, p. 83.

C. False Most major manufacturers use ceramic detector systems rather than the older xenon detectors. The former have higher photon detection efficiency and are more readily configured into multidetector arrays.
Ch. 4 Whole Body Computed Tomography: Recent Developments, p. 84.

D. True Unfortunately this definition has recently been changed by some manufacturers leading to confusion among radiologists.
Ch. 4 Whole Body Computed Tomography: Recent Developments, p. 83.

E. True The patient travels faster through the radiation beam. Image quality is reduced however.
Ch. 4 Whole Body Computed Tomography: Recent Developments, p. 84.

Q **1.13** Regarding the basic physics of magnetic resonance imaging (MRI)

A. Suitable nuclei for MRI have an even number of protons or neutrons.

B. Magnetic resonance occurs when an applied radiofrequency pulse is applied to protons at the same frequency at which they are precessing.

C. In human tissue T2 is usually ten times longer than T1.

D. Ear plugs are recommended when the peak noise from the gradient coils is 45 dB.

E. Cortical bone does not contain protons.

Q **1.14** Regarding angiography

A. Venography detects undescended testes.

B. Infrapopliteal arterial stenting is the definitive treatment for short below-knee stenoses.

C. Direct injection of bovine thrombin is used to treat fusiform arterial aneurysms.

D. The fovea of the femoral head is a useful radiographic landmark for common femoral artery puncture.

E. Inferior vena caval filters should be placed above the renal veins for maximum efficacy.

(Answers overleaf)

A **1.13**   **Regarding the basic physics of magnetic resonance imaging (MRI)**

A. False   An odd number of protons or neutrons confers a net charge and angular momentum. The hydrogen nucleus with one proton is ubiquitous in tissue and suitable for MRI. Other naturally occurring nuclei that can be studied are phosphorous, carbon, and potassium.
Ch. 5 Magnetic Resonance Imaging: Basic Principles, p. 102.

B. True   This allows radiofrequency energy to be absorbed and the net magnetization to be deviated through an angle that is dependent on the strength and duration of the radiofrequency pulse.
Ch. 5 Magnetic Resonance Imaging: Basic Principles, p. 102.

C. False   T1 (the time taken for nuclei to return to thermal equilibrium) is considerably longer than T2 (the time it takes nuclei to dephase after an RF pulse).
Ch. 5 Magnetic Resonance Imaging: Basic Principles, p. 102.

D. False   When peak noise reaches or exceeds 85 dB ear plugs are required.
Ch. 5 Magnetic Resonance Imaging: Basic Principles, p. 104.

E. False   The protons in cortical bone are bound to large molecules. This renders them immobile and unable to contribute to the MR signal.
Ch. 5 Magnetic Resonance Imaging: Basic Principles, p. 107.

A **1.14**   **Regarding angiography**

A. True   If cross-sectional imaging fails to locate an undescended testis, gonadal venography will demonstrate the pampiniform plexus of veins at the appropriate site. This can be anywhere between ipsilateral kidney and scrotum, but is usually around the inguinal canal.
Ch. 7 Principles, Techniques and Complications of Angiography, p. 164.

B. False   Currently there is no indication for the use of infrapopliteal stents owing to their tendency to early occlusion.
Ch. 7 Principles, Techniques and Complications of Angiography, p. 169.

C. False   Iatrogenic femoral arterial pseudoaneurysms may be occluded by injecting 500–1000 units of thrombin. These lesions lend themselves to this technique by virtue of their relatively small size and tiny communication with the superficial femoral artery.
Ch. 7 Principles, Techniques and Complications of Angiography, p. 177.

D. True
Ch. 7 Principles, Techniques and Complications of Angiography, p. 151.

E. False   Placement below the renal veins is recommended to prevent renal vein thrombosis.
Ch. 7 Principles, Techniques and Complications of Angiography, p. 183.

Q **1.15**   Regarding contrast agent pharmacokinetics

A.   Gadolinium chelate diffuses into the extracellular fluid compartment.

B.   Ultrasound microbubble agents are completely intravascular.

C. ^{99m}Tc-labelled red blood cells are poor blood pool markers.

D.   Gadolinium chelates are suitable agents for measuring transit times through the vessels of various organs.

E.   Hyperpolarized xenon gas is a suitable agent for functional imaging studies in MR.

Q **1.16**   Concerning measurement of tracer concentration

A.   In CT, an increase in iodine density of 1 mg/ml will increase attenuation in a voxel by 25–30 Hounsfield units (HU).

B.   In CT, there is an exponential relationship between the increase in iodine concentration and increase in attenuation in the absence of significant artefacts.

C.   In MR, with a high dose of gadolinium, there is a linear relationship between the increase in T1-weighted signal intensity and parenchymal gadolinium concentration.

D.   Ultrasound microbubbles increase the intensity of spectral Doppler or power Doppler signals.

E.   The fractional vascular volume of a tissue can be measured using microbubbles and the 'flash-reperfusion' technique.

(Answers overleaf)

A **1.15** Regarding contrast agent pharmacokinetics

A. True

Ch. 9 Functional and Physiological Imaging, p. 198.

B. True Thus making them highly suitable for measuring indices of the blood volume and perfusion in all organs.
Ch. 9 Functional and Physiological Imaging, p. 198.

C. False This agent has similar properties to ultrasound microbubble agents and remains only in the intravascular space.
Ch. 9 Functional and Physiological Imaging, p. 198.

D. False These agents are not purely intravascular.
Ch. 9 Functional and Physiological Imaging, p. 198.

E. True

Ch. 9 Functional and Physiological Imaging, p. 198.

A **1.16** Concerning measurement of tracer concentration

A. True There is a linear relationship between iodine concentration and attenuation values (HU).
Ch. 9 Functional and Physiological Imaging, p. 198.

B. False

Ch. 9 Functional and Physiological Imaging, p. 198.

C. False At high gadolinium concentrations, T2* effects start to counteract the positive contrast effects of the T1 shortening. Relative concentration measurements and thus quantitative measurement are only possible at a well-defined, relatively low concentration in which the relationship is linear.
Ch. 9 Functional and Physiological Imaging, p. 198.

D. True

Ch. 9 Functional and Physiological Imaging, p. 199.

E. True The 'flash' or transient pulse of high acoustic power destroys the microbubbles and refilling rates are then observed using a low acoustic power technique; this allows the assessment of microcirculatory flow speeds and the fractional vascular volume of a tissue.
Ch. 9 Functional and Physiological Imaging, p. 199.

Q **1.17** **Regarding functional measurements of vascularity of tissue**

    A. In the body, perfusion is conventionally defined as flow per unit volume.

    B. For 'wash-in' studies, it is important that the tracer agent does not filter into the capillary tissue bed.

    C. In 'wash-out' studies, the time concentration curve declines linearly, provided there is no significant arrival of additional tracer in time.

    D. In functional CT, perfusion through an organ is accurately calculated by taking the ratio of the peak gradient of the tissue time–concentration curve to the peak height of the arterial concentration curve.

    E. The gradient method of calculating tissue perfusion by Miles is limited because it assumes a single type of input vessel.

Q **1.18** **Regarding functional indices**

    A. The fractional vascular volume (FVV) is the fraction of tissue occupied by blood and corresponds to the vascularity of the tissue.

    B. Provides good correlation with conventional methods of GFR measurements.

    C. The transit time of a microbubble through the liver is typically prolonged (>30 s) in patients with hepatic metastatic deposits.

    D. The time intensity profile of the Doppler signal from hepatic vein, after an injection of microbubbles in patients with cirrhosis is shifted to the left in comparison with normal subjects in microbubble studies.

    E. In microbubble studies the initial gradient of a plot of echogenicity against triggering interval is proportional to fractional vascular volume of tissue insonated.

(Answers overleaf)

A **1.17** **Regarding functional measurements of vascularity of tissue**

A. True It is more correctly defined as flow per unit mass of tissue.
Ch. 9 Functional and Physiological Imaging, p. 199.

B. True It is important that the tracer is wholly intravascular.
Ch. 9 Functional and Physiological Imaging, p. 199.

C. False The time concentration curve declines exponentially.
Ch. 9 Functional and Physiological Imaging, p. 199.

D. True This technique reduces significant errors due to venous outflow before peak tissue enhancement occurs.
Ch. 9 Functional and Physiological Imaging, p. 200.

E. False The technique described by Miles allows it to be extended to tissues with two types of input vessel, e.g. the liver with its dual supply from the hepatic artery and portal vein.
Ch. 9 Functional and Physiological Imaging, p. 200.

A **1.18** **Regarding functional indices**

A. True
Ch. 9 Functional and Physiological Imaging, p. 200.

B. True This plot measures contrast clearance per unit volume of kidney, which is closely related to GFR.
Ch. 9 Functional and Physiological Imaging, p. 201.

C. False The early transit times < 24 s in these patients is due to shunts and arterialization of the liver blood supply.
Ch. 9 Functional and Physiological Imaging, p. 200.

D. True
Ch. 9 Functional and Physiological Imaging, p. 200.

E. False This provides a measure of the microcirculatory flow speed. The asymptote of this is proportional to FVV.
Ch. 9 Functional and Physiological Imaging, p. 200.

Q **1.19**   **Regarding litigation in clinical radiology in the UK**

A. In a major reported series one of the three most commonly missed fractures was that of the scaphoid bone.

B. Trauma cases are the commonest cause for litigation in radiology.

C. The definition of clinical negligence takes into account the experience and seniority of the practising doctor.

D. Since 1991, the cost and awards for medical negligence cases in the UK became the responsibility of the hospital trust and directly managed units.

E. After an interventional procedure, responsibility for the patient once back on the ward, reverts to the team that requested the procedure.

(Answers overleaf)

A **1.19**   Regarding litigation in clinical radiology in the UK

A. True

> *Ch. 10A Medico-legal Issues in Diagnostic Radiology: Litigation in Clinical Radiology in the United Kingdom, p. 207.*

B. True   In a recent series, this accounted for 25% of cases. However, vascular and interventional radiology cases are rising and constitute 14% of cases.
Ch. 10A Medico-legal Issues in Diagnostic Radiology: Litigation in Clinical Radiology in the United Kingdom, p. 208.

C. True

> *Ch. 10A Medico-legal Issues in Diagnostic Radiology: Litigation in Clinical Radiology in the United Kingdom, p. 206.*

D. True

> *Ch. 10A Medico-legal Issues in Diagnostic Radiology: Litigation in Clinical Radiology in the United Kingdom, p. 206.*

E. False   Although the patient is returned to the ward, it is the duty of the radiologist to see that relevant instructions are given to the appropriate staff and he/she has ongoing responsibility for the patients on the ward.
Ch. 10A Medico-legal Issues in Diagnostic Radiology: Litigation in Clinical Radiology in the United Kingdom, p. 209.

Q **1.20**　**Regarding consent**

    A.　It is adequate for consent for a radiological procedure to be obtained by the referring colleague.

    B.　There are two forms of consent, i.e. written or oral.

    C.　Consent should be obtained just before the radiological procedure.

    D.　Complications of the procedure should be disclosed to the patient even if the patient does not wish to be informed of them.

    E.　Consent cannot be delegated to a non-medically-qualified colleague.

Q **1.21**　**Regarding medico-legal aspects of radiology**

    A.　The purpose of the law is to diminish that component of human misery caused by conflict.

    B.　Tort is the legal consequence when one person feels injured by the actions of another.

    C.　The standard of care accepted by most courts is that which is a reasonably responsible and prudent physician would do under the same or similar circumstances.

    D.　Disclosure of an abnormality to the patient is the duty of the referring physician rather than the radiologist.

    E.　A radiologist cannot be found negligent if a mistaken radiological interpretation had no effect on the patient outcome.

(Answers overleaf)

A **1.20** Regarding consent

A. **False** It cannot be too strongly enforced that the radiologist has a prime duty to obtain consent, and fully informed consent, for the procedures he/she is undertaking.
Ch. 10A Medico-legal Issues in Diagnostic Radiology: Litigation in Clinical Radiology in the United Kingdom, p. 211.

B. **False** There are three forms of consent including **implied** consent, which infers that the patient has agreed to an intervention by the doctor, e.g. presenting an arm for an intravenous injection.
Ch. 10A Medico-legal Issues in Diagnostic Radiology: Litigation in Clinical Radiology in the United Kingdom, p. 211.

C. **False** The period between consent and procedure should allow enough time for the patient to consider the procedure adequately.
Ch. 10A Medico-legal Issues in Diagnostic Radiology: Litigation in Clinical Radiology in the United Kingdom, p. 211.

D. **False** If this is the case, this should be recorded in the notes as well as a record of obtaining adequate consent from the patient.
Ch. 10A Medico-legal Issues in Diagnostic Radiology: Litigation in Clinical Radiology in the United Kingdom, p. 211.

E. **False** It is not advisable to delegate to a non-medically-qualified colleague but, as long as this colleague is fully aware of all the issues involved in the procedure, e.g. its details and complications and the alternatives, and can answer any questions posed by the patient, then he or she may obtain consent.
Ch. 10A Medico-legal Issues in Diagnostic Radiology: Litigation in Clinical Radiology in the United Kingdom, p. 211.

A **1.21** Regarding medico-legal aspects of radiology

A. **True** It is not to invite conflict.
Ch. 10D Medico-legal Issues in Diagnostic Radiology: Rule Making and the Common Law, p. 225.

B. **True** The major tort in the practice of medicine is negligence.
Ch. 10D Medico-legal Issues in Diagnostic Radiology: Rule Making and the Common Law, p. 227.

C. **True**
Ch. 10D Medico-legal Issues in Diagnostic Radiology: Rule Making and the Common Law, p. 227.

D. **False** In Daly v United States (1991), the court found that disclosure of the abnormality falls within the scope of the duty owed by the radiologist to the patient.
Ch. 10D Medico-legal Issues in Diagnostic Radiology: Rule Making and the Common Law, p. 228.

E. **True**
Ch. 10D Medico-legal Issues in Diagnostic Radiology: Rule Making and the Common Law, p. 229.

Q **1.22** **Regarding radiation protection and patient dose in diagnostic imaging**

A. The dose equivalent is measured in Grays.

B. The effective dose is proportional to a quality factor (Q).

C. Stochastic effects are dose dependent.

D. The period when the fetus is most sensitive to irradiation is within the first 8 weeks of gestation.

E. Five per cent of lung cancers are attributable to background radon gas.

Q **1.23** **Regarding protection of staff involved with radiation**

A. The walls of an X-ray room are of equal thickness of shielding material all round.

B. High kV techniques reduce both patient and staff doses.

C. Nuclear medicine staff may record significant higher exposure readings because radio-nuclide such as ^{99m}Tc, have higher energies than diagnostic X-rays.

D. The dose limit recommended by the IRR 99 to the surface of the abdomen of a pregnant woman during the declared term of pregnancy is 13 mSv.

E. The Ionising Radiation Regulations in 1999 stipulated the need for an appropriate and administrative organization at local level for use of ionizing radiation for radiology.

(Answers overleaf)

A **1.22** **Regarding radiation protection and patient dose in diagnostic imaging**

A. False It is measured in sieverts (Sv).
Ch. 11 Radiation Protection and Patient Doses In Diagnostic Imaging, p. 231.

B. True The effective dose is calculated by multiplying the dose equivalent received by each individual organ or tissue by an appropriate tissue weighting and summing this for all tissues involved.
As the dose equivalent is proportional to a quality (Q) factor then the effective dose is also proportional to Q.
Ch. 11 Radiation Protection and Patient Doses in Diagnostic Imaging, p. 232.

C. False These describe long-term, low-dose effects that are of a random statistical nature and in which the severity is unrelated to the dose.
Ch. 11 Radiation Protection and Patient Doses in Diagnostic Imaging, p. 233.

D. False This is 8–15 weeks' gestation when the rate of proliferation of DNA is at a maximum. It is now believed that the fetus is relatively insensitive to radiation in the early stages of pregnancy; any deleterious effect is likely to lead to a spontaneous abortion within the few weeks after conception.
Ch. 11 Radiation Protection and Patient Doses in Diagnostic Imaging, p. 233.

E. True
Ch. 11 Radiation Protection and Patient Doses in Diagnostic Imaging, p. 233.

A **1.23** **Regarding protection of staff involved with radiation**

A. False The primary beam will be of higher intensity and also a higher mean energy and thus it will require larger thicknesses of shielding material than the walls, which are not within the primary beam, thus the walls are not of equal thickness.
Ch. 11 Radiation Protection and Patient Doses in Diagnostic Imaging, p. 241.

B. True
Ch. 11 Radiation Protection and Patient Doses in Diagnostic Imaging, p. 241.

C. True Also, it is difficult to add shielding whilst handling the nuclides and performing the scans.
Ch. 11 Radiation Protection and Patient Doses in Diagnostic Imaging, p. 241.

D. False It is limited to 2 mSv in pregnancy with a limit of 1 mSv to the fetus.
Ch. 11 Radiation Protection and Patient Doses in Diagnostic Imaging, p. 240.

E. True
Ch. 11 Radiation Protection and Patient Doses in Diagnostic Imaging, p. 239.

Q **1.24**   **Regarding the protection of the patient in radio nuclide radiology**

    A. Women are advised to avoid becoming pregnant within 8 months of an ^{131}I iodide scan, for thyroid metastases.

    B. Free pertechnetate crosses the placenta and accumulates in the fetal thyroid gland.

    C. Women who need to undergo a MAG3 study whilst breast feeding are required to interrupt breast feeding their infant for 24 hours.

    D. The ARSAC guidance notes state that any radiation dose to the fetus requires particular justification.

    E. During early lactation when colostrum is being secreted, all breast feeding should be interrupted after a nuclear medicine study, despite the nature of the pharmaceutical agent.

Q **1.25**   **Regarding clinical governance**

    A. The national institute of clinical excellence (NICE) was commissioned with the aim to provide an external check that local NHS organizations are complying with predetermined quality standards.

    B. In mammography screening, a minimum detection rate of small cancers (less than 15 mm) of greater than 1.35/1000 is a recognized outcome standard.

    C. The British Society of Interventional Radiology standards for interventional procedures states that the complication of haematoma (requiring treatment or delaying discharge) should occur in less than 1% of cases in diagnostic angiography.

    D. The suggested work load level for a radiologist per notional half-day session is 70 general radiology reporting examinations.

    E. The main aim of clinical governance is to guide doctors and to protect patients.

(Answers overleaf)

25

A **1.24**   Regarding the protection of the patient in radio nuclide radiology

A. False   The recommended delay is 4 months.
Ch. 11 Radiation Protection and Patient Doses in Diagnostic Imaging, Table 11.9, p. 246.

B. True   This occurs in the last two trimesters of pregnancy.
Ch. 11 Radiation Protection and Patient Doses in Diagnostic Imaging, p. 246.

C. False   No interruption of feeding time is needed following a MAG3 study.
Ch. 11 Radiation Protection and Patient Doses in Diagnostic Imaging, Table 11.11, p. 247.

D. False   Only doses over 1 mGy requires particular justification. A dose up to 1 mGy represents a level of risk comparable to variations in national background radiation.
Ch. 11 Radiation Protection and Patient Doses in Diagnostic Imaging, p. 246.

E. True

Ch. 11 Radiation Protection and Patient Doses in Diagnostic Imaging, p. 247.

A **1.25**   Regarding clinical governance

A. False   NICE *sets* the standards and these are checked by the commission for health improvement (CHI).
Ch. 12A Clinical Governance in Radiology, p. 254.

B. True

Ch. 12A Clinical Governance in Radiology, p. 256.

C. False   This has been set at 3% for diagnostic angiography and 4% for interventional vascular procedures (PTA/stenting).
Ch. 12A Clinical Governance in Radiology, Table 12a.2, p. 256.

D. True

Ch. 12A Clinical Governance in Radiology, Table 12a.3, p. 256.

E. False   This is the job of the GMC. Clinical governance is defined as 'a frame work through which any NHS organisations are accountable for continuously improving the quality of their services safeguarding high standards of care by creating an environment in which excellence in care will flourish'.
Ch. 12A Clinical Governance in Radiology, p. 253.

Q **1.26**   **Regarding audit**

   A.   In the UK medical audit is a requirement within all doctors job plans.

   B.   Audit identifies the best medical practice.

   C.   The appropriate gold standard for an audit should be based upon research evidence.

   D.   An audit cycle accepts or rejects the nul hypothesis that a certain standard is being implemented adequately with a probability value of less than 0.05.

   E.   The 'indicator' of an audit is linked with the set standard and is a particular variable or item that is easily measured.

(Answers overleaf)

A **1.26** **Regarding audit**

A. True

> *Ch. 12B Clinical Governance and Audit, p. 264.*

B. False Research identifies what is best practice. Audit determines if this has been put into practice.

> *Ch. 12B Clinical Governance and Audit, p. 264.*

C. True

> *Ch. 12B Clinical Governance and Audit, p. 265.*

D. False Audit does not have to reach statistical significance as opposed to research.

> *Ch. 12B Clinical Governance and Audit, p. 264.*

E. True

> *Ch. 12B Clinical Governance and Audit, p. 265.*

2 The respiratory system

Q **2.1** **The following statements are true regarding lymph nodes in the thorax**

A. The hilar shadows on a chest radiograph are mostly due to vascular markings.
B. Fifty per cent of normal lymph nodes are less than 10 mm in diameter.
C. A 10-mm lymph node in the retrocrural region is a normal finding.
D. Aortopulmonary window nodes are generally larger than subcarinal nodes.
E. A lymph node greater than 12 mm in diameter can be regarded as pathological.

Q **2.2** **The following statements are true**

A. A lateral chest radiograph is more sensitive than an erect PA chest radiograph in the detection of free intraperitoneal air.
B. It is possible to detect a pleural effusion as small as 50 ml on a chest radiograph.
C. In a correctly exposed lateral chest radiograph, there is a progressive descending increase in opacity of the retrocardiac lung and lower thoracic vertebral bodies.
D. Boerhaave's syndrome is a recognized cause of a pneumomediastinum.
E. Volume loss generally observed in lobar consolidation.

(Answers overleaf)

A **2.1** **The following statements are true regarding lymph nodes in the thorax**

A. True

    Ch. 14 The Hila, p. 288.

B. False   Ninety-five per cent of normal lymph nodes are less than 10 mm whilst some can be less than 15 mm in diameter.
Ch. 14 Lymph Nodes, p. 291.

C. False   Normal lymph nodes in the retrocrural region are less than 6 mm.
Ch. 14 Lymph Nodes, p. 291.

D. False   Lymph nodes in the region of the paraspinal area, brachiocephalic veins and retrocrurally are smaller (<6 mm in diameter) in size than AP window, subcarinal, pre- and paratracheal lymph nodes that are often 6–10 mm in diameter.
Ch. 14 Lymph Nodes, p. 291.

E. False   Normal lymph nodes can be up to 15 mm in diameter. Increased nodal size does not always imply significant pathology as some reactionary nodes can be large. It is then that clinical correlation or further 'functional' imaging is necessary.
Ch. 14 Lymph Nodes, p. 291.

A **2.2** **The following statements are true**

A. True

    Ch.15 The Lateral Projection, p. 304.

B. True

    Ch. 15 The Detection of Pleural Effusions, p. 304.

C. False   The reverse is T and this is known as the 'spine sign' on lateral chest radiographs.
Ch. 15 The Lateral Projection, p. 309.

D. True

    Ch. 15 Pneumomediastinum, p. 307.

E. False   There is generally, no significant loss of volume with consolidated lung.
Ch. 15 Consolidation, p. 311.

Q **2.3** Expansive consolidation is commonly associated with

    A. Bronchogenic carcinoma.
    B. Staphyloccocal pneumonia.
    C. *Klebsiella* pneumonia.
    D. Non-Hodgkins lymphoma.
    E. *Pneumocystis carinii* pneumonia.

Q **2.4** Regarding pleural effusions

    A. Occur in 10% of cases of pulmonary embolism.
    B. Antimigraine drugs cause pleural effusions.
    C. They are predominantly right-sided in Meigs syndrome.
    D. Lamellar effusions are a feature of ARDS.
    E. Chylous effusions can be distinguished from non-chylous effusions on CT because they are of lower density owing to their fat content.

(Answers overleaf)

A **2.3** **Expansive consolidation is commonly associated with**

A. **True**

Ch. 15 Consolidation, p. 311.

B. **False**

Ch. 15 Consolidation, p. 311.

C. **True**

Ch. 15 Consolidation, p. 311.

D. **True** Also known as 'drowned' lung, it has no relation to drowning but is associated with consolidation secondary to neoplasm.
Ch. 15 Consolidation, p. 311.

E. **False**

Ch. 15 Consolidation, p. 311.

A **2.4** **Regarding pleural effusions**

A. **False** This is seen in 25–50% of pulmonary embolism.
Ch. 16 Exudates and Transudates, p. 331.

B. **True** A whole host of drugs can cause this reaction, commonly chemotherapeutic drugs.
Ch. 16 Exudates and Transudates, p. 331.

C. **True** Meigs' syndrome has four features: ascites, pleural effusion, a benign ovarian tumour (fibroma commonly), and resolution of the ascites and effusions following removal of the tumour. The effusions are predominantly right-sided but may be bilateral and rarely left-sided only.
Ch. 16 Exudates and Transudates, p. 331.

D. **False** In patients with ARDS the primary pathology is capillary leakage that permits leakage of fluid into the alveoli. The fact that the pulmonary venous pressure and the capillary wedge pressure are not elevated accounts for the relative absence of septal lines and lamellar effusions.
Ch. 27 ARDS, p. 553.

E. **False** Whilst chylous effusions do contain fat, they also contain proteinaceous material that gives it an attenuation on CT similar to other types of effusions.
Ch. 16 Chylothorax, p. 332.

Q **2.5** In conventional chest radiography

A. Mediastinal structures are better visualized using a high kV exposure.

B. Normal vascular markings are better demonstrated using standard low kV method.

C. Pleural plaques or calcified nodules are best seen using a high kVp.

D. The spatial resolution is better than digital chest radiography.

E. A subpulmonary effusion cannot easily be distinguished from a high diaphragm.

Q **2.6** With regard to CT of the chest

A. The sensitivity of pulmonary nodule detection is improved with spiral CT scanning.

B. Differential densities are best displayed using a narrow collimation of 6 mm or less.

C. The patient should always be scanned prone for a HRCT exam.

D. A narrow window width of approx 600 HU may improve the characterization of airways disease.

E. Owing to the narrow slice thickness in HRCT, breath holding is not necessary during scan acquisition.

A 2.5 In conventional chest radiography

A. True

> *Ch. 13 Chest Radiography, p. 275.*

B. False

> *Ch. 13 Chest Radiography, p. 275.*

C. False Ribs, calcified nodules and pleural plaques are poorly defined.
> *Ch. 13 Chest Radiography, p. 275.*

D. True

> *Ch. 13 Table 13.1, p. 276.*

E. False A lateral decubitus view readily distinguishes between a high diaphragm and a non-loculated subpulmonary effusion.
> *Ch. 13 Radiographic Views, p. 276.*

A 2.6 With regard to CT of the chest

A. True

> *Ch. 13 Computed Tomography, p. 277.*

B. False < 3 mm.
> *Ch. 13 Computed Tomography, p. 277.*

C. False

> *Ch. 13 HRCT, p. 279.*

D. True May emphasize subtle densities that characterize emphysema or diffuse lung disease.
> *Ch. 13 HRCT, p. 279.*

E. False Breath holding to reduce movement artefact is essential.
> *Ch. 13 HRCT, p. 279.*

Q 2.7 In nuclear medicine studies of the chest

A. $^{99\,m}$Technetium-labelled macroaggregates should be used for perfusion scanning in patients with Eisenmenger syndrome.

B. Krypton-81m used in ventilation imaging has a long half-life.

C. A normal perfusion scan excludes pulmonary embolism.

D. An unmatched perfusion defect is specific for pulmonary embolism.

E. ^{18}F-fluorodeoxyglucose (FDG) is taken up by malignant cells owing to their increased cellular metabolism.

Q 2.8 In a normal patient

A. On a chest radiograph an azygos vein diameter of 10 mm is normal.

B. The left pulmonary artery arches over the left main bronchus while the right pulmonary artery passes anterior to the major bronchi.

C. On the right, the superior pulmonary vein is separated from the central bronchi by a lower division of the right pulmonary artery whereas on the left, the superior pulmonary vein is separated from the pulmonary artery by the bronchial tree.

D. The CT density of thymus above the age of 40 years is that of fat.

E. The aortic nipple is formed from the junction of the left superior intercostal vein and the azygos vein.

(Answers overleaf)

A **2.7 In nuclear medicine studies of the chest**

A. False Microspheres should be used owing to the larger size of macroaggregates which may cause embolization of medium sized systemic vessels in the presence of a right-to-left shunt.
Ch. 13 Ventilation – Perfusion Scintigraphy, p. 279.

B. False It has a short half-life and is this a disadvantage.
Ch. 13 Ventilation – Perfusion Scintigraphy, p. 279.

C. True
Ch. 13 Ventilation – Perfusion Scintigraphy, p. 280.

D. False It can be the result of many vascular diseases.
Ch. 13 Ventilation – Perfusion Scintigraphy, p. 280.

E. True
Ch. 13 PET, p. 280.

A **2.8 In a normal patient**

A. True
Ch. 14 The Mediastinum, p. 293.

B. True
Ch. 14 The Mediastinum, p. 289.

C. True
Ch. 14 The Mediastinum, p. 289.

D. True Fatty replacement occurs after puberty.
Ch. 14 The Mediastinum, p. 291.

E. False The nipple represents the left superior intercostal vein passing round the aortic knuckle.
Ch. 14 The Mediastinum, p. 298.

Q **2.9**   **In the normal radiograph of the chest**

A.   There are three lobes in each lung.
B.   The accessory fissure is seen in up to 1% of the population.
C.   A superior accessory fissure may be seen separating the anterior segment of the upper lobe from the apical segment of the lower lobe.
D.   Tracheal cartilage calcification is commonly appears between 20 and 30 years of age.
E.   The inferior pulmonary ligaments are pleural reflections.

Q **2.10**   **The following statements are true**

A.   Discernible calcification of breast tissue on a chest radiograph usually denotes a benign process.
B.   Nipples on a chest radiograph have ill-defined lateral margins.
C.   Poland's syndrome is associated with syndactyly.
D.   The commonest benign chest wall tumour is a neurofibroma.
E.   Unilateral transradiancy and an abnormal anterior axillary fold is pathognomonic of Poland's syndrome.

Q **2.11**   **The following are true regarding chest wall soft-tissue tumours**

A.   Neurofibromas give a high signal on T2-weighted images.
B.   Lymphangiomas can appear as septated cysts.
C.   Askin tumours are the commonest malignant soft-tissue chest wall tumours.
D.   Askin tumours frequently haemorrhage.
E.   Chest wall tumours seen in profile on the chest radiograph have sharp margins convex to the lung.

(Answers overleaf)

A 2.9   In the normal radiograph of the chest

A. False   The left has two lobes only.
Ch. 14 The Lungs, p. 283.

B. True
Ch. 14 The Lungs, p. 284.

C. False   This separates the apical segment of the lower lobe from the basal segments.
Ch. 14 The Lungs, p. 284.

D. False   Common after 40 years.
Ch. 14 The Lungs, p. 284.

E. True
Ch. 14 The Lungs, p. 285.

A 2.10   The following statements are true

A. True
Ch. 16 The Chest Wall, p. 316.

B. False   Nipples usually have sharp lateral margins and ill-defined medial ones.
Ch. 16 The Chest Wall, p. 316.

C. True
Ch. 16 The Chest Wall, p. 317.

D. False   Commonest chest wall tumours are lipomas.
Ch. 16 Soft Tissue Tumours, p. 317.

E. False   This is also a feature of mastectomy.
Ch. 16 The Chest Wall, p. 317.

A 2.11   The following are true regarding chest wall soft-tissue tumours

A. True
Ch. 16 Soft-Tissue Tumours, p. 318.

B. True   Can appear as fluid-filled cysts with or without septation.
Ch. 16 Soft-Tissue Tumours, p. 319.

C. False   These are rare tumours of children or young adults. Lipo- or fibro-sarcomas are the commonest.
Ch. 16 Soft-Tissue Tumours, p. 319.

D. True
Ch. 16 Soft-Tissue Tumours, p. 319.

E. True
Ch. 16 Sof-Tissue Tumours, p. 317.

Q 2.12 The following are true regarding the ribs

A. Cervical ribs occur in 5% of the population.
B. Cartilaginous tumours are the commonest benign primary rib tumours.
C. Chondrosacromas are the commonest malignant rib tumours.
D. The costal cartilages can be seen to calcify centrally in men.
E. Sprengel's deformity is associated with rib abnormalities.

Q 2.13 Concerning pleural tumours

A. Hypertrophic osteoarthropathy is a well-recognized complication of localized mesothelioma.
B. Pleural tumours usually make an acute angle with the chest wall on the chest radiograph.
C. The commonest pleural neoplasms are metastases from adenocarcinomas.
D. Liposarcomas exhibit homogeneous soft-tissue attenuation on CT.
E. Malignant pleural fibromas are typically of low signal intensity on T1- and T2-weighted images.

(Answers overleaf)

A **2.12** The following are true regarding the ribs

A. False From 1 to 2%.
Ch. 16 Ribs, p. 320.

B. True
Ch. 16 Ribs, p. 321.

C. False The commonest malignant rib tumours are metastases or myeloma.
Ch. 16 Ribs, p. 321.

D. False Calcification occurs peripherally in men and centrally in women.
Ch. 16 Ribs, p. 321.

E. True As are other syndromes, e.g. basal cell naevus syndrome.
Ch. 16 Ribs, p. 320.

A **2.13** Concerning pleural tumours

A. True Hypertrophic osteoarthropathy occurs in 10–30% of patients with this fibrous tumour, which occasionally also causes hypoglycaemia.
Ch. 16 Pleural Tumours, p. 339.

B. False Pleural tumours make an obtuse angle with the chest wall.
Ch. 16 Pleural Tumours, p. 339.

C. True The commonest pleural metastases are from adenocarcinomas of the ovary, stomach, breast and lung.
Ch. 16 Pleural Tumours, p. 340.

D. True When a pleural lesion displays a homogeneous fatty composition this represents a lipoma, if, however, any soft-tissue components are seen, then a liposarcoma should be suspected.
Ch. 16 Plural Tumours, p. 339.

E. True Pleural fibromas are typically of low signal intensity on T1- and T2-weighted images. A few cases, however, may display intermediate to high-signal intensity.
Ch. 16 Pleural Tumours, p. 339.

Q 2.14   Concerning the diaphragm

A. In the majority of normal people the right hemidiaphragm is higher than the left.

B. The excursions of the hemidiaphragms are unequal in 80% of normal people.

C. Herpes zoster is a recognized cause of a high diaphragm exhibiting paradoxical movement.

D. Diaphragmatic paralysis can be assumed when screening demonstrates paradoxical movements of the hemidiaphragm.

E. Bochdalek hernias can sometimes be difficult to differentiate from a low lying pericardial cyst.

Q 2.15   Regarding mediastinal masses

A. More than 50% of thymomas are malignant.

B. Calcification seen in a thymic tumour signifies a benign lesion.

C. On MRI, thymomas are isointense to muscle on T1-weighted images.

D. Thyrotoxicosis is a recognized association of thymic hyperplasia.

E. Within a mediastinal mass, the presence of fat, either as a focal collection or fluid fat, favours a diagnosis of benign cystic teratoma over other diagnoses.

(Answers overleaf)

A **2.14**   **Concerning the diaphragm**

A. True   This occurs in over 90% of normal people with a difference of 15–30 mm.
Ch. 16 The Diaphragm, p. 342.

B. True   This inequality of diaphragmatic excursion is usually less than 10 mm in most people.
Ch. 16 The Diaphragm, p. 344.

C. True   Phrenic palsy is normally caused by a tumour, usually a bronchial carcinoma, but can also be caused by trauma, irradiation, poliomyelitis, herpes zoster and cervical disc degeneration.
Ch. 16 The Diaphragm, p. 345.

D. False   An important mimic of phrenic paresis is eventration of the diaphragm usually on the left. In a small but significant number of normal individuals, no cause for phrenic paresis can be found. This usually occurs on the right and is thought by some to be the legacy of a previous neuritis.
Ch. 16 The Diaphragm, p. 345.

E. False   It is commonly the Morgagni hernia, which occurs anteriorly at the right cardiophrenic angle, and can be difficult to differentiate from a low-lying pericardial cyst.
Ch. 16 Diaphragmatic Hernias, p. 346.

A **2.15**   **Regarding mediastinal masses**

A. False   Approximately 10–40% are malignant.
Ch. 17 Thymic Tumours, p. 356.

B. False   Calcification may be seen in both benign and malignant forms of a thymoma.
Ch. 17 Thymic Tumours, p. 356.

C. True   On the T2-weighted images the signal intensity is increased and may make it difficult to distinguish it from the mediastinal fat.
Ch. 17 Thymic Tumours, p. 358.

D. True   Thymic hyperplasia is also associated, more commonly, with myasthenia gravis.
Ch. 17 Thymic Hyperplasia, p. 358.

E. True
Ch. 17 Teratoma/Germ-Cell Tumours of the Mediastinum, p. 358.

Q **2.16** **The following are true concerning mediastinal lymphadenopathy**

    A. Calcification in a lymph node always has a benign aetiology.

    B. Eggshell calcification in a lymph node is a feature of sarcoidosis.

    C. In Castleman's disease, the lymph nodes show a low-density centre with rim enhancement.

    D. Pleural effusions are a feature of angio immunoblastic lymphadenopathy

    E. PCP infection is a cause calification in lymph nodes in the mediastinum.

Q **2.17** **Concerning neurogenic tumours of the thorax**

    A. Five per cent of phaechromocytomas occur in the chest.

    B. Lateral thoracic meningoceles always communicate with the subarachnoid space.

    C. Mediastinal neural tumours commonly present as well-defined round or oval masses.

    D. Neurogenic tumours enhance avidly with IV contrast.

    E. Nerve sheath tumours commonly calcify.

(Answers overleaf)

A **2.16** The following are true concerning mediastinal lymphadenopathy

A. False Although lymph node calcification is rare in neoplasms it can occasionally be seen in metastatic lymph nodes and treated Hodgkin's lymphoma.
Ch. 17 Mediastinal Lymphadenopathy, p. 359.

B. True Eggshell calcification can also be seen in treated lymphoma and pneumoconiosis.
Ch. 17 Mediastinal Lymphadenopathy, p. 359.

C. False Rim enhancement of nodes tends to point toward tuberculous infection. Lymph nodes in Castleman's disease show strikingly uniform marked contrast enhancement.
Ch. 17 Mediastinal Lymphadenopathy, p. 359.

D. True This cause of mediastinal hilar lymph node enlargement can be confused with malignant lymphoma and, although it is a form of reactive hyperplasia of lymph nodes, it may be a precursor of malignant disease.
Ch. 17 Angioimmunoblastic Lymphadenopathy, p. 364.

E. True These have a strikingly foamy appearance.
Ch. 17 Mediastinal Lymphadenopathy, p. 359.

A **2.17** Concerning neurogenic tumours of the thorax

A. False Less than 2% are found in the thorax, these commonly occur in the posterior mediastinum closely related to the heart, in particular the wall of the left atrium.
Ch. 17 Mediastinal Paragangliomas, p. 368.

B. True The meningocele is an extension of the theca containing CSF within the subarachnoid space and will, therefore, fill with contrast medium during myelography, though MRI is now the investigation of choice. Lateral thoracic meningoceles are rare lesions, commonly associated with neurofibromatosis, and can present as asymptomatic masses causing pressure deformity of the bone.
Ch. 17 Lateral Thoracic Meningocele, p. 368.

C. True This is commonly the case except in some chemodectomas, phaeochomocytomes and the very rare neurofibroma of the vagus nerve.
Ch. 17 Neurogenic Tumours, p. 366.

D. True This can be a striking feature on CT particularly in the case of phaeochromocytoma.
Ch. 17 Neurogenic Tumours, p. 367.

E. False They rarely calcify. Calcification is more commonly seen in sympathetic nerve tumours both in the benign and malignant forms.
Ch. 17 Neurogenic Tumours, p. 367.

Q **2.18** The following statements are true regarding the mediastinum

A. In Boerhaave's syndrome a tear occurs in the upper oesophagus as a result of vomiting.

B. Histoplasmosis is a recognized cause of fibrosing mediastinitis.

C. Haemorrhage within the mediastinum frequently produces a well-defined apical cap.

D. Mediastinal emphysema is associated with a pneumoperitoneum in 5–10% of patients.

E. Discrete masses in the mediastinum are a CT feature of fibrosing mediastinitis.

Q **2.19** Regarding pneumonia

A. Lobar expansion is commonly a feature of *Klebsiella pneumoniae* infection.

B. *Pneumocystis carinii* pneumonia (PCP) is a cause of pneumatoceles.

C. Cavitation and abscess formation are seen in 20–30% of mycoplasma pneumonias.

D. Empyemas are commonly associated with *Streptococcus pneumonae* infection.

E. The appearance of a large irregular cavity containing an irregular intracavitary body is a recognized complication of *Klebsiella pneumoniae* infection.

(Answers overleaf)

45

A 2.18   The following statements are true regarding the mediastinum

A. False   Boerhaave's syndrome is the commonest cause of acute mediastinitis; the tears, however, commonly occur just above the gastro-oesophageal junction.
Ch. 17 Acute Mediastinitis, p. 371.

B. True   Histoplasmosis, tuberculosis and fungal infections are the commonest cause of fibrosing mediastinitis.
Ch. 17 Fibrosing Mediastinitis, p. 373.

C. True   Blood in the mediastinum frequently runs over the apex of the left lung producing an apical cap. This apical cap is usually smoother in outline than those caused by inflammatory disease and neoplasms.
Ch. 17 Mediastinal Haemorrhage, p. 373.

D. False   Pneumomediastinum is classically associated with retroperitoneal gas rather than intraperitoneal gas.
Ch. 17 Mediastinal Emphysema, p. 373.

E. False   The fibrosis obliterates the fat planes but does not normally form recognizable masses.
Ch. 17 Fibrosing Mediastinitis, p. 373.

A 2.19   Regarding pneumonia

A. True   This is considered to be a characteristic feature of infection by that organism.
Ch. 18 Volume Changes, p. 387.

B. True   Pneumatoceles are also a feature of pneumonia particularly in childhood.
Ch. 18 Pneumatocoele Formation, p. 387.

C. False   Cavitation can occur with *Mycoplasma*, viral or chlamydial infections but is rare in these conditions. It is seen more commonly in pneumonias caused by *Staphylococcus aureus*, Gram-negative bacteria and tuberculosis.
Ch. 18 Abscess Formation, p. 387.

D. True
Ch. 18 Pleural Effusion/emphasema, p. 387.

E. True   Rarely, *Klebsiella* or *Strep. pneumoniae* infections cause thrombosis of intrapulmonary vessels leading to pulmonary gangrene with the features described above.
Ch. 18 Pulmonary Gangrene, p. 387.

Q 2.20 Regarding pulmonary tuberculosis

A. Normal chest radiographs are seen in 5% of patients with pulmonary tuberculosis.

B. Bilateral pleural effusions are commonly seen in primary pulmonary tuberculosis.

C. In post primary tuberculosis, the initial lesion arises in the anterior segments of the upper lobe in 95% of patients.

D. Cavitary tuberculosis is associated with Rasmussen aneurysms.

E. In patients with miliary tuberculosis, calcification of the nodules is seen in approximately 10% of cases.

Q 2.21 Concerning pulmonary infection

A. In HSV pneumonia, approximately 50% of patients have pleural effusions.

B. From 20 to 30% of mycetomas completely fill the cavity in which they are seen.

C. In hydatid disease, lung cysts usually occur in the upper zones.

D. In mycoplasma pneumonia, multi-lobar consolidation is a frequent finding.

E. Cavitating mass like lesions are a feature of *Legionella* pneumonia.

(Answers overleaf)

A **2.20** **Regarding pulmonary tuberculosis**

A. True

Ch. 18 Pulmonary Tuberculosis, p. 288.

B. True Effusions are unilateral except when they are a complicating feature of miliary spread.
Ch. 18 Pleural Effusion, p. 390.

C. False These lesions tend to arise from the apical posterior segment of the upper lobe or the superior segment of the lower lobe. Isolated involvement of the anterior segment of an upper lobe, with few exceptions, virtually excludes tuberculosis.
Ch. 18 Major Radiological Findings, p. 390.

D. True These are rare, life-threatening complications of cavitating tuberculosis resulting from granulomatous weakening of the pulmonary arterial wall.
Ch. 18 Major Radiological Findings, p. 391.

E. False Calcification within miliary nodules is rare or virtually non-existent.
Ch. 18 Miliary Tuberculosis, p. 390.

A **2.21** **Concerning pulmonary infection**

A. True

Ch. 18 Viral Pneumonias, p. 385.

B. False This is rare.
Ch. 18 Mycetoma, p. 398.

C. False Most are situated in the mid and lower zones.
Ch. 18 Hydatid Disease, p. 400.

D. True Consolidation more commonly involves one lobe, but bilateral or multilobar involvement is frequently observed.
Ch. 1 Mycoplasma Pneumonias, p. 384.

E. True It is, however, only common in the immunocompromised patient.
Ch. 1 Legionella, p. 381.

Q 2.22   Regarding pulmonary involvement in AIDS

A. In *Pneumocystis carinii* pneumonia (PCP), the substantial gallium-67 uptake is a specific diagnostic feature.

B. Pneumatoceles are seen in 30% of patients with PCP.

C. In the late stages of AIDS, infection with *Mycobacterium tuberculosis* typically produces upper-lobe cavitating opacities.

D. *Mycobacterium kansasii* is the commonest non-tuberculosis mycobacterial infection complicating HIV infection.

E. Only 20% of patients with pulmonary Kaposi's sarcoma have cutaneous lesions.

Q 2.23   These following statements are true

The following are causes of tracheobronchial narrowing:

A. Sarcoidosis.

B. Amyloidosis.

C. Tracheobronchopathia osteochrondroplastica.

D. Upper-lobe lung fibrosis.

E. Relapsing polychondritis.

(Answers overleaf)

A **2.22**   Regarding pulmonary involvement in AIDS

A. False   Although uptake of gallium-67 does occur, this is a non-specific finding.
Ch. 1 Pneumocystis Carinii, p. 402.

B. False   This occurs in 10%.
Ch. 18 Pneumocystis Carinii, p. 402.

C. False   The conventional patterns of tuberculosis infection are not observed in the final stages of AIDS. Typically, diffuse, bilateral, reticulo-nodular opacities are seen.
Ch. 18 Mycobacterium Tuberculosis, p. 406.

D. False   *Mycobacterium avium intracellulae* is by far the commonest non-tuberculosis mycobacterial infection isolated.
Ch. 18 Other Non-tuberculous Mycobacteria, p. 408.

E. False   The majority of patients with pulmonary involvement exhibit skin lesions and 20% of patients with skin lesions are found at autopsy to have pulmonary involvement.
Ch. 18 Kaposi Sarcoma, p. 410.

A **2.23**   These following statements are true

A. True
Ch. 19 Table 19.1, p. 420.

B. True
Ch. 19 Table 19.1, p. 420.

C. True
Ch. 19 Table 19.1, p. 420.

D. False   Lung fibrosis may cause tracheal dilatations.
Ch. 19 Table 19.1, p. 421.

E. True
Ch. 19 Table 19.1, p. 420.

Q 2.24 Regarding large airway disease

A. Bronchial wall thickening is the commonest radiological finding in patients with asthma.

B. Churg-Strauss vasculitis is a chronic complication of asthma.

C. Bronchogenic cyst formation is a common feature.

D. Alpha$_1$-anti-trypsin deficiency is a cause of bronchiectasis.

E. Bronchiectasis gives rise to cysts.

Q 2.25 Regarding lobar collapse

A. In partial collapse, the more collapsed a lobe is, the more opaque it appears on the chest radiograph.

B. Hilar elevation is a well-recognized sign of upper-lobe collapse.

C. Hilar 'depression' is a more reliable sign for lower-lobe collapse on a PA chest radiograph than the 'small hilum' sign.

D. The 'Luftsichel' appearance is said to occur more commonly in left than in the right upper-lobe collapse and is a characteristic feature of upper-lobe collapse.

E. Rounded atelectasis can occur in the absence of pleural reaction/thickening or an effusion.

(Answers overleaf)

51

A **2.24** **Regarding large airway disease**

A. True This is seen in 48–71% of patients in one series.
Ch. 19 Bronchial Diseases, p. 122.

B. True
Ch. 19 Complications of Asthma, p. 423.

C. False This is a congenital anomaly that is not associated with large airways disease.
Ch. 17 Foregut Cysts, p. 364.

D. True
Ch. 19, Table 19.3, p. 424.

E. True Also known as cystic bronchiectasis, with the presence of cysts measuring 3–20 mm. Sometimes the cysts may contain air-fluid levels.
Ch. 19 Bronchiectasis, p. 425.

A **2.25** **Regarding lobar collapse**

A. False The opacity of a partially collapsed lobe depends on the amount of retained fluid/secretions in that lobe and not on the volume of the lobe.
Ch. 20A Opacity of the Collapsed Lobe, p. 439.

B. True
Ch. 20A Hilar Vascular Alterations, p. 440.

C. False When a lobe collapses, the opaque collapsed lobe obscures the lower-lobe artery that lies within it and the interlobar artery is usually rotated out of profile, neither vessel being recognizable. If this is the case, it is difficult to recognize the hilum as being depressed. However, at the expected position of the hilum, smaller vascular structures are noted. Thus the small hilum is a better indicator of lower-lobe collapse than hilar depression.
Ch. 20A Hilar Vascular Alterations, p. 440.

D. True The Luftsichel appearance is produced by the over-inflated superior segment of the ipsilateral lower lobe, located between the mediastinum and the medial surface of the collapsed upper lobe.
Ch. 20A Compensatory Overinflation, p. 442.

E. False Rounded atelectasis commonly occurs from one of two proposed mechanisms, one being a pleural effusion and the other pleural fibrosis and subsequent pleural contraction causing lung folding.
Ch. 20A Rounded Atelectasis, p. 443.

Q 2.26   Concerning emphysema

A. Centrilobular emphysema is associated with α_1-antitrypsin deficiency.

B. Panlobular emphysema is most severe in the lower lobes.

C. Paraseptal emphysema predominantly involves the air spaces located in the distal part of the secondary pulmonary lobule.

D. Paracicatricial emphysema occurs in patients with pulmonary fibrosis.

E. Focal areas of emphysema usually have distinct walls on CT images.

Q 2.27   Regarding small airway disease of the lung

A. HRCT features classically include the nodular and linear branching opacities known as the 'tree in bud' appearance.

B. Obliterative bronchiolitis is associated with inflammatory bowel disease.

C. Mosaic perfusion and expiratory air trapping are characteristic HRCT features of obliterative bronchiolitis.

D. In organizing pneumonia, the distribution of airspace consolidation is within a sub pleural or peribronchial distribution in more than 50% of cases.

E. Diffuse panbronchiolitis is commonly associated with connective tissue disorders.

(Answers overleaf)

A **2.26**   Concerning emphysema

A. False   Panlobular emphysema is classically associated with α_1-antitrypsin deficiency.
Ch. 21 Centrilobular Emphysema, p. 455.

B. True
Ch. 21 Panlobular Emphysema, p. 455.

C. True
Ch. 21 Paraseptal Emphysema, p. 455.

D. True
Ch. 21 Irregular Emphysema, p. 455.

E. False   Emphysematous areas lack distinct walls as opposed to lung cysts.
Ch. 21 CT Findings, p. 455.

A **2.27**   Regarding small airway disease of the lung

A. True
Ch. 21 Cellular Bronchiolitis, p. 458.

B. True   This is a rare finding. More commonly, the disorder results from childhood viral infection, *Mycoplasma pneumonia* or toxic fume inhalation. It also occurs in patients with rheumatoid arthritis, particularly those treated by pencillin and as a manifestation of chronic graft-versus-host disease.
Ch. 21 Obliterative (Constrictive) Bronchiolitis, p. 458.

C. False   Mosaic perfusion and air trapping, although seen in obliterative bronchiolitis, are not specific. For example, this manifestation can be seen in hypersensitivity pneumonitis.
Ch. 21 Specific Clinical Pathological Forms, p. 459.

D. True
Ch. 21 Bronchiolitis Obliterans, p. 458.

E. False   Diffuse panbronchiolitis is a condition of unknown aetiology but an important cause of progressive obstructive lung disease particularly within Japan and Korea. Follicular bronchiolitis, however, is an entity that is usually associated with a tissue disorder, in particular, rheumatoid arthritis and Sjögren's syndome.
Ch. 21 Specific Clinicopathological Forms, p. 459.

Q 2.28   Regarding pulmonary neoplasms

A. Squamous cell carcinomas compromise 15–20% of cases.

B. A 'corona radiata' appearance of a mass strongly suggests the presence of a bronchial carcinoma.

C. Calcification is seen in 10% of bronchogenic carcinomas on conventional chest radiographs.

D. The demonstration of a peripheral line shadow or tail is pathognomonic of malignancy.

E. In bronchial carcinoma, 40–60% of patients are asymptomatic at time of diagnosis.

Q 2.29   Concerning bronchogenic carcinoma

A. FDG-PET has a sensitivity greater than 80% in the detection of lymph-node invasion.

B. Tumour encircling the aorta with a contract area exceeding 150° is non-resectable.

C. Local chest wall pain is a more specific indicator of tumour spread to the chest wall than the CT findings.

D. CT is regarded as the optimal modality for demonstrating the extent of superior sulcus tumours.

E. A patient with a primary lung cancer with a pleural effusion is classified as having a T4 stage tumour.

(Answers overleaf)

A **2.28** **Regarding pulmonary neoplasms**

A. False This is commonly seen in 30–50% of cases.
Ch. 22 Bronchial Carcinoma, p. 463

B. True Although this sign is not specific, it is highly suggestive of a bronchial tumour.
Ch. 22 The Peripheral Tumour, p. 464.

C. False Although CT studies show calcification in approximately 6% of bronchogenic carcinomas, this is very rarely detected using conventional radiography, but it is more commonly seen on CT.
Ch. 22 The Peripheral Tumour, p. 465.

D. False A streak or tail shadow is a non-specific finding.
Ch. 22 The Peripheral Tumour, p. 464.

E. False The figure is closer to 25%.
Ch. 22 Bronchial Carcinoma, p. 463.

A **2.29** **Concerning bronchogenic carcinoma**

A. True The sensitivity and specificity of PET in the diagnosis of lymph node involvement in bronchogenic carcinoma is in excess of 80%; considerably better than either CT or MRI.
Ch. 22 Mediastinal Invasion, p. 472.

B. True Tumours showing less than 90° of circumferential contact with the aorta are deemed to be resectable.
Ch. 22 Mediastinal Invasion, p. 473.

C. True The assessment of chest wall involvement adjacent to the tumour is unreliable on CT, unless there is clear-cut bone invasion or a large soft-tissue mass.
Ch. 22 Chest Wall Invasion, p. 474.

D. False This is now thought to be better shown with MRI with its multi-planar imaging and its ability to display excellent tissue contrast between tumour and the soft tissues of the chest wall.
Ch. 22 Chest Wall Invasion, p. 475.

E. False Although a pleural effusion with an associated primary lung cancer suggests that a T4 stage is very probable, this has to be proven with cytology and other causes of pleural effusion eliminated (e.g. heart failure). Attempts to characterize the nature of pleural fluid based on density measurements on CT or intensity signals on MRI have not proved useful.
Ch. 22 Pleural Involvement, p. 475.

Q 2.30   Pulmonary metastases

A. Nodules with an irregular edge are suggestive of metastases from an adenocarcinoma.

B. Calcification is common when the primary tumour demonstrates calcific deposits.

C. Are a rare cause of an asymptomatic solitary pulmonary nodule in patients without a known extrathoracic primary neoplasm.

D. CT is the most cost-effective method of finding pulmonary metastases.

E. MRI is more sensitive in detecting metastases than CT.

Q 2.31   Regarding pulmonary tumours

A. Bronchial carcinoid tumours may present as Cushing's syndrome.

B. Carcinoid syndrome is common in patients with a solitary bronchial carcinoid tumour.

C. From 20 to 30% of bronchial carcinoid lesions calcify.

D. Pulmonary harmatomas may be in a recognized association with functioning extra adrenal paragangliomas and gastric smooth-muscle tumours.

E. 'Popcorn' calcification is diagnostic of a harmatoma.

(Answers overleaf)

A **2.30** **Pulmonary metastases**

A. True Metastases, however, are typically well defined and spherical.
Ch. 22 Metastases, p. 483.

B. False Calcification is very unusual except in metastases from osteosarcoma and chrondrosarcoma. Even if the primary tumour shows visible calcification it is rare in the pulmonary metastases.
Ch. 22 Pulmonary Neoplasms, p. 483.

C. True This comprised no more than 2–3% of cases in one series.
Ch. 22 Metastases, p. 483.

D. True
Ch. 22 Metastases, p. 484.

E. False Only one study has shown MRI to be as sensitive as CT. MRI does have its advantages, however, with its lack of radiation exposure and its ability to differentiate small, centrally-located metastases from adjacent normal blood vessels.
Ch. 22 Metastases, p. 484.

A **2.31** **Regarding pulmonary tumours**

A. True These tumours may secret ACTH in sufficient quantities for a patient to present with Cushing's syndrome.
Ch. 22 Bronchial Carcinoid, p. 477.

B. False Carcinoid syndrome is rare if the tumour is confined to the lung.
Ch. 22 Bronchial Carcinoid, p. 477.

C. True A third of lesions may calcify, a feature best demonstrated on CT.
Ch. 22 Benign Pulmonary Tumours, p. 477.

D. True
Ch. 22 Pulmonary Harmatomas, p. 477.

E. False Although virtually diagnostic, this feature can occasionally also be seen in chrondrosarcomas.
Ch. 22 Pulmonary Harmatomas, p. 478.

Q 2.32   Regarding pulmonary lymphoma

A. In Hodgkins lymphoma, isolated pulmonary involvement is common.

B. Lung involvement in malignant lymphoma occurs in 10–15% of cases at presentation.

C. Malignant lymphoma may present as reticular shadowing, which cannot be distinguished from lymphangitis carcinomatosa.

D. Pleural effusions are a common finding.

E. Lobar atelectasis caused by extrinsic compression of a bronchus an enlarged lymph node is common.

Q 2.33   Regarding sarcoidosis

A. Eighty per cent of patients with enlarged lymph nodes on the chest radiograph develop parenchymal opacities within 1 year.

B. Less than 20% of patients with the disorder have an abnormal chest radiograph.

C. Broncho vascular nodular beading is a highly specific feature of sarcoidosis on HRCT.

D. Twenty per cent of patients have concomitant pleural effusions.

E. In 20% of patients, lymphadenopathy persists indefinitely and can be confused with other subsequent incidental chest pathology.

(Answers overleaf)

A **2.32** Regarding pulmonary lymphoma

A. False This is only rarely seen with Hodgkins lymphoma but is not uncommonly seen with non-Hodgkins lymphoma.
Ch. 22 Malignant Lymphoma, p. 479.

B. True
Ch. 22 Malignant Lymphoma, p. 479.

C. True
Ch. 22 Malignant Lymphoma, p. 479.

D. True These are common except in MAL/lymphoma.
Ch. 22 Malignant Lymphoma, p. 481.

E. False This is mostly caused by endobronchial lymphoma. Compression by enlarged lymph nodes is rare; encasement rather than obstruction is the more usual pattern.
Ch. 22 Malignant Lymphoma, p. 481.

A **2.33** Regarding sarcoidosis

A. False This is closer to 40%. One-third will go on to have fibrotic, persistent shadowing.
Ch. 23 Sarcoidosis, p. 495.

B. False Ninety per cent of patients have an abnormal chest radiograph at some stage, featuring lymphadenopathy, parenchymal opacities or both.
Ch. 23 Sarcoidosis, p. 495.

C. True This sign is very sensitive and specific for sarcoidosis. The phenomenon is characterized by 1–5 mm nodules in the peri-lymphatic region along the broncho-vascular bundles, interlobular septa and subpleural spaces.
Ch. 23 Sarcoidosis, p. 497.

D. False The prevalence of effusions is about 2% and their presence should raise doubts about sarcoidosis.
Ch. 23 Sarcoidosis, p. 497.

E. False Only 5% of these nodes persist indefinitely. In 90% of patients nodal enlargement is maximal on the first radiograph and disappears within 6–12 months.
Ch. 23 Sarcoidosis, p. 495.

Q **2.34** The following are causes of eggshell nodal calcification

A. Sarcoidosis.
B. Histiocytosis.
C. Histoplasmosis.
D. Amyloidosis.
E. Tuberculosis.

Q **2.35** Concerning extrinsic allergic alveolitis (EAA)

A. The fibrosis resulting from repeated episodes is most severe in the mid and lower zones of the lung.
B. Air trapping is a feature of EAA on HRCT.
C. A 'ground glass' appearance is a common feature on both the chest radiograph and HRCT.
D. It is commonly associated with eosinophilia.
E. A normal chest radiograph taken during an acute episode excludes EAA.

Q **2.36** Regarding interstitial lung disease

A. Langerhans' cell histocytosis (LCH) is commoner in females than males.
B. The thin-walled cysts associated with lymphangioleiomyomatosis (LAM) are randomly distributed throughout the lungs with normal intervening parenchyma on HRCT.
C. Spontaneous pneumothoraces occur in about 20% of patients with LCH.
D. LAM is strongly associated with smoking.
E. In the context of cryptogenic fibrosing alveolitis (CFA), the presence of ground-glass opacities on HRCT suggests that the patients are unlikely to respond to treatment.

(Answers overleaf)

A 2.34 The following are causes of eggshell nodal calcification

A. True

Ch. 23 Table 23.3, p. 495.

B. False

Ch. 23, Lymphadenopathy, p. 495.

C. True

Ch. 23 Table 23.3, p. 495.

D. True

Ch. 23 Table 23.3, p. 495.

E. False

Ch. 23, Lymphadenopathy, p. 495.

A 2.35 Concerning extrinsic allergic alveolitis (EAA)

A. True

Ch. 23 Extrinsic Allergic Alveolitis, p. 497.

B. True This reflects the co-existing bronchiolitis caused by antigen deposition in the small airways.
Ch. 23, Extrinsic Allergic Alveolitis, p. 498.

C. True

Ch. 23 Extrinsic Allergic Alveolitis, p. 497.

D. False There is no such association.
Ch. 23, Extrinsic Allergic Alveolitis, p. 497.

E. False The chest radiograph can be normal in the acute phase.
Ch. 23, Extrinsic Allergic Alveolitis, p. 497.

A 2.36 Regarding interstitial lung disease

A. False There is a male to female ratio of 4:1.
Ch. 23 Langerhans Cell Histiocytosis, p. 499.

B. True

Ch. 23 Lymphangioleimyomatosis, p. 499.

C. True Spontaneous pneumothoraces occur in 20%.
Ch. 23 Langerhans Cell Histiocytosis, p. 499.

D. False This is true of Langerhans cell histiocytosis.
Ch. 23 Lymphangioleimyomatosis, p. 499.

E. False The reverse is true.
Ch. 23 Fibrosing Alveolitis, p. 500.

Q 2.37 Regarding collagen vascular diseases in the chest

A. Pulmonary haemorrhage is a recognized manifestation systemic lupus erythematosus (SLE).

B. Pleural effusion is the commonest radiographic manifestation of rheumatoid disease.

C. Fifty per cent of patients with rheumatoid arthritis develop pulmonary interstitial fibrosis.

D. Enlarged mediastinal lymph nodes are a frequent finding on CT in patients with collagen vascular diseases.

E. Caplan's nodules occur in patients who have been exposed to silicone.

Q 2.38 Concerning chest involvement with systemic vasculitis

A. Wegener's granulomatosis is associated with bronchial narrowing.

B. In Wegener's granulomatosis, cavitation is seen in approximately 50% of cases with pulmonary nodules or masses.

C. The most common radiographic finding in Churg-Strauss syndrome is patchy peripheral consolidation.

D. Pulmonary arterial aneurysms are associated with Behçet's disease.

E. A positive serum C-ANCA titre is specific for the diagnosis of Wegener's granulomatosis.

(Answers overleaf)

A **2.37**   Regarding collagen vascular diseases in the chest

A. True
   Ch. 23 Collagen Vascular Diseases, p. 501.

B. True   Effusions are five times more common in men then women.
   Ch. 23 Rheumatoid Disease, p. 501.

C. True   It is, however, more usually associated with penicillamine or gold therapy.
   Ch. 23 Rheumatoid Disease, p. 501.

D. True
   Ch. 23 Systemic Sclerosis, p. 503.

E. False   Caplan's syndrome, first described in Welsh miners, is a disease entity in which
   nodules rapidly appear in crops in some patients with rheumatoid arthritis
   following exposure to silica. Silicone is an unrelated prosthetic material.
   Ch. 21 Rheumatoid Disease, p. 501.

A **2.38**   Concerning chest involvement with systemic vasculitis

A. True   This may lead to sub-segmental or lobar atelectasis. It is also associated with
   subglottic and tracheal narrowing.
   Ch. 23 Wegener's Granulomatosis, p. 504.

B. True
   Ch. 23 Wegener's Granulomatosis, p. 504.

C. True   This is similar to that seen in chronic eosinophilic pneumonia.
   Ch. 23 Churg-Strauss Syndrome, p. 505.

D. True
   Ch. 23 Behçet's Disease, p. 505.

E. False   A small percentage of patients with microscopic polyangiitis and
   Churg-Strauss syndrome may also have positive serum C-ANCA titres.
   Ch. 23 Wegener's Granulomatosis, p. 505.

Q 2.39 Regarding lymphoid disorders of the lung

A. Lymphocytic interstitial pneumonia (LIP) is associated with Sjögren's syndrome.

B. Lymph node enlargement is common in LIP.

C. Lymphomatoid granulomatosis is a pre-malignant condition.

D. A normal chest radiograph is a common finding in patients with leukaemia.

E. In patients with acute myeloid leukaemia (AML), air space shadowing on a chest radiograph is likely to be secondary to infiltrative disease.

Q 2.40 Regarding industrial/occupational lung disease

A. In coal worker's pneumoconiosis (CWP), the severity of disease is dependent on the relative amount of silica in the dust inhaled.

B. In CWP, the chest radiograph may demonstrate large spiculated intrapulmonary masses up to 10 cm in diameter.

C. In CWP, centrilobular emphysema is a prominent feature.

D. Exposure to silica causes multiple small nodules located predominantly in the middle and upper zones.

E. Inhalation of silica (SiO_2) can lead to extensive fibrosis.

(Answers overleaf)

A **2.39** Regarding lymphoid disorders of the lung

A. True It also occurs in isolation and in children with AIDS.
Ch. 22 Lymphocytic Interstitial Pneumonitis, p. 481.

B. False The presence of lymph node enlargement should suggest the development of lymphoma.
Ch. 22 Lymphocytic Interstitial Pneumonitis, p. 481.

C. True Transformation to a malignant lymphoma occurs in up to 50% of patients.
Ch. 22 Lymphomatoid Granulomatosis, p. 481.

D. True
Ch. 22 Leukaemia, p. 482.

E. False In AML, the chest radiograph may be normal or show air-space shadowing, which is probably due to pulmonary oedema rather than directly to the accumulating leuaemic cells in the lungs.
Ch. 22 Leukaemia, p. 482.

A **2.40** Regarding industrial/occupational lung disease

A. True These particles contribute to the pathological and radiological signs. At low exposure levels, the matter deposited in the lungs can be cleared into sputum; at higher levels these mechanisms are overwhelmed and the phagocytosed particles deposited in the lung.
Ch. 24 Coal Workers Pneumoconiosis, p. 511.

B. True This is the description of progressive massive fibrosis.
Ch. 24 Progressive Massive Fibrosis, p. 512.

C. False This is seen pathologically, but is not a prominent radiological feature.
Ch. 24 Coal Workers Pneumoconiosis, p. 511.

D. True
Ch. 24 Silicosis, p. 512.

E. True The inhalation of silica may cause a marked fibrotic reaction including progressive massive fibrosis.
Ch. 24 Industrial Lung Silicosis, p. 513.

Q 2.41   Regarding asbestos-related lung disease

A. The commonest radiological feature of asbestos exposure is visceral pleural plaque.

B. The presence of asbestos bodies in the lungs indicates the presence of interstitial disease.

C. Ninety per cent of malignant malignant mesotheliomas are related to asbestos exposure.

D. In asbestosis the upper lunch zones are spared even in severe cases of pulmonary involvement, a feature distinguishing it from CWP.

E. Pulmonary pseudotumours are metabolically active on FDG-PET examination.

Q 2.42   Regarding the diagnosis of pulmonary thromboembolism

A. A ventilation–perfusion scan has a high sensitivity and specificity for the diagnosis of pulmonary embolism.

B. It is unlikely (false-negative rate < 5%), in patients with a low 'probability' ventilation–perfusion scan using the PIOPED criteria.

C. A normal ventilation–perfusion scan excludes pulmonary embolism with a probability of approximately 60%.

D. Pulmonary angiography remains the gold standard for diagnosis of pulmonary embolism.

E. In the PIOPED study, 50% of chest radiographs in patients with pulmonary embolism were normal.

(Answers overleaf)

A **2.41** Regarding asbestos-related lung disease

A. False Although pleural plaques are the commonest feature, these are well-defined soft-tissue sheets originating on the *parietal* pleural surface. The extent of the plaques is related to the severity of exposure
Ch. 24 Silicate Pneumoconiosis, Asbestosis, p. 513.

B. False The presence of asbestos bodies (asbestos fibres coated in proteinaceous material) which coats the asbestos fibres (asbestos bodies) indicates exposure to asbestos rather than the presence of disease.
Ch. 24 Silicate Pneumoconiosis, p. 513.

C. True The risk is most pronounced with blue asbestos (crocidolite).
Ch. 24 Silicate Pneumoconiosis, p. 514.

D. True This occurs in even severe cases.
Ch. 24 Silicate Pneumoconiosis Pulmonary Changes, p. 515.

E. False They are inactive. A fibrotic atelectasis occurs in the lung periphery, usually in the lower zone adjacent to an area of pleural thickening. It has the classic 'comet tail' appearance.
Ch. 24 Silicate Pneumoconiosis, pp. 515/516.

A **2.42** Regarding the diagnosis of pulmonary thromboembolism

A. False The high sensitivity is not matched by a high specificity.
Ch. 25 Radionuclide Studies in Pulmonary Thromboembolism, p. 523.

B. False The F negative rate was 15% in the PIOPED study.
Ch. 25 Radionuclide Studies in Pulmonary Thromboembolism, p. 524.

C. False This is closer to 95%.
Ch. 25 Radionuclide Studies in Pulmonary Thromboembolism, p. 523.

D. True In experienced hands, the mortality is negligible with a death rate well below 1%.
Ch. 25 Radionuclide Studies in Pulmonary Thromboembolism, p. 524.

E. False The chest radiograph was abnormal in 88%, the most common findings being areas of atelectasis, areas of parachymal opacifications and pleural effusions.
Ch. 25 Imaging of Pulmonary Thromboembolism, p. 521.

Q **2.43** Regarding drug-induced lung disease

 A. In the blood film eosinophilia is a common finding.
 B. Pleural effusions are a feature of most drug-induced reactions.
 C. Methotrexate causes hilar lymphadenopathy.
 D. The severity of chronic reactions is dose related.
 E. Penicillamine is a recognized cause of obliterative bronchiolitis.

Q **2.44** Concerning pulmonary thromboembolism

 A. Chest pain is a presenting symptom in more than 80% of patients.
 B. Distal blood flow is compromised in a pulmonary artery when its lumen is reduced by 50%.
 C. The classical ECG findings of pulmonary embolism include sinus tachycardia, right axis deviation, an $S_1Q_3T_3$ pattern and ST changes.
 D. The D-dimer test is an effective exclusion test with a negative predictive value approaching 100%.
 E. Right-sided cardiac failure occurs when more then 50% of the pulmonary vasculature has been occluded acutely by emboli.

(Answers overleaf)

A **2.43** **Regarding drug-induced lung disease**

A. **True**
   Ch. 23 Drug-Induced Lung Disease, p. 506.

B. **False** These are not seen in association with most acute or even chronic pulmonary reactions except in drug-induced lupus.
   Ch. 23 Drug-Induced Lung Disease, p. 507.

C. **True** Anticonvulsants and methotrexate do cause enlargement of the hilar lymph nodes.
   Ch. 23 Drug-Induced Lung Disease, p. 507.

D. **True**
   Ch. 23 Drug-Induced Lung Disease, p. 506.

E. **True** Penicillamine and gold therapy are recognized causes.
   Ch. 23 Table 23.7, p. 506.

A **2.44** **Concerning pulmonary thromboembolism**

A. **False** This symptom is less common than acute dyspnoea and a feeling of anxiety. Chest pain occurred in approximately 43% in one series.
   Ch. 25 Clinical Features and Physiological Effects of Pulmonary Thromboembolism, p. 520.

B. **False** There needs to be a reduction of 80% in the luminal diameter before distal blood flow is reduced.
   Ch. 25 Clinical Features and Physiological Effects of Pulmonary Thromboembolism, p. 520.

C. **True**
   Ch. 25 Imaging Tests for Pulmonary Embolism, p. 521.

D. **True** D-dimers have a high sensitivity but low specificity.
   Ch. 25 Non-imaging Tests for Pulmonary Embolism, p. 521.

E. **True** The maximum pressure that the right normal ventricle can withstand is 45 mm Hg, values above this will produce rapid-onset, right-sided cardiac failure.
   Ch. 25 Pulmonary Embolism, p. 520.

Q **2.45**   **Regarding the imaging of pulmonary thromboembolism**

> **A.** Emboli confined to the sub-segmental pulmonary arteries can result in a false-negative diagnosis on spiral CT.
> **B.** The optimum concentration of contrast medium is 350 mg/ml of iodine for a CT pulmonary angiogram.
> **C.** 'Hampton's hump' describes a typical plain-film appearance of a pulmonary infarct.
> **D.** Sterile cavitation of pulmonary infarcts occurs in 10% of cases.
> **E.** Consolidation involving an entire lobe is unlikely and should suggest an infective aetiology.

Q **2.46**   **Regarding traumatic injury to the chest**

> **A.** Lung contusions occur in 70–80% of cases with severe blunt chest trauma.
> **B.** Rib fractures in children are common following accidental injury.
> **C.** Sternal fractures are associated with a high incidence of mortality.
> **D.** The radiographic changes associated with pulmonary contusion are seen within 6 hours and clear within 1–2 days.
> **E.** Worsening consolidation on a CXR in a case of lung contusion is a feature of fat embolism.

(Answers overleaf)

A **2.45** Regarding the imaging of pulmonary thromboembolism

A. True An there are several other causes of a false-negative diagnosis on CT.
Ch. 25 Table 25.3, p. 529.

B. False A high concentration such as this, may produce a marked streak artefact from the superior vena cava that can obscure the adjacent right main and right upper-lobe pulmonary arteries. A concentration of 150–240 mg/ml of iodine injected at 4–5 ml is optimal.
Ch. 25 Imaging of Pulmonary Thromboembolism, p. 527.

C. True This is a shallow hump-shaped lesion with its base applied to a pleural surface. Many pulmonary infarcts do not resemble humps, however, and can have a variety of shapes depending on their orientation and the mask of surrounding haemorrhage.
Ch. 25 Radiographic Signs of Pulmonary Emboli, p. 522.

D. False Data from various studies suggest that it is less than 5%. It usually occurs within 2 weeks of the radiographic appearance of an infarct and is more common in lesions greater than 4 cm in diameter.
Ch. 25 Aseptic Cavitation, p. 523.

E. True
Ch. 25 Radiographic Signs of Pulmonary Emboli, p. 522.

A **2.46** Regarding traumatic injury to the chest

A. True
Ch. 26 Pulmonary Contusion, p. 537.

B. False These are rare and when present should raise the possibility of non-accidental injury.
Ch. 26 Chest Trauma, p. 536.

C. True There is a 25% mortality rate in patients who have sternal fractures owing to associated injuries including cardiac contusion, pulmonary contusion, haemothorax.
Ch. 26 Chest Trauma, p. 536.

D. False Although the opacities appear within 6 hours, they clear within 3–10 days.
Ch. 26 Pulmonary Contusion, p. 537.

E. True Other possibilities include infection, aspiration or ARDS.
Ch. 26 Pulmonary Contusion, p. 537.

Q **2.47**   **Concerning diaphragmatic rupture due to abdominal trauma**

A. This occurs in approximately 10% of patients with major blunt abdominal trauma.

B. Left-sided diaphragmatic tears are more common than right-sided tears.

C. A normal chest radiograph excludes diaphragmatic rupture.

D. Ultrasound should not be used to detect acute diaphragmatic tears.

E. When using magnetic resonance imaging T1-weighted images are the most useful sequence for the accurate diagnosis of diaphragmatic tear.

Q **2.48**   **Concerning the mediastinal structures and trauma**

A. Tracheobronchial tear is located within a main-stem bronchus in 90% of patients.

B. Aortic ruptures occur just distal to the origin of the left subclavian artery in 90% of cases.

C. On a chest radiograph, the presence of a left apical pleural cap in the context of trauma should raise the possibility of aortic rupture.

D. Helical CT can obviate the need for angiography in the assessment of aortic tears in the majority of patients.

E. Rupture of the oesophagus is most frequently due to blunt or external penetrating trauma.

(Answers overleaf)

A **2.47** **Concerning diaphragmatic rupture due to abdominal trauma**

A. False This occurs in 0.8–5% of patients. The impact leads to a sudden rise in intra-abdominal pressure, which results in the rupture.
Ch. 26 The Diaphragm, p. 538.

B. True Most series show tears to be more common on the left than the right in 70–90% of cases.
Ch. 26 The Diaphragm, p. 538.

C. False The chest radiograph has been shown to be diagnostic in less than 50% of patients.
Ch. 26 The Diaphragm, p. 538.

D. False Ultrasound has been shown to be of value. The diaphragm can be directly visualized especially if there is free fluid above and below the diaphragm. Direct visualization of the tear is possible, appearing often as a 'flapping' free edge.
Ch. 26 The Diaphragm, p. 538.

E. True The diaphragm appears as a low signal intensity line with high intensity mediastinal and abdominal fat on either side. Tears can be clearly seen and occasionally fat or upper abdominal organs may be seen herniating through.
Ch. 26 The Diaphragm, p. 538.

A **2.48** **Concerning the mediastinal structures and trauma**

A. True The remaining 10% are located within the trachea, within 2 cm of the carina. Tracheobroncheal tears are commonly associated with upper rib, sternal and thoracic spine fractures.
Ch. 26 The Mediastinum, p. 540.

B. True These figures are true in a clinical series; in autopsy series, however, 20–25% of aortic injuries occur in the ascending aorta.
Ch. 26 The Mediastinum, p. 540.

C. True The cap is due to an extra-pleural haematoma and occasionally a left pleural effusion can be seen as well.
Ch. 26 The Mediastinum, p. 541.

D. True Catheter angiography need only be used in a minority of patients with small or indeterminate tears or those with tears involving the origins of the great vessels.
Ch. 26 The Aorta, p. 541.

E. False Most oesophageal perforations are iatrogenic, being due to endoscopy with or without dilatation.
Ch. 26 The Oesophagus, p. 543.

Q **2.49**   **Regarding the chest radiograph in the post-operative patient**

A.   Lower-lobe consolidation is more common than Fleischner's plate atelectases in the lower lung fields after major abdominal surgery.
B.   Aspiration pneumonitis typically shows resolution within 72 hours.
C.   In adult respiratory distress syndrome (ARDS), the chest radiograph can be normal for up to 12 hours following the onset of the condition.
D.   In the presence of a pulmonary capillary wedge pressure below 15 mmHg, air-space shadowing is unlikely to be due to cardiac failure.
E.   Discrete nodules appearing on the chest radiograph in the post-operative or critically ill patient suggest lung infection.

Q **2.50**   **Regarding external therapeutic radiation**

A.   Symptomatic reactions are uncommon when less than 25% of the lung volume is irradiated.
B.   Cyclophosphamide potentiates the lung reaction to chest radiation.
C.   More than 50% of patients with acute radiation pneumonitis, progress to chronic fibrosis.
D.   The fibrotic stage tends to stabilize within 2 years.
E.   Radiation-induced sarcoma usually occurs within 5 years of radiation therapy.

(Answers overleaf)

75

A **2.49** **Regarding the chest radiograph in the post-operative patient**

A. False Plate atelectasis occurs in more than 50% of patients soon after surgery and patchy, segmental or complete lobar consolidation is less common.
Ch. 27 Atelectasis, p. 548.

B. False One to 2 days: progression of airspace shadowing; 5–7 days: stabilization and regression; 7–14 days: complete clearance.
Ch. 27 Aspiration Pneumonitis, p. 549.

C. True Microemboli and small haemorrhage may be visible microscopically but essentially the chest radiograph is normal. Until interstitial oedema occurs followed by inhomogeneous shadowing and areas of atelectasis.
Ch. 27 ARDS, p. 553.

D. True The first signs of interstitial pulmonary oedema are peri-hilar haze, peribronchial cuffing and fluid in the interlobular septa (Kerley A and B lines). These features tend to occur at pulmonary capillary wedge pressures of 18–22 mmHg.
Ch. 27 Pulmonary Oedema, p. 550.

E. True Lung infection due to septicaemia may appear as either discrete nodules, diffuse patchy consolidation or diffuse oedema.
Ch. 27 Pneumonia, p. 551.

A **2.50** **Regarding external therapeutic radiation**

A. True The field size and dose should be kept to a minimum.
Ch. 27 Radiation Therapy, p. 559.

B. True Chemotherapeutic agents such as cyclophosphamide, actinomycin D, bleomycin and adriamycin all potentiate the lung reaction to radiation changes whether given simultaneously or sequentially.
Ch. 27 Radiation Therapy, p. 559.

C. True
Ch. 27 Radiation Therapy, p. 559.

D. True From time to time, the fibrotic stage can be difficult to differentiate from tumour recurrence or lymphangitis. In these cases CT may be helpful.
Ch. 27 Radiation Therapy, p. 560.

E. False This entity is rare but when present occurs more than 16 years after radiation treatment, in patients receiving over 30 Gy.
Ch. 27 Radiation Therapy, p. 561.

Q **2.51**   **Concerning the chest radiograph in the critically ill patient**

A.   Tracheostomy is a frequent cause of a pneumomediastinum.
B.   In a patient with a suspected pneumothorax, a negative supine film does not effectively exclude the diagnosis.
C.   The absence of mediastinal shift in the presence of a pneumothorax excludes a tension pneumothorax.
D.   Ultrasound and CT are both valuable techniques in the assessment of loculated collections.
E.   In patients who have undergone coronary artery bypass surgery, sub-diaphragmatic air in the immediate post-operative period suggests perforation of an intra-abdominal viscus.

Q **2.52**   **Regarding lung volume reduction surgery (LVRS)**

A.   Patients with emphysema in the upper lobes and relative sparing of the lower lungs are the best candidates for LVRS.
B.   There is a lack of correlation between pathological and HRCT determinations of the severity of emphysema.
C.   Patients with a diffuse emphysema have a better prognosis after LVRS than those with heterogeneous or focal emphysema.
D.   Five percent of patients being evaluated for LVRS or lung transplantation also have primary bronchogenic carcinoma.
E.   The residual volume of the contralateral, non-LVRS lung is seen to decrease following unilateral surgery.

(Answers overleaf)

77

A **2.51** **Concerning the chest radiograph in the critically ill patient**

A. **True** Other causes include oesophageal or tracheal perforation, interstitial emphysema and mediastinitis due to gas-forming organisms.
Ch. 27 Extrapulmonary Air, p. 555.

B. **True** If a pneumothorax is suspected, an upright or decubitus film (or a CT scan) must be obtained.
Ch. 27 Extrapulmonary Air, p. 555.

C. **False** In the presence of a densely consolidated lung pleural adhesions, total collapse or mediastinal shift may be absent. The most reliable sign in these cases is a depression of the diaphragm.
Ch. 27 Extrapulmonary Air, p. 555.

D. **True**
Ch. 27 Pleural Effusion, p. 556.

E. **False** This finding is usually caused by inadvertent disruption of the xiphisternal attachment of the diaphragm. It is benign and self-limiting.
Ch. 27 Cardiac Surgery, p. 557.

A **2.52** **Regarding lung volume reduction surgery (LVRS)**

A. **True**
Ch. 28A Patient Selection for LVRS, p. 569.

B. **False** Many studies have shown an excellent correlation, using both visual scoring systems and quantitative analysis.
Ch. 28A Computed Tomography, p. 566.

C. **False** The reverse is true, the more heterogeneous the emphysema, the better the improvement in FEV_1 3 months after LVRS.
Ch. 28A Patient Outcome After LVRS, p. 569.

D. **True** There is an associated risk of lung cancer with severe emphysema and several studies have detected an approximately 5% incidence of incidental bronchogenic carcinoma at time of evaluation.
Ch. 28A Incidental Lung Cancer, p. 570.

E. **False** There is no alteration of severity of air-flow obstruction in the non-LVRS lung.
Ch. 28A Post Operative Imaging, p. 574.

Q 2.53   Regarding lung transplantation

A. Acute rejection is the first demonstrable complication following a lung transplant on a chest X-ray (CXR).

B. There is an association with the Epstein Barr virus and post-transplantation lymphoproliferative disease.

C. Primary graft failure is the commonest cause of early mortality following lung transplantation.

D. Transbronchial lung biopsy remains the gold standard technique for the diagnosis of obliterative bronchiolitis and, hence, chronic rejection.

E. Sarcoidosis may recur after lung transplantation.

Q 2.54   Regarding pulmonary oedema

A. Plain readiography is more sensitive than clinical evaluation at detecting pulmonary oedema on a chest radiograph.

B. Kerley B lines are diagnostic of pulmonary oedema.

C. Unilateral air space consolidation would not be consistent with pulmonary oedema on the chest radiograph.

D. Upper lobe blood diversion on the chest radiograph is invariably present.

E. A peripheral distribution of oedema is consistent with ARDS (non-cardiogenic oedema) rather than a cardiogenic cause.

(Answers overleaf)

A **2.53** **Regarding lung transplantation**

A. **False** Reperfusion oedema is normally seen in the absence of acute rejection and is not a common feature of that condition.
Ch. 28B Acute Complications, p 578

B. **True** There is a very strong association. LPD after lung transplantation is twice that seen after the transplantation of other organs.
Ch. 28B Post-transplantation Malignancies, p. 585.

C. **False** Pulmonary graft failure ranks secondly to infection as a cause of mortality.
Ch. 28B Primary Graft Failure, p. 578.

D. **False** The transbronchial biopsy is only 15–18% sensitive in making the diagnosis of OB, due to its patchy nature and difficulty in adequate samplings. Chronic rejection is a clinical diagnosis based on FEV_1 and changes secondary to a progressive airways disease that cannot be otherwise explained by infection, acute rejection or anastomotic complications.
Ch. 28B Obliterative BronChiolitis, p. 584.

E. **True** The other diseases that can recur include diffuse pan-bronchiolitis, alveolar proteinosis, giant-cell pneumonia, DIP and LAM.
Ch. 28B Recurrence of Disease, p. 585.

A **2.54** **Regarding pulmonary oedema**

A. **True**
Ch. 29 Chest Radiographic Signs of Pulmonary Oedema, p. 592.

B. **False** There can be seen in any case of interlobular septal thickening, e.g. lymphagitis carcinomatosis interstitial lung disease.
Ch. 29 Chest Radiographic Signs of Pulmonary Oedema, p. 592.

C. **False** Pulmonary oedema can be positional and infrequently assymetrical.
Ch. 29 Chest Radiographic Signs of Pulmonary Oedema, p. 592.

D. **False**
Ch. 29 Chest Radiographic Signs of Pulmonary Oedema, p. 592.

E. **False** Although one study claimed this was the case, others have refuted this. Chest radiography is unreliable at distinguishing the cause of pulmonary oedema.
Ch. 29 Chest Radiographic Signs of Pulmonary Oedema, p. 592.

Q 2.55   Regarding pulmonary haemorrhage

    A. A normal chest radiograph in the presence of an increased K_{co}, is sufficient evidence to suggest early alveolar haemorrhage.

    B. Air-space consolidation commonly resolves within a few days.

    C. There is an association with autoimmune renal disease.

    D. On the chest radiograph, air-space consolidation is most pronounced in the mid and lower zones.

    E. The presence of reticulo-nodular opacities on the chest radiograph suggests repeated episodes of pulmonary haemorrhage.

Q 2.56   Regarding wegener's granulomatosis

    A. The disorder is characterized by a necrotizing vasculitis of large vessels.

    B. It is most prevalent in the second to fourth decades.

    C. In adults, cavitating nodules are more common than consolidation or ground-glass opacities on CT.

    D. The disorder is a cause of bronchiectasis.

    E. Mediastinal lymph node enlargement is common.

(Answers overleaf)

A **2.55**   **Regarding pulmonary haemorrhage**

A. True   Rise in K_{co} may proceed overt radiographic changes. The measurement of K_{co} is considered to be a sensitive non-invasive indicator of fresh alveolar blood.
Ch. 29 Diffuse Pulmonary Haemorrhage, p. 596.

B. True   Pulmonary oedema may clear within 24–48 hours; pulmonary infections tend to clear within 5–30 days.
Ch. 29 Diffuse Pulmonary Haemorrhage, p. 596.

C. True   This entity is referred to as Goodpasture's syndrome in which antibodies are directed against components of the basement membrane in the lungs and kidneys.
Ch. 29 Antibasement Membrane Antibody Disease, p. 596.

D. True
Ch. 29 The Radiology of DPH Syndromes, p. 596.

E. True
Ch. 29 Diffuse Pulmonary Haemorrhage, p. 597.

A **2.56**   **Regarding wegener's granulomatosis**

A. False   It is a necrotizing vasculitis, but of medium and small-sized vessels.
Ch. 29 Wegener's Granulomatosis, p. 597.

B. False   Patients present at any age from childhood to the eighth decade.
Ch. 29 Wegener's Granulomatosis, p. 597.

C. True   Interestingly, the converse is apparently the case in children in when nodules are less frequent.
Ch. 29 Wegener's Granulomatosis, p. 597.

D. True   Bronchial vascular thickening and bronchiectasis have all been reported.
Ch. 29 Wegener's Granulomatosis, p. 598.

E. False   This is a rare finding. More commonly, atelectasis, pleural effusions or thickening arc the ancillary features of Wegener's Granulomatosis.
Ch. 29 Wegener's Granulomatosis, p. 598.

Q **2.57**   Concerning eosinophilic lung disease

A. In Löffler's syndrome air-space consolidation resolves between 1–2 months.

B. There is an association with bronchoceles.

C. Phenytoin is associated with pulmonary eosinophilia.

D. Fleeting, peripheral, air-space opacities are a characteristic feature.

E. A restrictive defect with impaired gas transfer on lung function tests is a common finding in chronic eosinophilic pneumonia.

Q **2.58**   Concerning the diagnosis and staging of lung cancer

A. A negative CXR with positive cytology carries a better prognosis than a positive CXR with positive cytology.

B. The TNM classification applies to small-cell cancer of the lung.

C. MRI is more sensitive then CT at detecting hilar node involvement.

D. Mediastinoscopy and lymph-node sampling should be performed on nodes greater than 10 mm in size.

E. Using the TNM classification for staging, stage IIIA denotes non-resectable intra-thoracic disease with hilar lymphadenopathy.

(Answers overleaf)

A **2.57**   **Concerning eosinophilic lung disease**

A. False   The resolution of the opacities occurs within a period of days and, by
definition, within a month is the rule.
Ch. 29 Simple Pulmonary Eosinophilia, p. 600.

B. True   Bronchoceles are a characteristic finding in patients with advanced allergic
bronchopulmonary aspergillosis (ABPA).
Ch. 29 Allergic Bronchopulmonary Aspergillosis, p. 601.

C. True
Ch. 29 Table 29.4, p. 599.

D. True   These seem to parallel the chest wall, a finding that has been termed the
'photographic negative of pulmonary oedema'.
Ch. 29 Chronic Eosinophilic Pneumonia, p. 600.

E. True
Ch. 29 Chronic Eosinophilic Pneumonia, p. 600.

A **2.58**   **Concerning the diagnosis and staging of lung cancer**

A. True   This is probably a reflection of the small size of the tumour, though the true
reason for this phenomenon is unknown.
Ch. 22 Early Diagnosis of Bronchial Carcinoma, p. 470.

B. False   TNM is used for all non-small-cell pulmonary cancers.
Ch. 22 Spread of Tumour, p. 470.

C. True   The multiplanar imaging capability of MRI also helps with AP window and
subcarinal nodes when doubt exists on CT.
Ch. 22 Spread of Tumour, p. 470.

D. True   Preoperative nodal sampling should be undertaken in patients whom the
transaxial node diameter is greater than 10 mms.
Ch. 22 Spread of Tumour, p. 470.

E. False   Stage IIIA indicates locally extensive intra-thoracic disease, with or without
hilar and ipsilateral lymph node involvement, which is surgically resectable.
Ch. 22 Spread of Tumour, p. 470.

Q **2.59** **Concerning alveolar proteinosis**

  A. Is associated with an abnormality of surfactant metabolism.
  B. There is an association with lymphoma in adult patients.
  C. On HRCT, a striking geographical distribution of ground-glass opacification and thickened interlobular septa resembling 'crazy-paving' is highly suggestive of the diagnosis.
  D. The most effective treatment is bronchoalveolar lavage.
  E. The condition in adults has a worse prognosis, than in children.

Q **2.60** **Regarding therapeutic pulmonary arterial embolization**

  A. The occlusion of a pulmonary artery results in pulmonary infarction.
  B. The principal indication for pulmonary arterial embolization is the occlusion of pulmonary arteriovenous malformations.
  C. Ninety per cent of patients with Osler-Weber-Rendu disease have associated pulmonary arterio-venous malformations that can be successfully treated by embolization.
  D. PAVM embolization can be safely performed using either steel coils or particulate material.
  E. The arterial oxygen saturation returns to normal after successful PAVM embolization.

(Answers overleaf)

85

A **2.59** Concerning alveolar proteinosis

A. True The aetiology of primary alveolar proteinosis, however, is unclear.
Ch. 29 Alveolar Proteinosis, p. 601.

B. True There is a recognized link between alveolar proteinosis and haematological malignancies.
Ch. 29 Alveolar Proteinosis, p. 601.

C. True These features are highly suggestive of, but not pathognomonic of, alveolar proteinosis.
Ch. 29 Alveolar Proteinosis, p. 601.

D. True Spontaneous resolution has been reported but significant improvement occurs with therapeutic bronchoalveolar lavage.
Ch. 29 Alveolar Proteinosis, p. 601.

E. False
Ch. 29 Alveolar Proteinosis, p. 601.

A **2.60** Regarding therapeutic pulmonary arterial embolization

A. False Although flow has ceased, the presence of a bronchial artery supply will usually prevent lung infarction.
Ch. 30A Pulmonary Arterial Embolization, p. 613.

B. True
Ch. 30A Pulmonary Arterial Embolization, p. 613.

C. False
Ch. 30A Pulmonary Arterial Embolization, p. 613.

D. False The only safe agents are detachable balloon catheters or steel coils. Fluid or particulate emboli can be disastrous if these are carried into any systemic vessel especially the coronary or cerebral arteries.
Ch. 30A Pulmonary Arteriovenous Malformation, p. 613.

E. False It is not possible to restore the arterial oxygen saturation value to complete normality in many patients. After a successful embolization procedure, radionuclide shunt measurements show residual shunts in these patients. These findings suggest that microscopic PAVMs are present in most patients even after successful treatment of the macroscopic lesions.
Ch. 30A Pulmonary Arterial Embolization, p. 613.

Q 2.61 Regarding thoracic drainage procedures

A. Ultrasound is superior to CT in demonstrating loculated pleural collections.
B. Empyemas are adequately drained using an 18 Fr catheter.
C. A 14 Fr catheter is a more effective than a small-bore 7 Fr catheter in the treatment of pneumothorax.
D Mediastinal abscesses can be successfully drained transoesophageally.
E. When draining an empyema, it is important not to flush the catheter as this may induce septicaemia.

Q 2.62 Regarding neonatal radiographs

A. The optimum position for an endotracheal tube is approximately 1–1.5 cms above the carina.
B. The umbilical arterial line should ideally be placed above the renal arteries at the L1/2 level.
C. A typical course for an umbilical vein catheter is cephalad through the right side of the abdomen via the right portal vein and into the inferior vena cava.
D. The normal cardiothoracic ratio is less than 50%.
E. Air in the distal oesophagus and marked gaseous distension of the gastrointestinal tract is a clue to malposition of a ET tube.

(Answers overleaf)

A **2.61** Regarding thoracic drainage procedures

A. True

> *Ch. 30B Pleural Collections, p. 627.*

B. False Thick pus often requires 12–14 Fr drains.

> *Ch. 30B Pleural Collections, p. 627.*

C. False There is no evidence that these larger drains offer any advantage over small-bore catheters.

> *Ch. 30B Pleural Collections, p. 628.*

D. True This is particularly effective when there is an anastomotic leak or other post-surgical problem, or when the patient is unlikely to survive primary surgical treatment.

> *Ch. 30B Mediastinal Collections, p. 629.*

E. False The tube must be regularly irrigated with saline to prevent clogging with fibrinous debris.

> *Ch. 30 Pleural Collections, p. 628.*

A **2.62** Regarding neonatal radiographs

A. True

> *Ch. 31A Evaluation of Tubes and Lines, p. 632.*

B. False The tip should, ideally, lie either well above the level of the coeliac axis and superior mesenteric vessels (T6 to T10) but below the aortic arch or, alternatively, below the level of the renal arteries L3-L5.

> *Ch. 31A Evaluation of Tubes and Lines, p. 633.*

C. False The umbilical vein catheter enters the *left* portal vein, at which point it may enter the ductus venosus and then the inferior vena cava.

> *Ch. 31A Evaluation of Tubes and Lines, p. 633.*

D. False The normal cardiothoracic ratio can be as large as 65% owing to the presence of the thymus.

> *Ch. 31A The Neonatal Chest, p. 631.*

E. True

> *Ch. 31A Evaluation of Tubes and Lines, p. 633.*

Q **2.63**   Regarding respiratory distress syndrome in the neonate

A. Fifty per cent of premature babies born between 26 and 28 weeks develop RDS.

B. The chest radiograph is usually normal at 6 hours.

C. Bronchopulmonary dysplasia (BPD) can occur as a result of respiratory distress syndrome.

D. It can be distinguished from transient tachypnoea of the new born on CXR.

E. Uncomplicated RDS is a bilaterally symmetrical disease.

Q **2.64**   Concerning pulmonary agenesis and hypoplasia

A. There is an association with Potter's syndrome which comprises renal agenesis, abnormal facies, pulmonary hypoplasia and truncus arteriosus.

B. On clinical and radiological examination, unilateral agenesis presents with a symmetrically developed thorax.

C. It is commonly an isolated abnormality.

D. It is more common in females than males.

E. A left-sided primary pulmonary hypoplasia maybe indistinguishable from left upper lobe collapse.

(Answers overleaf)

A **2.63** Regarding respiratory distress syndrome in the neonate

A. True   This percentage reduces to 20–30% at 30–31 weeks of gestation.
Ch. 31A Respiratory Distress Syndrome, p. 634.

B. False
Ch. 31A Respiratory Distress Syndrome, p. 634.

C. True   RDS not uncommonly requires ventilation and this can lead to bronchopulmonary dysplasia.
Ch. 31A Late Effects of Ventilation and Respiratory Distress Syndrome, p. 637.

D. True   There is normal to decreased aeration of the lungs in RDS in comparison with TTN, in which there is increased aeration.
Ch. 31A Respiratory Distress Syndrome, p. 634.

E. True   Asymmetrical changes may be seen, however, in areas which have been differentially aerated (e.g. by a misplaced endotracheal tube and where there is localized pathology such as interstitial emphysema, pulmonary haemorrhage or superimposed infection.
Ch. 31A Respiratory Distress Syndrome, p. 635.

A **2.64** Concerning pulmonary agenesis and hypoplasia

A. False   Truncus arteriosus is not a feature of Potter's syndrome.
Ch. 31A Pulmonary Agenesis and Hypoplasia, p. 637.

B. True   The radiographic appearance is indistinguishable from that of total lung collapse. The chest wall is normal.
Ch. 31A Pulmonary Agenesis and Hypoplasia, p. 637.

C. False   There are commonly associated anomalies including anomalous pulmonary venous retur, absence of pulmonary arteries and pulmonary sequestration.
Ch. 31A Pulmonary Agenesis and Hypoplasia, p. 638.

D. False   There is no known sex predominance.
Ch. 31A Pulmonary Agenesis and Hypoplasia, p. 638.

E. True   A helpful feature in the differentiation of the two conditions is the presence of a wedge of tissue orientated towards the hilum.
Ch. 31A Pulmonary Agenesis and Hypoplasia, p. 638.

Q 2.65   Congenital diaphragmatic hernia

A.   Involves the left diaphragm in the majority of cases.
B.   The radiological appearances can be confused with cystic adenomatoid malformation.
C.   Is associated with pulmonary hypoplasia.
D.   Is associated with bronchopulmonary sequestration.
E.   On a chest radiograph, cannot be distinquished from a pneumatocoele.

Q 2.66   The following may appear on the chest radiograph as multiple lung cysts in children

A.   Pulmonary seqestration.
B.   Basal bronchopmonary dysplasia.
C.   Bronchiectasis.
D.   Bronchogenic cysts.
E.   Morgagni hernia.

Q 2.67   Regarding congenital cystic adenomatoid malformation (CAM)

A.   The cysts of CAM commonly communicate with the bronchial tree.
B.   CAMs have their own blood supply which originates directly from the thoracic aorta.
C.   CAMs can be indistinguishable from bronchopulmonary sequestration radiographically.
D.   The mass of CAM is always predominantly cystic.
E.   Appears similar to congenital diaphragmatic hernia (congenital diaphragmatic hernias) on chest X-ray.

(Answers overleaf)

A **2.65** Congenital diaphragmatic hernia

A. True   This occurs in 70% of cases.
Ch. 31A Congenital Diaphragmatic Hernia, p. 639.

B. True   The differential diagnosis of a multi-loculated cystic mass in the lung should include a Bochdalek hernia, cystic adenomatoid malformation and pneumatocele formation.
Ch. 31A Congenital Diaphragmatic Hernia, p. 639.

C. True
Ch. 31A Congenital Diaphragmatic Hernia, p. 639.

D. True
Ch. 31A Congenital Diaphragmatic Hernia, p. 639.

E. True   Radiographically, the differential diagnosis includes congenital cystic adenomatoid malformation and pneumatocele formation. Ultrasound may help in distinguishing these entities.
Ch. 31A Congenital Diaphragmatic Hernia, p. 639.

A **2.66** The following may appear on the chest radiograph as multiple lung cysts in children

A. True
Ch. 31B Table 31B.3, p. 654.

B. True
Ch. 31B Table 31B.3, p. 654.

C. True   The cystic variety of bronchiectasis.
Ch. 31B Table 31B.3, p. 654.

D. False   They are generally single.
Ch. 17 Foregut Cysts, p. 364

E. True
Ch. 31B Table 31B.3, p. 654.

A **2.67** Regarding congenital cystic adenomatoid malformation (CAM)

A. True   The cysts may or may not communicate with the bronchial tree but most do.
Ch. 31A Congenital Cystic Adenomatoid Malformation, p. 639.

B. False   They receive their blood supply from a normal pulmonary artery and vein.
Ch. 31A Congenital Adenomatoid Malformation, p. 639.

C. True   As both CAM and BPS commonly occur at the lung bases, the clinical presentation and radiographic features also overlap.
Ch. 31A Congenital Adenomatoid Malformation, p. 654.

D. False   CAM contains both solid and cystic components that vary in their relative proportions and may present with differing radiological pictures.
Ch. 31A, Congenital Adenomatoid Malformation, p. 639.

E. True
Ch. 31A, CDH, p. 639.

Q **2.68**　Regarding congenital lobar emphysema (CLE)

    A.　Involves the upper lobes in more than 50%.

    B.　May present with complete opacification of the affected lobe.

    C.　A neonate with patent ductus arteriosus can present with similar appearances on the chest radiograph.

    D.　There is an association with ventricular septal defects.

    E.　Requires surgical treatment in most neonate cases.

Q **2.69**　Concerning bronchopulmonary sequestration (BPS)

    A.　Occurs in the right lung in more than 50% of cases.

    B.　Intra-lobar sequestration usually drains into the portal vein.

    C.　In extra-lobar sequestration, presentation is commonly between 8 and 12 years.

    D.　BPS can be readily distinguished from lower-lobe collapse on the chest radiograph.

    E.　Colour Doppler ultrasound is sufficient work-up prior to surgery in 80% of cases.

(Answers overleaf)

A **2.68**   Regarding congenital lobar emphysema (CLE)

A. True
>   *Ch. 31B Congenital Lobar Emphysema, p. 652.*

B. True   Although the precise cause of CLE has not been fully established, it is believed that there is some defect in the bronchial supporting structures. This theory is supported by the occasional case in which fetal lung fluid is trapped within the lobe resulting in an opaque, expanded lobe that converts to the classical form when the fluid is drained or absorbed.
>   *Ch. 31A Congenital Lobar Emphysema, p. 640.*

C. True   This is because there may be secondary compression of the bronchial tree though, the degree of overinflation is less severe in the case of PDA.
>   *Ch. 31A, Congenital Lobar Emphysema, p. 640.*

D. True   There is a well established association between congenital heart disease and infantile lobar emphysema, particularly ventricular septal defects and tetralogy of Fallot.
>   *Ch. 31A Congenital Lobar Emphysema, p. 640.*

E. False   In most cases treatment is expectant in the hope of improvement with time and growth.
>   *Ch. 31A Congenital Lobar Emphysema, p. 640.*

A **2.69**   Concerning bronchopulmonary sequestration (BPS)

A. False   It is most commonly left sided.
>   *Ch. 31B Bronchopulmonary Sequestration, p. 655.*

B. False   Intra lobular sequestration drains into the left atrium and extra-lobar sequestration into to systemic veins.
>   *Ch. 31B Table 31B.4, p. 655.*

C. False   Sixty per cent of patients with extra-lobar sequestation present below the age of 1 year.
>   *Ch. 31B Bronchopulmonary Sequestration, p. 655.*

D. False   Serial radiography typically mimics lower-lobe collapse/consolidation or cavitation. This also overlaps with CAM.
>   *Ch. 31B Bronchopulmonary Sequestration, p. 654.*

E. False   Ultrasound may not visualize an arterial supply from the thoracic aorta. Vascular imaging of the heart and aorta either by DSA or MRI is commonly employed.
>   *Ch. 31B Bronchopulmonary Sequestration, p. 655.*

Q **2.70**   **The following features occur with approximately equal frequency in patients with intra-lobar and extra-lobar pulmonary sequestration**

  A. No connection to the tracheal bronchial tree.
  B. Recurrent pneumonias.
  C. A similar blood supply.
  D. Lower lobe predominance.
  E. Other associated congenital anomalies.

Q **2.71**   **Regarding Scimitar Syndrome**

  A. The affected lung has no connection with the bronchial tree.
  B. Affects the left lower lobe in most cases.
  C. Localized bronchiectasis is a common feature.
  D. The anomalous vein drains into the left atrium.
  E. A small ipsilateral lung with mediastinal shift to the affected side is a characteristic feature on the chest radiograph.

(Answers overleaf)

95

A **2.70** **The following features occur with approximately equal frequency in patients with intra-lobar and extra-lobar**

A. True

Ch. 31A Congenital Cystic Adenomatoid Malformation and Bronchopulmonary Sequestration, p. 640.

B. False This occurs more frequently in intra-lobar pulmonary sequestration. Extra-lobar sequestration typically presents with a mass.
Ch. 31B Table 31B.4, p. 655.

C. True Both intra and extra-lobar pulmonary sequestrations are supplied by a systemic artery, usually from the aorta.
Ch. 31B Table 31B.4, p. 655.

D. True The condition is very rare in the middle, lingula and upper lobes.
Ch. 31B Table 31B.4, p. 655.

E. False It is rare for intra-lobar sequestration to be associated with other congenital abnormalities.
Ch. 31B Table 31B.4, p. 655.

A **2.71** **Regarding Scimitar Syndrome**

A. False The lung is normally connected to the bronchial tree.
Ch. 31B Scimitar Syndrome, p. 655.

B. False

Ch. 31B Scimitar Syndrome, p. 655.

C. True Localized bronchiectasis is common.
Ch. 31B Scimitar Syndrome, p. 655.

D. False The vein draining the lobe drains into the IVC or portal vein.
Ch. 31B Scimitar Syndrome, p. 655.

E. True

Ch. 31B Scimitar Syndrome, p. 655.

Q **2.72** **The following cause for a mediastinal mass are appropriate for the compartments in the chest**

    A. Thyroid tumour and middle mediastinum.
    B. Plexiform neurofibroma and anterior (superior) mediastinum.
    C. Bronchogenic cyst and middle mediastinum.
    D. Bronchopulmonary sequestration and anterior (inferior) mediastinum.
    E. Phaeochromocytoma and posterior mediastinum.

Q **2.73** **The following statements are true regarding paediatric chest tumours**

    A. Primary lung tumours are commoner than chest-wall tumours.
    B. Askin tumours are associated with pleural effusions.
    C. Peripheral pulmonary metastases are often seen in the posterior inferior recess.
    D. Pulmonary metastases are a common presentation of malignancy.
    E. Rhabdomyosarcomas metastasize to the lungs.

Q **2.74** **Regarding airway obstruction in children**

    A. The right main bronchus is the commonest site for a foreign body to lodge.
    B. Pneumomediastinum is commonly caused by inhaled foreign bodies.
    C. Pneumothorax is a common occurrence in childhood asthma.
    D. Air trapping in the lung causes mediastinal shift towards the affected side.
    E. Pulmonary agenesis or hypoplasia causes mediastinal shift towards the affected side.

(Answers overleaf)

97

A **2.72**   **The following cause for a mediastinal mass are appropriate for the compartments in the chest**

A. **False**   This is typically in the anterior (superior mediastinum).
Ch. 31B Table 31.5, p. 657.

B. **True**   These also occur in the middle and posterior mediastinum.
Ch. 31B Table 31.5, p. 657.

C. **True**

Ch. 31B Table 31.5, p. 657.

D. **False**   This is seen in the posterior mediastinum.
Ch. 31B Table 31.5, p. 657.

E. **True**

Ch. 31B Table 31.5, p. 657.

A **2.73**   **The following statements are true regarding paediatric chest tumours**

A. **False**   Primary bronchial and pulmonary tumours are rare in paediatric practice.
Ch. 31B Tumours, p. 659.

B. **True**   These are sarcomas arising from the chest wall, often with rib involvement and a pleural effusion.
Ch. 31B Tumours, p. 659.

C. **True**

Ch. 31B Tumours, p. 659.

D. **False**   Presentation of malignancy by the finding of multiple pulmonary metastases is rare in comparison with adults.
Ch. 31B Tumours, p. 659.

E. **True**

Ch. 31B Tumours, p. 659.

A **2.74**   **Regarding airway obstruction in children**

A. **True**   Though an FB may lodge in any bronchus in the trachea.
Ch. 31B Inhaled Foreign Bodies, p. 651.

B. **False**   Pneumothorax and pneumomediastinum are rarely caused by inhaled foreign bodies.
Ch. 31B Tumours, p. 651.

C. **False**   Pneumothorax is a rare occurrence in childhood asthma.
Ch. 31B Asthma, p. 650.

D. **False**

Ch. 31B Mediastinal Shift, p. 650.

E. **True**

Ch. 31B Mediastinal Shift, p. 650.

Q **2.75** **Regarding pulmonary Kaposi's sarcoma**

   A. Most patients do not have Kaposi's lesions elsewhere in the body.
   B. Cavitation is commonly seen with nodular Kaposi's sarcoma.
   C. Lymphadenopathy is seen in 90% of cases.
   D. May present as a solitary nodule.
   E. Kaposi's sarcoma is believed to be caused by human herpes virus 8 (IIHV8).

Q **2.76** **The following are causes of an 'interstitial' pattern of abnormalities on imaging in the paediatric chest**

   A. Neurofibromatosis.
   B. *Mycoplasma* pneumonia.
   C. Gaucher's disease.
   D. Non-cardiogenic pulmonary oedema.
   E. Staphylococal pneumonia.

(Answers overleaf)

A **2.75**   **Regarding pulmonary Kaposi's sarcoma**

A. False   Most patients have obvious disease in the skin or elsewhere.
Ch. 18 Kaposi's Sarcoma, p. 410.

B. False   This is a distinguishing feature from septic emboli.
Ch. 18 Kaposi's Sarcoma, p. 410.

C. True   Lymphadenopathy is seen in 10–30%.
Ch. 18 Kaposi's Sarcoma, p. 410.

D. True   Bilateral, multiple lesions are, however, more typical.
Ch. 18 Kaposi's Sarcoma, p. 410.

E. True   Theraputic measures are directed against this virus; these incorporate anti-angiogenesis agents and chemotherapeutic agents such as paclitaxel.
Ch. 18 Kaposi's Sarcoma, p. 410.

A **2.76**   **The following are causes of an 'interstitial' pattern of abnormalities on imaging in the paediatric chest**

A. True
Ch. 31B Table 31B.9, p. 661.

B. True
Ch. 31B Table 31B.9, p. 661.

C. True
Ch. 31B Table 31B.9, p. 661.

D. True
Ch. 31B Table 31B.9, p. 661.

E. False   Typically airspace shadowing and not an 'interstitial' lung pattern.
Ch. 31B Table 31B.9, p. 661.

The cardiovascular system

Q **3.1** Regarding normal cardiac anatomy

Cardiac anatomy and enlargement

A. The superior vena cava enters the upper anterior aspect of the right atrium.
B. The right ventricle forms most of the anterior surface of the heart.
C. The atrial and ventricular septa both lie in the left anterior oblique plane.
D. The right coronary artery lies in the anterior atrio-ventricular grove.
E. The left coronary artery lies in the posterior atrio-ventricular grove.

Q **3.2** Regarding individual heart chambers

A. The coronary sinus enters the posterior wall of the right atrium between the tricuspid value and the inferior vena cava.
B. The crista terminalis separates the body of right atrium from the right atrial appendage.
C. The left ventricle forms the posterior border of the heart below the mitral valve on the lateral chest X-ray.
D. The membranous part of the ventricular septum lies immediately below the aortic valve.
E. Enlargement of the left atrium causes an indentation in the anterior wall of the oesophagus on barium swallow.

Q **3.3** Concerning cardiac enlargement

A. In 90% of normal adult males the transverse cardiac diameter, measured on the standard 6 feet (2 m) PA radiograph is less than 15.5 cm.
B. The lateral border of an enlarged left atrium is effaced by overlying IVC on a postero-anterior chest X-radiograph.
C. The confluence of the pulmonary veins may cause a double heart border on the right.
D. An enlarged left atrium usually displaces the descending aorta to the left.
E. The cardiac: thoracic ratio may exceed 60% in the normal neonate.

(Answers overleaf)

A **3.1 Regarding normal cardiac anatomy**

A. False It enters the upper posterior aspect of the right atrium.
Ch. 32 Cardiac Anatomy and Enlargement, p. 673.

B. True
Ch. 32 Cardiac Anatomy and Enlargement, p. 673.

C. True
Ch. 32 Cardiac Anatomy and Enlargement, p. 673.

D. True
Ch. 32 Cardiac Anatomy and Enlargement, p. 675.

E. False
Ch. 32 Cardiac Anatomy and Enlargement, p. 674.

A **3.2 Regarding individual heart chambers**

A. True
Ch. 32 Cardiac Anatomy and Enlargement, p. 675.

B. True Due to the lack of any conus or infundibulum.
Ch. 32 Cardiac Anatomy and Enlargement, p. 679.

C. True
Ch. 32 Cardiac Anatomy and Enlargement, p. 679.

D. True The ventricular system is studied most effectively by applying cranial
angulation to the X-ray beam in addition to left anterior obliquity.
Ch. 32 Cardiac Anatomy and Enlargement, p. 679.

E. True
Ch. 32 Cardiac Anatomy and Enlargement, p. 679.

A **3.3 Concerning cardiac enlargement**

A. True Normal adult males transverse cardiac diameter is less then 15.5 cm in 90%
and in normal adult females is less than 12.5 cm.
Ch. 32 Cardiac Anatomy and Enlargement, p. 682.

B. False The right atrial border is limited below by the entry of the inferior vena cava.
Ch. 32 Cardiac Anatomy and Enlargement, p. 683.

C. True
Ch. 32 Cardiac Anatomy and Enlargement, p. 684.

D. False An enlarged left atrium rarely displaces the descending aorta to the left. When
is displaces the oesophagus this is usually to the right-hand side, but, rarely, to
the left when dysphagia may result.
Ch. 32 Cardiac Anatomy and Enlargement, p. 684.

E. True
Ch. 32 Cardiac Anatomy and Enlargement, p. 682.

Q 3.4   Causes of a large left atrium include

A. Right atrial myxoma.
B. Hypertrophic obstructive cardiomyopathy.
C. Patent ductus arteriosus.
D. Atrial septal defect.
F. Mitral regurgitation.

Q 3.5   Signs of left ventricular enlargement on a chest X-ray

A. Rounding of the apex of the heart.
B. Elongation of the long axis of the left ventricle.
C. Rotation of the left atrial appendage.
D. Posterior displacement of the inferior vena cava on the lateral chest X-ray.
E. Double left heart border.

Q 3.6   Causes of an enlarged right ventricle include

A. Left heart failure.
B. Right to left shunt.
C. Chronic thrombo-embolic disease.
D. Pulmonary arterio-venous malformation.
E. Pulmonary regurgitation.

(Answers overleaf)

A **3.4 Causes of a large left atrium include**

A. False Left atrial myxoma causes left atrial enlargement.
Ch. 32 Cardiac Anatomy and Enlargement, p. 684.

B. True
Ch. 32 Cardiac Anatomy and Enlargement, p. 684.

C. True
Ch. 32 Cardiac Anatomy and Enlargement, p. 685.

D. True Often with left ventricular failure.
Ch. 32 Cardiac Anatomy and Enlargement, p. 685.

E. True Often with left ventricular failure.
Ch. 32 Cardiac Anatomy and Enlargement, p. 684.

A **3.5 Signs of left ventricular enlargement on a chest X-ray**

A. True This may be the only sign and is often seen before overall cardiac enlargement has developed. It may be due to muscular hypertrophy.
Ch. 32 Cardiac Anatomy and Enlargement, p. 685.

B. True This is the earliest sign of left ventricular cavity dilation. The cardiac apex may descend below the diaphragm where it may be difficult to recognize.
Ch. 32 Cardiac Anatomy and Enlargement, p. 685.

C. False
Ch. 32 Cardiac Anatomy and Enlargement, p. 685.

D. False
Ch. 32 Cardiac Anatomy and Enlargement, p. 685.

E. False
Ch. 32 Cardiac Anatomy and Enlargement, p. 685.

A **3.6 Causes of an enlarged right ventricle include**

A. True This is the commonest cause of right ventricular enlargement particularly associated with mitral valve disease.
Ch. 32 Cardiac Anatomy and Enlargement, p. 687.

B. False
Ch. 32 Cardiac Anatomy and Enlargement, p. 687.

C. True
Ch. 32 Cardiac Anatomy and Enlargement, p. 687.

D. True Due to high volume shunting through these lesions.
Ch. 32 Cardiac Anatomy and Enlargement, p. 687.

E. True
Ch. 32 Cardiac Anatomy and Enlargement, p. 687.

Q **3.7**   **Causes of a large right atrium include**

  A. Endomyocardial fibrosis.
  B. Pulmonary hypertension.
  C. Restrictive cardiomyopathy.
  D. Right atrium myxoma.
  E. Acquired tricuspid stenosis.

Q **3.8**   **Signs of pectus excavatum on chest X-ray include**

  A. Prominent right heart border.
  B. Increased convexity of the left heart border.
  C. Reduced prominence of the main pulmonary artery.
  D. Reduced slope of posterior rib ends.
  E. Prominent right lower zone vessels.

Q **3.9**   **Regarding echocardiography**

  A. Deep inspiration improves imaging in the subcostal plane.
  B. The parasternal long axis view is useful for examining the left ventricular outflow tract.
  C. Peak maximal aortic velocity in adults is 10–17 metres per second.
  D. Ultrasound is better than angiography at assessing left ventricular aneurysms.
  E. Assessment of the entire aortic arch with echocardiography is possible in adults.

(Answers overleaf)

A **3.7** Causes of a large right atrium include

A. **True**
Ch. 32 Cardiac Anatomy and Enlargement, p. 688.

B. **True** Usually with a degree of tricuspid regurgitation.
Ch. 32 Cardiac Anatomy and Enlargement, p. 688.

C. **True** Especially in diabetes mellitus.
Ch. 32 Cardiac Anatomy and Enlargement, p. 688.

D. **True** Or any tumour causing tricuspid valve obstruction.
Ch. 32 Cardiac Anatomy and Enlargement, p. 688.

E. **True** Carcinoid syndrome more commonly causes tricuspid regurgitation.
Ch. 32 Cardiac Anatomy and Enlargement, p. 688.

A **3.8** Signs of pectus excavatum on chest x-ray include

A. **False**
Ch. 32 Cardiac Anatomy and Enlargement, p. 688.

B. **True** Straightening and increased convexity of the left heart border are signs of pectus excavatum.
Ch. 32 Cardiac Anatomy and Enlargement, p. 688.

C. **False**
Ch. 32 Cardiac Anatomy and Enlargement, p. 688.

D. **False** Increased slope of the anterior rib ends is a feature.
Ch. 32 Cardiac Anatomy and Enlargement, p. 688.

E. **True**
Ch. 32 Cardiac Anatomy and Enlargement, p. 688.

A **3.9** Regarding echocardiography

A. **True**
Ch. 33 Echocardiography Including Doppler, p. 699.

B. **True**
Ch. 33 Echocardiography Including Doppler, p. 703.

C. **False** It is 1–1.7 metres per second.
Ch. 33 Echocardiography Including Doppler, p. 713.

D. **True** Because contrast medium within a large aneurysm or areas of impaired function may be superimposed on normally functionally myocardium.
Ch. 33 Echocardiography Including Doppler, p. 716.

E. **True**
Ch. 33 Echocardiography Including Doppler, p. 717.

Q **3.10**   Regarding myocardial perfusion imaging with ^{201}thallium

A. ^{201}Thallium decays by electron capture to ^{201}strontium.
B. ^{201}Thallium is administered intravenously as thallous bisulphate.
C. Twenty per cent of the injected dose localizes in the myocardium.
D. Myocardial extraction efficiency is inhibited by hypoxia.
E. Distribution within the myocardium is proportional to perfusion.

Q **3.11**   Regarding stress techniques of myocardial imaging

A. Dipyridamole is a potent coronary arteriolar dilator.
B. Dipyridamole activates adenosine deaminase.
C. Dipyridamole causes chest pain in approximately 50% of patients.
D. Aminophylline is administered to reverse the adverse effects of dipyridamole.
E. Adenosine may cause chest pain in normal volunteers.

(Answers overleaf)

A **3.10**   **Regarding myocardial perfusion imaging with ²⁰¹thallium**

A. **False**   It decays be electron capture to ²⁰¹mercury emitting mainly X-rays of energy 67–82 keV.
Ch. 34 Nuclear Cardiology, p. 722.

B. **False**   It is administered as thallous chloride.
Ch. 34 Nuclear Cardiology, p. 722.

C. **False**   Four per cent of the injected dose is localized in the myocardium.
Ch. 34 Nuclear Cardiology, p. 722.

D. **False**
Ch. 34 Nuclear Cardiology, p. 722.

E. **True**
Ch. 34 Nuclear Cardiology, p. 722.

A **3.11**   **Regarding stress techniques of myocardial imaging**

A. **True**   It is relatively specific for myocardium, although it dilates arterioles in a number of other organs including the skin and gastro-intestinal tract.
Ch. 34 Nuclear Cardiology, p. 725.

B. **False**   It reduces the deactivation of adenosine by inhibiting adenosine deaminase.
Ch. 34 Nuclear Cardiology, p. 725.

C. **False**   This happens in approximately 20% of patients. Headache, dizziness, nausea and epigastric pain are observed in one-third of patients.
Ch. 34 Nuclear Cardiology, p. 725.

D. **True**
Ch. 34 Nuclear Cardiology, p. 725.

E. **True**
Ch. 34 Nuclear Cardiology, p. 725.

Q 3.12 Regarding cardiac MRI

A. Spin-echo imaging is particularly useful for anatomical imaging of the heart and great vessels.

B. Gradient echo sequences are used to eliminate irregular flow caused by valve dysfunction.

C. Imaging of coronary arteries is performed in mid-systole.

D. The fast low-angled shot technique (Flash) has a lower signal to noise ratio than echo-planar imaging.

E. Intra-cardiac lipomas return high T1 weighted signal on cardiac MRI.

Q 3.13 Regarding left-to-right shunts

A. Enlarged pulmonary veins are more conspicuous than enlarged pulmonary arteries on the postero-anterior chest radiograph.

B. Ostium secundum involves the tricuspid valve in over 50% of cases.

C. Patent foramen ovale is in the same position as ostium primum ASD.

D. In ASD the left atrium is usually enlarged.

E. The ascending aorta often appears small in ASD.

(Answers overleaf)

109

A **3.12** **Regarding cardiac MRI**

A. True   Fast spin echo imaging significantly reduces the total imaging time and reduces the phase-encode artefacts.
Ch. 35 Magnetic Resonance Imaging of the Heart and Circulation, p. 742.

B. False   These sequences accentuate irregular flow in circumstances where there is valvular disease.
Ch. 35 Magnetic Resonance Imaging of the Heart and Circulation, p. 743.

C. False   Mid-diastole.
Ch. 35 Magnetic Resonance Imaging of the Heart and Circulation, p. 751.

D. True   It is also slower than the EPI method, however, it is less dependent on gradient performance and may be implemented on unmodified machines.
Ch. 35 Magnetic Resonance Imaging of the Heart and Circulation, p. 745.

E. True
Ch. 35 Magnetic Resonance Imaging of the Heart and Circulation, p. 754.

A **3.13** **Regarding left-to-right shunts**

A. False   The pulmonary veins are often enlarged but tend to be less conspicuous on the plain radiograph.
Ch. 36B Congenital Heart Disease: Left-to-Light Shunts, p. 786.

B. False   The ostium secundum or fossa ovalis defect is situated in the upper part of the atrial septum, behind the coronary sinus, well above the tricuspid valve.
Ch. 36B Congenital Heart Disease: Left-to-Light Shunts, p. 787.

C. False   The patent foramen ovale is in the same position as the ostium secundum defect and may transmit a right-to left (paradoxical) embolism to the brain in the systemic circulation.
Ch. 36B Congenital Heart Disease: Left-to-Light Shunts, p. 787.

D. False   Only rarely in some cases of endocardial cushion defect and Lutembacher's syndrome.
Ch. 36B Congenital Heart Disease: Left-to-Light Shunts, p. 787.

E. True   The arch may also appear small possibly due to rotation.
Ch. 36B Congenital Heart Disease: Left-to-Light Shunts, p. 788.

Q 3.14   Regarding septal defects

A. In ASD the chest X-ray may closely simulate pulmonary valve stenosis.

B. In ASD the Eisenmenger reaction develops in the majority of untreated patients.

C. In ASD Kerley B lines suggest associated mitral valve pathology.

D. Echocardiography easily differentiates ostium primum from ostium secundum defects.

E. On the postero-anterior chest X-ray ventricular septal defect (VSD) is usually distinguishable from atrial septal defect (ASD) by the cardiac shape.

Q 3.15   Regarding aorto-pulmonary shunts

A. The ductus arteriosus has a central valve.

B. Demonstration of 'filling in' of the aorta-pulmonary window is seen on chest X-ray in over 50% of cases of patent ductus arteriosus.

C. Calcification of the proximal pulmonary arteries complicates patent ductus arteriosus.

D. Surgical closure of a patent ductus arteriosus is mandatory if Eisenmenger reaction is present.

E. The chest X-ray in aorto-pulmonary window simulates patent ductus arteriosus and ventricular septal defect.

(Answers overleaf)

A **3.14** Regarding septal defects

A. True This occurs on CXR in ASD with a modest shunt because, in common with pulmonary stenosis, there is slightly enlarged right ventricle, enlarged main pulmonary artery and the lungs appear normal.
Chapter 36B Congenital Heart Disease: Left-to-Right Shunts, p. 788.

B. False Eisenmenger reaction occurs in a small minority of patients with a large ASD usually after the age of 30.
Ch. 36B Congenital Heart Disease: Left-to-Right Shunts, p. 788.

C. True
Ch. 36B Congenital Heart Disease: Left-to-Right Shunts, p. 788.

D. True
Ch. 36B Congenital Heart Disease: Left-to-Right Shunts, p. 788.

E. False
Ch. 36B Congenital Heart Disease: Left-to-Right Shunts, p. 791.

A **3.15** Regarding aorto-pulmonary shunts

A. False
Ch. 36B Congenital Heart Disease: Left-to-Right Shunts, p. 794.

B. False Not often shown.
Ch. 36B Congenital Heart Disease: Left-to-Right Shunts, p. 795.

C. True Curvilinear calcification in the wall of enlarged central pulmonary arteries and in the ductus is a characteristic appearance occurring in long-standing severe patent ductus arteriosus with Eisenmenger's reaction.
Ch. 36B Congenital Heart Disease: Left-to-Right Shunts, p. 795.

D. False This may prove to be fatal.
Ch. 36B Congenital Heart Disease: Left-to-Right Shunts, p. 795.

E. True It may be identical.
Ch. 36B Congenital Heart Disease: Left-to-Right Shunts, p. 796.

Q 3.16 Regarding tetralogy of Fallot

    A. The ventricular septal defect is large.
    B. Cyanotic spells in Fallot's tetralogy are caused by infundibular spasm.
    C. The ascending aorta is always enlarged in Fallot's tetralogy.
    D. The aortic arch is usually left-sided in Fallot's tetralogy.
    E. In Fallot's tetralogy with right sided aortic arch the descending aorta remains right-sided below the diaphgram in over 50% of patients.

Q 3.17 Concerning the treatment of congenital heart disease

    A. Fallot's tetralogy may be surgically corrected by a synthetic graft linking the left pulmonary artery with the ipsilateral subclavian artery.
    B. The main pulmonary artery is surgically joined to the right atrium in the treatment of tricuspid atresia.
    C. Transposition of the great arteries is surgically corrected by transecting the aorta and pulmonary artery and switching them.
    D. Rashkind balloon septostomy tears a hole in the interatrial septum.
    E. In transposition of the great arteries, the Mustard procedure directs pulmonary venous return to the right atrium.

(Answers overleaf)

A **3.16** **Regarding tetralogy of fallot**

A. True The infundibular septum fails to fuse with the top of the interventricular septum producing a large, high-ventricular septal defect.
Ch. 36B Congenital Heart Disease: Left-to-Right Shunts, p. 801.

B. True
Ch. 36B Congenital Heart Disease: Left-to-Right Shunts, p. 801.

C. True
Ch. 36B Congenital Heart Disease: Left-to-Right Shunts, p. 801.

D. True In about 25% of patients the aortic arch is on the right (with mirror imaging branching – left innominate, right carotid, right subclavian arising from proximal to distal off the aortic arch).
Ch. 36B Congenital Heart Disease: Left-to-Right Shunts, p. 801.

E. False The descending aorta usually crosses to the left of the spine in the lower thorax.
Ch. 36B Congenital Heart Disease: Left-to-Right Shunts, p. 801.

A **3.17** **Concerning the treatment of congenital heart disease**

A. True This is the modified Blalock-Taussig shunt.
Chapter 36C Cyanotic Congenital Heart Disease, p. 803.

B. True This is the Fontan procedure.
Ch. 36C Cyanotic Congenital Heart Disease, p. 805.

C. True
Ch. 36C Cyanotic Congenital Heart Disease, p. 810.

D. True
Ch. 36C Cyanotic Congenital Heart Disease, p. 810.

E. True
Ch. 36C Cyanotic Congenital Heart Disease, p. 810.

Q **3.18** In persistent truncus arteriosus

    A. The truncal valve fails to separate into aortic and mitral valve.
    B. There is a VSD.
    C. Pulmonary arterial stenosis limits the flow through the shunt.
    D. The heart shape resembles Fallot's tetralogy.
    E. A right-sided aortic arch is associated.

Q **3.19** In uncorrected transposition of the great arteries

    A. The superior mediastinum is narrow on the frontal film and wide on the lateral view.
    B. The lungs are usually plethoric.
    C. Treatment is best undertaken after the 2nd year of life.
    D. Pulmonary stenosis is associated with 20%.
    E. The ascending aorta, aortic arch and descending aorta lie in the mid sagittal plane.

(Answers overleaf)

115

A **3.18** **In persistent truncus arteriosus**

A. False The truncal valve fails to separate into aortic and pulmonary valves.
Ch. 36C Cyanotic Congenital Heart Disease, p. 806.

B. True Both ventricles discharge into the truncus.
Ch. 36C Cyanotic Congenital Heart Disease, p. 806.

C. False They limit flow to the lungs producing cyanosis.
Ch. 36C Cyanotic Congenital Heart Disease, p. 807.

D. True
Ch. 36C Cyanotic Congenital Heart Disease, p. 807.

E. True Persistent truncus arteriosus has the highest incidence (30–50%) of right-sided aortic arch of any congenital heart abnormality.
Ch. 36C Cyanotic Congenital Heart Disease, p. 807.

A **3.19** **In uncorrected transposition of the great arteries**

A. True Because both the ascending aorta (anterior) and pulmonary artery (posterior) tend to lie in the midline.
Ch. 36C Cyanotic Congenital Heart Disease, p. 808.

B. True Because left ventricular output is generally greater than right ventricular output.
Ch. 36C Cyanotic Congenital Heart Disease, p. 809.

C. False Ninety per cent die if a correcting procedure is not performed within 1 year.
Ch. 36C Cyanotic Congenital Heart Disease, p. 809.

D. True
Ch. 36C Cyanotic Congenital Heart Disease, p. 809.

E. True
Ch. 36C Cyanotic Congenital Heart Disease, p. 808.

Q **3.20** **Regarding anomalous pulmonary venous drainage**

A. Produces a right-to-left shunt.
B. Scimitar syndrome is associated with bronchiectasis.
C. Supracardiac drainage of the pulmonary veins is the commonest type of total anomalous pulmonary venous drainage.
D. In total anomalous venous drainage, the right atrium is the only chamber of the heart to receive a venous return.
E. Kerley A lines occur in infra-diaphragmatic total anomalous pulmonary venous drainage.

Q **3.21** **Cardiac valvular calcification visible on chest X-ray is a recognized feature of**

A. Bacterial endocarditis.
B. Dermatomyositis.
C. Syphilis.
D. Ankylosing spondylitis.
E. Sarcoidosis.

(Answers overleaf)

A **3.20** Regarding anomalous pulmonary venous drainage

A. False It produces a left-to-right shunt of small-to-moderate size.
Ch. 36D Other Congenital Heart Lesions, p. 818.

B. True
Ch. 36D Other Congenital Heart Lesions, p. 818.

C. True The right and left pulmonary veins meet behind the left atrium with a venous confluence from that a large vertical vein passes upwards in front of the left hilum to meet the left innominate vein.
Ch. 36D Other Congenital Heart Lesions, p. 819.

D. True
Ch. 36D Other Congenital Heart Lesions, p. 819.

E. True In this condition there is intense venous congestion, alveolar oedema and septal lines which are more frequently of the central A type than the costophrenic parallel Kerley B type.
Ch. 36D Other Congenital Heart Lesions, p. 820.

A **3.21** Cardiac valvular calcification visible on chest X-ray is a recognized feature of

A. True An old vegetation may calcify and become visible.
Ch. 37 Acquired Valvular Heart Disease, p. 827.

B. False
Ch. 37 Acquired Valvular Heart Disease, p. 827.

C. True
Ch. 37 Acquired Valvular Heart Disease, p. 827.

D. True
Ch. 37 Acquired Valvular Heart Disease, p. 827.

E. False
Ch. 37 Acquired Valvular Heart Disease, p. 827.

Q **3.22**   Regarding mitral valve disease

A. Mitral stenosis is almost always rheumatic in origin.
B. Mitral regurgitation is an association of systemic lupus erythematosus.
C. A floppy mitral valve is the commonest cause of mitral prolapse.
D. Papillary muscle rupture as a consequence of myocardial infarction results in massive mitral regurgitation.
E. Severe mitral stenosis and severe mitral regurgitation cannot co-exist.

Q **3.23**   Radiographic changes seen in rheumatic mitral valve disease include

A. Dilatation of lower lobe veins.
B. Increased iron deposition in the lungs.
C. Pulmonary ossification primarily affecting upper lobes.
D. Peripheral vascular pruning.
E. Kerley A lines.

(Answers overleaf)

A **3.22** Regarding mitral valve disease

A. True
   Ch. 37 Acquired Valvular Heart Disease, p. 828.

B. True
   Ch. 37 Acquired Valvular Heart Disease, p. 828.

C. True
   Ch. 37 Acquired Valvular Heart Disease, p. 829.

D. True
   Ch. 37 Acquired Valvular Heart Disease, p. 830.

E. True
   Ch. 37 Acquired Valvular Heart Disease, p. 832.

A **3.23** Radiographic changes seen in rheumatic mitral valve disease include

A. False
   Ch. 37 Acquired Valvular Heart Disease, p. 833.

B. True Pulmonary haemosiderosis is seen as fine punctate densities throughout the lungs because repeated pulmonary haemorrhage leaves iron-containing deposits in lung tissue.
   Ch. 37 Acquired Valvular Heart Disease, p. 833.

C. False Pulmonary ossified nodules are seen as discrete calcified densities of up to 1 cm in diameter which occur at the lung bases as the result of longstanding pulmonary hypertension in mitral valve disease.
   Ch. 37 Acquired Valvular Heart Disease, p. 833.

D. True This is a sign of pulmonary arterial hypertension.
   Ch. 37 Acquired Valvular Heart Disease, p. 833.

E. True Interstitial oedema causes Kerley B septal costophrenic lines and also central A lines.
   Ch. 37 Acquired Valvular Heart Disease, p. 833.

Q 3.24   Regarding tricuspid valve disease

A.   A large right atrium bulging to the right and increase in the curvature of the right heart border always suggests tricuspid valve involvement.
B.   Rheumatic tricuspid valve calcification is almost unknown.
C.   Endomyocardial fibrosis causes severe tricuspid regurgitation.
D.   In carcinoid syndrome there is thickening of the valve cusps causing tricuspid regurgitation.
E.   There is subendocardial fibrosis of the right ventricle in carcinoid syndrome.

Q 3.25   Regarding aortic valve disease

A.   Valvular calcification causes the stenosis.
B.   Echocardiography is used to assess the valve area accurately.
C.   Post-stenotic dilatation of the aorta commonly occurs in rheumatic aortic stenosis.
D.   Aortic valve calcification is higher and more horizontal on the chest X-ray than mitral valve calcification.
E.   Acute aortic regurgitation may result from acute dissecting aneurysms of the aorta.

Q 3.26   Regarding bicuspid aortic valve

A.   It is associated with co-arctation of the aorta.
B.   There are usually three sinuses of Valsalva.
C.   Progressive aortic valve stenosis usually begins in the second decade.
D.   The presence of a murmur implies stenosis has developed.
E.   The two aortic cusps are the same size.

(Answers overleaf)

A **3.24** Regarding tricuspid valve disease

A. True
> *Ch. 37 Acquired Valvular Heart Disease, p. 853.*

B. True
> *Ch. 37 Acquired Valvular Heart Disease, p. 835.*

C. True This happens when the papillary muscles become scarred and retracted.
> *Ch. 37 Acquired Valvular Heart Disease, p. 835.*

D. True Carcinoid syndrome may also cause tricuspid stenosis.
> *Ch. 37 Acquired Valvular Heart Disease, p. 835.*

E. True
> *Ch. 37 Acquired Valvular Heart Disease, p. 835.*

A **3.25** Regarding aortic valve disease

A. True Unlike calcification in the mitral valve where calcium is deposited on an already stenosed valve.
> *Ch. 37 Acquired Valvular Heart Disease, p. 836.*

B. False Echocardiography cannot estimate aortic valve area because of limited resolution and multiple reverberations within the abnormal cusps especially when calcification is present.
> *Ch. 37 Acquired Valvular Heart Disease, p. 836.*

C. False Although the aorta may be dilated if there is also aortic regurgitation.
> *Ch. 37 Acquired Valvular Heart Disease, p. 838.*

D. True
> *Ch. 37 Acquired Valvular Heart Disease, p. 838.*

E. True
> *Ch. 37 Acquired Valvular Heart Disease, p. 839.*

A **3.26** Regarding bicuspid aortic valve

A. True
> *Ch. 37 Acquired Valvular Heart Disease, p. 841.*

B. False Usually only two sinuses of Valsalva, one much larger than the other.
> *Ch. 37 Acquired Valvular Heart Disease, p. 841.*

C. False Bicuspid aortic valve rarely causes symptoms before the third and fourth decade when thickening, irregularity and calcification cause progressive stenosis.
> *Ch. 37 Acquired Valvular Heart Disease, p. 841.*

D. True
> *Ch. 37 Acquired Valvular Heart Disease, p. 841.*

E. False The two cusps are unequal in size – the larger usually being divided by a raphe.
> *Ch. 37 Acquired Valvular Heart Disease, p. 841.*

Q 3.27   Concerning left ventriculography technique

A. A power injector is always used.
B. An end-hole only catheter is preferable.
C. The tip of the catheter is placed at the apex of the left ventricle.
D. A zero-second rate rise is advisable.
E. Very rapid (30–50 ml/s) delivery of the contrast medium is required.

Q 3.28   Regarding coronary artery anatomy

A. The right coronary sinus on Valsalva lies posteriorly.
B. The circumflex artery lies at the left atrio-ventricular grove.
C. The sinus node artery arises from the right coronary artery in 90% of people.
D. The commonest congenital variant of coronary anatomy is a circumflex artery that arises from the right coronary artery.
E. There is a risk of sudden death if the left coronary artery arises from the right coronary artery as a congenital variant.

(Answers overleaf)

A **3.27** Concerning left ventriculography technique

A. True
> *Ch. 38 Ischaemic Heart Disease, p. 846.*

B. False
> *Ch. 38 Ischaemic Heart Disease, p. 846.*

C. False It needs to be positioned away from the apex of the ventricle to avoid extrasystoles.
> *Ch. 38 Ischaemic Heart Disease, p. 846.*

D. False A rise time is important as it minimizes the possibility of ectopic beats.
> *Ch. 38 Ischaemic Heart Disease, p. 846.*

E. False A slower injection rate of 8–12 ml per second allows adequate opacification without ectopic beats.
> *Ch. 38 Ischaemic Heart Disease, p. 846.*

A **3.28** Regarding coronary artery anatomy

A. False It lies anteriorly and slightly to the right.
> *Ch. 38 Ischaemic Heart Disease, p. 847.*

B. True It passes backwards and leftwards within the left AV grove where it gives rise to one or more obtuse marginal branches to the free wall of the ventricle.
> *Ch. 38 Ischaemic Heart Disease, p. 848.*

C. False This anatomy pertains in about two-thirds of the population.
> *Ch. 38 Ischaemic Heart Disease, p. 849.*

D. True *Ch. 38 Ischaemic Heart Disease, p. 849.*

E. True This is because the left coronary artery passes through the aortic wall and between aorta and pulmonary artery allowing it to be compressed leading to angina or sudden death.
> *Ch. 38 Ischaemic Heart Disease, p. 849.*

Q 3.29 Regarding coronary artery pathology

A. Arteries which go into spontaneous spasm have no atheromatous narrowing in their relaxed state.
B. Coronary artery spasm almost never responds to administration of nitrates or calcium channel blockers.
C. Catheter-induced spasm occurs most commonly in the left coronary artery.
D. Coronary artery spasm causes collaterals to develop.
E. Coronary arteries are large in hypertrophic cardiomyopathy.

Q 3.30 Regarding septal lines on the chest radiograph

A. Kerley A lines usually abut the lateral pleural surface.
B. Kerley A lines generally indicate a chronic degree of pulmonary hypertension.
C. Kerley A lines usually disappear after reduction of pulmonary venous pressure.
D. Persistent septal lines may be seen in fibrotic lung disease.
E. Septal lines are subpleural bands of atelectasis.

Q 3.31 Causes of asymmetrical pulmonary oedema include

A. Bullous emphysema.
B. Scimitar syndrome.
C. Fibrosing mediastinitis.
D. Re-expansion of contralateral pneumothorax.
E. Ipsilateral lung infarction.

(Answers overleaf)

125

A **3.29** **Regarding coronary artery pathology**

A. **False** The characteristic finding in coronary artery spasm is that the relaxed artery shows a minor but definite area of atheromatous narrowing on angiography.
Ch. 38 Ischaemic Heart Disease, p. 856.

B. **False** These agents usually reverse spasm.
Ch. 38 Ischaemic Heart Disease, p. 856.

C. **False** This occurs at the catheter tip most commonly in the right coronary artery. It rarely produces symptoms or ECG changes and it chief importance is the potential for confusion with atheromatous coronary artery disease.
Ch. 38 Ischaemic Heart Disease, p. 856.

D. **True** *Ch. 38 Ischaemic Heart Disease, p. 856.*

E. **True**

Ch. 38 Ischaemic Heart Disease, p. 857.

A **3.30** **Regarding septal lines on the chest radiograph**

A. **False** They are central.
Ch. 39 Pulmonary Circulation, p. 875.

B. **False**

Ch. 39 Pulmonary Circulation, p. 875.

C. **True**

Ch. 39 Pulmonary Circulation, p. 875.

D. **True**

Ch. 39 Pulmonary Circulation, p. 875.

E. **False** They are caused be accumulation of fluid in interlobular septa or lymphatics.
Ch. 39 Pulmonary Circulation, p. 875.

A **3.31** **Causes of asymmetrical pulmonary oedema include**

A. **True**

Ch. 39 Pulmonary Circulation, p. 875.

B. **False**

Ch. 39 Pulmonary Circulation, p. 875.

C. **True**

Ch. 39 Pulmonary Circulation, p. 875.

D. **False** Ipsilateral pneumothorax re-expansion may cause unilateral pulmonary oedema.
Ch. 39 Pulmonary Circulation, p. 875.

E. **True**

Ch. 39 Pulmonary Circulation, p. 875.

Q **3.32**   **Causes of peripheral pulmonary arterial pruning include**

   A. Beri-Beri.
   B. Schistosomiasis.
   C. Bronchopulmonary dysplasia.
   D. Takayasu's arteritis.
   E. Sarcoidosis.

Q **3.33**   **Pulmonary arterial stenosis is a feature of**

   A. Ankylosing spondylitis.
   B. Rubella syndrome.
   C. Tetralogy of Fallot.
   D. Williams syndrome.
   E. Ehlers Danlos syndrome.

(Answers overleaf)

A **3.32**   **Causes of peripheral pulmonary arterial pruning include**

A. **False**   This causes a high-output state with pulmonary plethora.
Ch. 39 Pulmonary Circulation, p. 878.

B. **True**   Due to peripheral pulmonary artery thrombosis/stenosis.
Ch. 39 Pulmonary Circulation, p. 878.

C. **True**
Ch. 39 Pulmonary Circulation, p. 878.

D. **True**
Ch. 39 Pulmonary Circulation, p. 878.

E. **True**
Ch. 39 Pulmonary Circulation, p. 878.

A **3.33**   **Pulmonary arterial stenosis is a feature of**

A. **False**   Aortitis in this condition causes aortic root thickening and dilation leading to regurgitation.
Ch. 39 Pulmonary Circulation, p. 882.

B. **True**
Ch. 39 Pulmonary Circulation, p. 882.

C. **True**
Ch. 39 Pulmonary Circulation, p. 882.

D. **True**   This is a combination of supravalvar aortic stenosis, elfin facies, mental retardation and hypercalcemia.
Ch. 39 Pulmonary Circulation, p. 882.

E. **True**
Ch. 39 Pulmonary Circulation, p. 882.

Q **3.34**   Concerning disease of cardiac muscle

A. Sarcoidosis causes papillary muscle dysfunction.

B. Involvement of the base of the left ventricle helps to distinguish cardiac sarcoid from ischaemia.

C. Cardiac failure caused by Diphtheria toxin is usually followed by complete recovery if the patient survives the toxaemic phase.

D. Cardiomyopathy caused by Chagas's disease is suspected if there is a history of recent travel to Patagonia.

E. Doxorubicin causes reversible cardiac muscle dysfunction.

Q **3.35**   Regarding cardiac tumours

A. An enlarged left atrial appendage indicates left atrial myxoma.

B. Left atrial myxoma is attached to the lower part of the interatrial septum.

C. Ventricular fibroma may be diagnosed on chest X-ray.

D. Lymphoma of the heart usually affects the right ventricular outflow tract.

E. Rhabdomyomas in tuberous sclerosis require early surgical excision.

(Answers overleaf)

A **3.34** Concerning disease of cardiac muscle

A. True

> *Ch. 40 Cardiomyopathies, Cardiac Tumours, Trauma and Cardiac Transplantation, p. 891.*

B. True Coronary artery ischaemic disease involves the apex more and tends to spare the base. These changes may be evident on echocardiography or cardiac MRI.
> *Ch. 40 Cardiomyopathies, Cardiac Tumours, Trauma and Cardiac Transplantation, p. 891.*

C. True

> *Ch. 40 Cardiomyopathies, Cardiac Tumours, Trauma and Cardiac Transplantation, p. 891.*

D. False Chagas's disease is endemic in rural, central and South America. The initial infection takes place in childhood and after a latent period of 10–20 years the patient becomes symptomatic. Recent travel to South America is not a risk factor for the development of cardiomyopathy.
> *Ch. 40 Cardiomyopathies, Cardiac Tumours, Trauma and Cardiac Transplantation, p. 891.*

E. True

> *Ch. 40 Cardiomyopathies, Cardiac Tumours, Trauma and Cardiac Transplantation, p. 891.*

A **3.35** Regarding cardiac tumours

A. False In a patient with signs of mitral valve disease an enlarged left atrial appendage suggests a rheumatic aetiology.
> *Ch. 40 Cardiomyopathies, Cardiac Tumours, Trauma and Cardiac Transplantation, p. 897.*

B. True

> *Ch. 40 Cardiomyopathies, Cardiac Tumours, Trauma and Cardiac Transplantation, p. 897.*

C. True It may show characteristic whorls of calcium allowing a plain film diagnosis.
> *Ch. 40 Cardiomyopathies, Cardiac Tumours, Trauma and Cardiac Transplantation, p. 897.*

D. True

> *Ch. 40 Cardiomyopathies, Cardiac Tumours, Trauma and Cardiac Transplantation, p. 898.*

E. False These tumours are basically inoperable because they are so deep-seated, poorly demarcated and multiple.
> *Ch. 40 Cardiomyopathies, Cardiac Tumours, Trauma and Cardiac Transplantation, p. 898.*

Q 3.36 Regarding normal pericardial anatomy and imaging

A. Epicardial fat lies between visceral and parietal pericardium.
B. Pericardium usually extends along the right and left pulmonary arteries.
C. Parietal pericardium is thinner than the visceral layer.
D. Normal pericardium usually appears as a hyperintense line on T1 weighted images.
E. The inferior pericardium is attached to the diaphragm.

Q 3.37 Concerning pericardial anomalies

A. The heart is more mobile when there is a pericardial defect.
B. The left lung can surround intrapericardial structures when the left pericardium is absent.
C. Complete absence of the left pericardium is associated with bronchogenic cysts.
D. Pericardial defects are usually symptomatic.
E. They are commoner in females.

(Answers overleaf)

A **3.36** Regarding normal pericardial anatomy and imaging

A. False It lies deep to the visceral pericardium.
Ch. 42 The Pericardium, p. 927

B. False It extends along the main pulmonary artery as far as its bifurcation.
Ch. 42 The Pericardium, p. 927.

C. False The normal visceral layer is a monolayer of mesothelium whereas parietal pericardium is approximately 1 mm thick.
Ch. 42 The Pericardium, p. 927.

D. False It is hypointense. Rarely is hyperintense due to motion of pericardial fluid caused by cardiac pulsation.
Ch. 42 The Pericardium, p. 927.

E. True
Ch. 42 The Pericardium, p. 928.

A **3.37** Concerning pericardial anomalies

A. True This is said to allow partial incarceration of the heart through the defect during exercise and to allow torsion of great vessels due to lack of fixation.
Ch. 42 The Pericardium, p. 929.

B. True The most common pericardial anomaly is complete absence of the left pericardium.
Ch. 42 The Pericardium, p. 929.

C. True It is also associated with ASD, patent ductus arteriosus, Fallot's tetralogy and pulmonary sequestration.
Ch. 42 The Pericardium, p. 929.

D. False
Ch. 42 The Pericardium, p. 929.

E. False
Ch. 42 The Pericardium, p. 929.

Q 3.38   Concerning pericardial effusion

A. Haemopericardium occurs in primary mesothelioma of the pericardium.
B. Bilateral hilar overlay is seen on the lateral chest X-ray.
C. The epicardial fat pad sign is positive.
D. Epicardial fat simulates pericardial fluid on echocardiography.
E. CT readily allows differentiation of pericardial thickening from fluid.

Q 3.39   Regarding pericardial disease

A. Most cases of constrictive pericarditis in the Western world are tuberculous in aetiology.
B. Focal pericardial thickening is usually post-operative.
C. Acromegaly causes pericardial constriction.
D. Chronic renal failure causes constrictive pericarditis.
E. Pericardial thickening is always present when there is symptomatic pericardial constriction.

Q 3.40   Regarding the normal thoracic aorta

A. Most of the thickness of the wall is the adventitia.
B. The media contains nerves, lymphatics and vasae vasorum.
C. Immediately below the normal aortic isthmus there is a mild local dilation.
D. The descending thoracic aorta is the same diameter as the ascending aorta in most young adults.
E. The innominate artery and left common carotid artery have a common origin in 40% of patients.

(Answers overleaf)

A **3.38** **Concerning pericardial effusion**

A. **True**

    Ch. 42 The Pericardium, p. 931.

B. **False** This is a sign on the PA chest X-ray.
    Ch. 42 The Pericardium, p. 932.

C. **True** This sign occurs when an anterior pericardial strip bordered by epicardial fat posteriorly and mediastinal fat anteriorly is thicker than 2 mm. It is diagnostic of pericardial thickening or fluid.
    Ch. 42 The Pericardium, p. 932.

D. **True**

    Ch. 42 The Pericardium, p. 932.

E. **False**

    Ch. 42 The Pericardium, p. 933.

A **3.39** **Regarding pericardial disease**

A. **False** Most are of unknown aetiology, presumably viral aetiology.
    Ch. 42 The Pericardium, p. 934.

B. **True**

    Ch. 42 The Pericardium, p. 934.

C. **False** Pericardial thickening, calcification and constriction occurs in Mulibrey nanism, which is an autosomal recessive disorder associated with dwarfism.
    Ch. 42 The Pericardium, p. 935.

D. **True**

    Ch. 42 The Pericardium, p. 934.

E. **False**

    Ch. 42 The Pericardium, p. 936.

A **3.40** **Regarding the normal thoracic aorta**

A. **False** Most of the thickness of the thoracic aorta wall is the media which contains concentric elastic lamella, smooth muscle and connective tissue. The adventitia is the thin outer layer.
    Ch. 43 The Thoracic Aorta, p. 943.

B. **False** The adventitia contains these structures.
    Ch. 43 The Thoracic Aorta, p. 943.

C. **True** This is known as the aortic spindle.
    Ch. 43 The Thoracic Aorta, p. 943.

D. **False** It is smaller by a ratio of 3:2.
    Ch. 43 The Thoracic Aorta, p. 945.

E. **False** This anomaly occurs in 20%
    Ch. 43 The Thoracic Aorta, p. 943.

Q 3.41   Concerning aortic co-arctation

A. It is commoner in females.
B. It is associated with male pattern baldness.
C. The lesion is concentric.
D. The lesion carries an increased risk of dissection and rupture.
E. It is associated with retrograde flow in the internal mammary artery

Q 3.42   Regarding rib notching

A. It is commoner in children.
B. It often spares the first two ribs.
C. It may be seen in chronic severe vena caval obstruction.
D. It is left sided only if there is an aberrant right subclavian artery.
E. Notches usually have a corticated margin.

(Answers overleaf)

A **3.41** **Concerning aortic co-arctation**

A. **False** About 80% of patients are male.
Ch. 43 The Thoracic Aorta, p. 948.

B. **True** Co-arctation is common in Turner's syndrome.
Ch. 43 The Thoracic Aorta, p. 948.

C. **False** The lesion is usually asymmetric and preceded by some tapering of the aortic lumen.
Ch. 43 The Thoracic Aorta, p. 948.

D. **True**
Ch. 43 The Thoracic Aorta, p. 948.

E. **True**
Ch. 43 The Thoracic Aorta, p. 949.

A **3.42** **Regarding rib notching**

A. **False** It is rare below the age of 10 years.
Ch. 43 The Thoracic Aorta, p. 949.

B. **True**
Ch. 43 The Thoracic Aorta, p. 949.

C. **True**
Ch. 43 The Thoracic Aorta, p. 949.

D. **True**
Ch. 43 The Thoracic Aorta, p. 949.

E. **True**
Ch. 43 The Thoracic Aorta, p. 949.

4 The gastrointestinal system

Q 4.1 Regarding the plain abdominal radiograph

A. Valvulae conniventes are commonly seen in the normal patient.
B. A caecal fluid level is seen in the erect/decubitus position in around 20% of normal patients.
C. An ill-defined psoas muscle is an abnormal finding in more than 50% of cases.
D. It is unusual for large bowel calibre to be less than 5 cm in severe large bowel obstruction.
E. The outline of the spleen can be identified in 60% of normal individuals.

Q 4.2 The following are recognized causes of hepatic calcification

A. Cavernous haemangioma.
B. Cholangiocarcinoma.
C. Focal nodular hyperplasia.
D. Hepatic adenoma.
E. *Armillifer armillatus* infestation.

Q 4.3 The following are recognized causes of pancreatic calcification

A. Insulinoma.
B. Cavernous lymphangioma.
C. Acute pancreatitis.
D. Pseudohypoparathyroidism.
E. Hyperthyroidism.

(Answers overleaf)

137

A **4.1** Regarding the plain abdominal radiograph

A. False There is rarely sufficient gas to outline more than a short length of small bowel. The thin bands of the valvulae conniventes are rarely seen.
Ch. 45 Normal Appearances, p. 977.

B. True
Ch. 45 Normal Appearances, p. 978.

C. False Nineteen per cent of normal individuals have a blurred right psoas outline.
Ch. 45 Normal Appearances, p. 978.

D. True This is helpful when trying to distinguish between small and large bowel dilatation as it is unusual for obstructed small bowel to measure more than 5 cm. An exception to this is long-standing complete obstruction.
Ch. 45 The Distinction Between Small and Large Bowel Dilatation, p. 980.

E. True This cannot be identified in 42% of normal subjects.
Ch. 45 Normal Appearances, p. 978.

A **4.2** The following are recognized causes of hepatic calcification

A. True Phleboliths and septal calcification may occur in these tumours.
Ch. 45 Abdominal Calcification, p. 978.

B. True
Ch. 45 Abdominal Calcification, p. 978.

C. False
Ch. 45 Abdominal Calcification, p. 978.

D. False
Ch. 45 Abdominal Calcification, p. 978.

E. True
Ch. 45 Abdominal Calcification, p. 978.

A **4.3** The following are recognized causes of pancreatic calcification

A. True Calcification can be seen in islet cell tumours.
Ch. 45 Table 45.4, p. 979.

B. True
Ch. 45 Table 45.4, p. 979.

C. True This occurs uncommonly after pancreatic fat is broken down by pancreatic enzymes: 'saponification'.
Ch. 45 Table 45.4, p. 979.

D. False Hyperparathyroidism is a recognized cause.
Ch. 45 Table 45.4, p. 979.

E. False
Ch. 45 Table 45.4, p. 979.

Q **4.4**   Causes of adrenal calcification in adults include

A.   Addison's disease.
B.   Adrenal adenoma.
C.   Wolman's disease.
D.   Sarcoidosis.
E.   Adrenal hyperplasia.

Q **4.5**   Regarding dilatation of bowel

A.   A gastric volvulus may mimic a caecal volvulus.
B.   The 'string of beads' sign is diagnostic of small bowel obstruction.
C.   Strangulated hernias are the commonest cause of mechanical small bowel obstruction in the UK.
D.   A normal erect and supine AXR excludes small bowel obstruction.
E.   Gallstone ileus accounts for 10% of cases of small bowel obstruction.

(Answers overleaf)

139

A **4.4** Causes of adrenal calcification in adults include

A. True Calcification is frequent when Addison's disease is due to TB of the adrenals, but this is now an uncommon cause of Addison's disease.
Ch. 45 Table 45.5, p. 979.

B. True
Ch. 45 Table 45.4, p. 979.

C. False This lipidosis is a cause of adrenal calcification but affected infants die within a few months of birth.
Ch. 45 Table 45.4, p. 979.

D. False This granulomatous disease of the adrenal is not a cause of calcification unlike TB or histoplasmosis.
Ch. 45 Table 45.4, p. 979.

E. False Calcification is not a feature. Bilateral hyperplasia is usually smooth but occasionally nodular.
Ch. 45 Table 45.4, p. 979.

A **4.5** Regarding dilatation of bowel

A. True These two viscera may be positioned beneath the left hemidiaphragm but it is unusual for a gastric volvulus to have dilated loops of small bowel.
Ch. 45 Gastric Dilatation, p. 980.

B. True This is due to bubbles of gas trapped between the valvulae conniventes and is seen only when very dilated small bowel is almost completely filled with fluid.
Ch. 45 Small Bowel Obstruction, p. 982.

C. False In Western countries, the commonest cause in 75% of cases is adhesions.
Ch. 45 Table 45.4, p. 979.

D. False In a proportion of patients with small bowel obstruction, normal or equivocal initial radiographs are obtained. No gas or fluid visible in the small bowel of patients with high jejunal obstruction because of vomiting.
Ch. 45 Table 45.4, p. 982.

E. False This accounts for 2% of cases.
Ch. 45 Gallstone Ileus, p. 984.

Q 4.6   Regarding intussusception

A. Usually frequently seen in children under the age of 2 years.

B. In children, a barium enema is frequently required to establish a definitive diagnosis.

C. In adults, it is commonly idiopathic.

D. In the best centres surgical reduction is still required in over 50% of cases.

E. Mesenteric fat within the intussusception suggests that pneumatic reduction is futile.

Q 4.7   Regarding large bowel obstruction

A. In the presence of generalized gaseous bowel distension, decubitus radiographs may help distinguish between obstruction and ileus.

B. After carcinoma of the colon, volvulus is the most common cause of large bowel obstruction in the Western world.

C. Right-sided large bowel obstruction is almost as common as left-sided obstruction.

D. The proximal small bowel is not dilated in 30–40% of patients.

E. Massive colonic distension invariably indicates a distal obstructing lesion.

(Answers overleaf)

A **4.6** Regarding intussusception

A. True

Ch. 45 Intussusception, p. 984.

B. False This is commonly performed using ultrasound, which has nearly 100% sensitivity.
Ch. 45 Intussusception, p. 984.

C. False This is typically either secondary to a tumour of the bowel or as a result of surgery.
Ch. 45 Intussusception, p. 984.

D. False The intussusception can be reduced using barium enema, gas or Hartman's solution using US or fluoroscopic guidance. Certain precautions are needed.
Ch. 45 Intussusception, p. 984.

E. False This is a characteristic feature for the diagnosis of intussusception.
Ch. 45 Intussusception, p. 984.

A **4.7** Regarding large bowel obstruction

A. True This radiograph may allow the demonstration of absence of gas in the rectum, indicting large bowel obstruction instead of a paralytic ileus.
Ch. 45 Mechanical Large Bowel Obstruction, p. 987.

B. False Diverticulitis is the second commonest cause of large bowel obstruction in the USA and Great Britain.
Ch. 45 Mechanical Large Bowel Obstruction, p. 986.

C. False Left-sided obstruction is much more common.
Ch. 45 Mechanical Large Bowel Obstruction, p. 986.

D. False Only in a minority of patients is there a competent ileocaecel valve and thus in marked distension of the caecum, the small bowel is not distended.
Ch. 45 Mechanical Large Bowel Obstruction, p. 986.

E. False This can occur with paralytic ileus.
Ch. 45 Mechanical Large Bowel Obstruction, p. 987.

Q **4.8** Regarding caecal volvulus

A. It is the cause of 20–30% of cases mechanical large bowel obstruction in the UK.

B. Caecal or right colonic volvulus can only occur when there is a degree of malrotation.

C. Occurs more frequently in the 60–80 year age group.

D. A haustral pattern is usually present.

E. The distended caecum may be anywhere in the abdomen.

Q **4.9** Plain radiographic signs supporting a diagnosis of sigmoid volvulus include

A. A dilated viscus with the top of the apex reaching T10 or above.

B. The margin of the dilated loop overlapping the soft-tissue shadow of the inferior border of the liver.

C. The apex of the loop usually underlies the right hemidiaphragm.

D. 'Shouldering' is present on a barium enema.

E. An 'inferior convergence' sign in the left lower quadrant.

(Answers overleaf)

A **4.8** **Regarding caecal volvulus**

A. False Volvulus is the cause of mechanical large bowel obstruction in only 10% of cases in USA and up to 85% in Africa.
Ch. 45 Large Bowel Volvulus, p. 987.

B. True This is liable to occur only if the caecum and ascending colon are on a mesentery.
Ch. 45 Large Bowel Volvulus, p. 987.

C. False From 30 to 60 years is common – a younger age group then seen in sigmoid volvulus.
Ch. 45 Large Bowel Volvulus, p. 987.

D. True This is a distinguishing feature for sigmoid volvulus where haustra folds are absent.
Ch 45 Caecal Volvulus, p. 987.

E. True
Ch. 45 Large Bowel Volvulus, p. 987.

A **4.9** **Plain radiographic signs supporting a diagnosis of sigmoid volvulus include**

A. True
Ch. 45 Sigmoid Volvulus, p. 988.

B. True This is also known as the liver overlap sign.
Ch. 45 Sigmoid Volvulus, p. 988.

C. False The apex typically lies underneath the left hemidiaphragm.
Ch. 45 Sigmoid Volvulus, p. 988.

D. True This is seen in chronic volvulus, the point of torsion has features resembling a 'hooked beak'.
Ch. 45 Sigmoid Volvulus, p. 988.

E. True
Ch. 45 Sigmoid Volvulus, p. 988.

Q **4.10** **Regarding acute colitis**

A. Perforation occurs in 20% of patients with Crohn's disease.
B. Gaseous distension of small bowel in the presence of a toxic megacolon indicates a poor prognosis.
C. Pseudomembranous colitis commonly affects the descending and sigmoid colon.
D. The right side of the colon tends to be dilated in ischaemic colitis.
E. 'Thumb-printing' on the plain abdominal radiograph is a sign of bowel necrosis from ischaemia.

Q **4.11** **Regarding imaging of acute appendicitis**

A. A scoliosis concave to the right is a recognised sign on plain radiography.
B. On ultrasound, an appendix with a diameter of 3 mm is normal.
C. On ultrasound, a compressible appendix excludes appendicitis.
D. The normal appendix is visualized in nearly the same proportion of patients on ultrasound and CT.
E. On CT contrast medium or air in the caecum pointing towards the obstructed appendix (arrowhead sign) is present in over 50% of cases.

(Answers overleaf)

145

A **4.10**   Regarding acute colitis

A. False   Perforation in Crohn's is rare, whilst it is far more common in ulcerative colitis where the sigmoid is the usual site.
Ch. 45 Acute Colitis, p. 989.

B. True   This tends to predict a poor response to medical treatment.
Ch. 45 Acute Colitis, p. 989.

C. False   The right transverse colon are more likely to appear abnormal then the left side.
Ch. 45 Acute Colitis, p. 989.

D. True
Ch. 45 Acute Colitis, p. 989.

E. False   This term describes the appearance of submucosal thickening with its cresentic margins and is not specific for bowel ischaemia.
Ch. 45 Acute Colitis, p. 989.

A **4.11**   Regarding imaging of acute appendicitis

A. True
Ch. 45 Table 45.20, p. 994.

B. True   The signs of acute appendicitis include visualization of a blind ending tubular structure that is non-compressible with a diameter of 7 mm or greater.
Ch. 45 Ultrasound in Acute Appendicitis, p. 994.

C. False   The appendix may be compressible when it has perforated. This has been reported in 38% of children and 55% of adult operations.
Ch. 45 Ultrasound in Acute Appendicitis, p. 994.

D. False   The normal appendix is visualized more frequently on CT and this is a key advantage of CT over ultrasound.
Ch. 45 Ultrasound in Acute Appendicitis, p. 995.

E. False   This is present in approximately 30% of cases. CT has a reported overall accuracy of 93–98% for diagnosis of appendicitis.
Ch. 45 Ultrasound in Acute Appendicitis, p. 996.

Q **4.12**   **The following are causes of pneumoperitoneum without peritonitis**

    A. Perforated jejunal diverticulosis.
    B. Perforated cyst of pneumatosis intestinalis.
    C. A sealed perforation of a sigmoid diverticulum in an elderly patient.
    D. Hysterosalpingogram.
    E. Endoscopy.

Q **4.13**   **The following statements are true**

    A. Forty per cent of gallstones are visible on plain AXR.
    B. A left-sided pleural effusion in a patient with acute pancreatitis indicates a worse prognosis.
    C. Linear intramural gas shadows in a patient with cystic pneumatosis is a normal finding.
    D. Chronic obstructive airways disease is strongly associated with pneumatosis cystoides intestinalis.
    E. A paralytic ileus is commonly found in association with a leaking abdominal aortic aneurysm.

(Answers overleaf)

A **4.12** The following are causes of pneumoperitoneum without peritonitis

A. True This is the most common cause of pneumoperitoneum without peritonitis.
Ch. 45 Pneumoperitoneum, p. 993

B. True There is a wide spectrum of severity in this condition. An asymptomatic pneumoperitoneum may persists for months following perforation of the cyst with no apparent sequelae.
Ch. 45 Pneumoperitoneum, p. 993.

C. True Silent perforation of a viscus, which has sealed itself in elderly patients, patients on steroids, or the unconscious patient can cause pneumoperitoneum without peritonitis.
Ch. 45 Pneumoperitoneum, p. 993.

D. True Other iatrogenic causes of fallopian tube insufflation will cause pneumoperitoneum without peritonitis.
Ch. 45 Pneumoperitoneum, p. 993.

E. True Leakage of air through a distended stomach after endoscopic inflation can cause pneumoperitoneum without peritonitis.
Ch. 45 Pneumoperitoneum, p. 993.

A **4.13** The following statements are true

A. False Only about 20% of gallstones contain sufficient calcium to be visible on plain radiographs.
Ch. 45 Acute Cholecystitis, p. 997.

B. True
Ch. 45 Acute Pancreatitis, p. 997.

C. False Cystic pneumatosis is usually a relatively benign condition but the presence of linear gas shadows in the bowel wall is usually a sign of necrosis.
Ch. 45 Intramural Gas, p. 998.

D. True The cause of pneumatosis cystoides is unknown but there is a strong association with COPD.
Ch. 45 Cystic Pneumatosis, p. 999.

E. True The loops of bowel may completely obscure the signs of a leaking aneurysm on a plain AXR and US.
Ch. 45 Leaking Abdominal Aortic Aneurysm, p. 1001.

Q **4.14**   **The following are normal features of the oesophagus on a barium swallow**

A.   The cervical oesophagus starts at the cricopharyngeous impression, usually at the C3/C4 level.

B.   The post-cricoid impression is a small, posterior, web-like indentation.

C.   An anterior indentation in the mid oesophagus is related to the left main bronchus.

D.   The A ring (tubulovestibular junction) varies in calibre during the examination.

E.   The mucosal gastro-oesophageal junction cannot be identified on double contrast studies.

Q **4.15**   **Regarding oesophageal pathology**

A.   The HIV virus can cause oesophageal ulceration.

B.   Oral candidiasis usually gives rise to infections within the mid and distal oesophagus.

C.   Oesophageal intramural pseudodiverticulosis is associated with oesophageal carcinoma.

D.   Adenocarcinoma is the commonest malignancy of the lower third of the oesophagus.

E.   A dilated oesophagus with a 'bird beak' shaped gastro-oesophageal junction is a presentation of an oesophageal carcinoma.

(Answers overleaf)

149

A **4.14** The following are normal features of the oesophagus on a barium swallow

A. **False** The cricopharyngeal impression is usually at the C5 – C6 level.
Ch. 46 Normal Anatomy, p. 1005.

B. **False** An anterior impression (as opposed to the posteriorly-placed cricopharyngeous impressions) that is like a web but changes shape with swallowing.
Ch. 46 Normal Anatomy, p. 1005.

C. **True** The thoracic part, its main anterior relationship is the left main bronchus and inferior to this lies the pericardium and heart.
Ch. 46 Normal Anatomy, p. 1006.

D. **True** This ring is visible only if the vestibule and tubular oesophagus are adequately distended.
Ch. 46 Function, p. 1006.

E. **False** This normal feature is occasionally visible as a thin, slightly radiolucent line. It is also known as the Z line or oraserrata.
Ch. 46 Function, p. 1006.

A **4.15** Regarding oesophageal pathology

A. **True** Other infective agents causing ulceration include herpes simplex virus and cytomegalovirus.
Ch. 46 Miscellaneous Conditions, p. 1028.

B. **True** Surprisingly, in many cases of mid and distal oesophageal candidiasis there is no evidence of disease in the throat or mouth.
Ch. 46 Miscellaneous Conditions, p. 1028.

C. **True**
Ch. 46 Benign Strictures, p. 1030.

D. **False** Adenocarcinoma only represents 30% of the oesophageal carcinoma that commonly occurs in the lower third of the oesophagus. Squamous cell carcinoma is by far the commonest malignancy and is found commonly in the mid oesophagus.
Ch. 46 Malignant Tumours, p. 1017.

E. **True** This is an uncommon manifestations of tumours at the gastro-oesophageal junction, which can give rise to achalasia-like picture. It is unclear whether this is caused by actual destruction of the myenteric plexus or results from some unknown paraneoplastic process.
Ch. 46 Malignant Tumours, p. 1018.

Q **4.16** Regarding motility of the oesophagus

A. Achalasia is the commonest motility disorder of the oesophagus.

B. Heller's myomectomy is a better treatment than pneumatic dilatation of the gastro-oesophageal junction in achalasia.

C. Scleroderma is the commonest systemic disease to cause motor dysfunction.

D. Oesophageal dismotility due to scleroderma cannot be reliably distinguished from achalasia.

E. In patients with a 'corkscrew' oesophagus, dysphagia is the commonest symptom.

Q **4.17** Regarding inflammatory disease of the stomach

A. Virtually all gastric ulceration is benign and commonly due to *Helicobacter pylori* infection.

B. An ulcer in the fundus of the stomach should always be considered suspicious for malignancy.

C. Atrophic gastritis is associated with pernicious anaemia.

D. In 20% of patients with Crohn's disease affecting the stomach, there is sparing of the duodenum.

E. Menetrier's disease is a triad of achlorhydria, hypoproteinaemia and hypertrophy of the gastric glands.

(Answers overleaf)

151

A **4.16**   Regarding motility of the oesophagus

A. False   Gastro-oesophageal reflux disease is the commonest cause of disorder of oesophageal motility.
Ch. 46 Motility Disorders, p. 1025.

B. False   They appear to have equal success.
Ch. 46 Achalasia, p. 1025.

C. True   Scleroderma when it involves the gastrointestinal tract, affects the oesophagus most frequently.
Ch. 46 Systemic Disorders Associated with Motor Dysfunction, p. 1025.

D. False   In achalasia the gastro-oesophageal junction is narrowed whereas it is patulous in scleroderma.
Ch. 46 Motility Disorders, p. 1026.

E. False   In diffuse oesophageal spasm, this is associated with chest pain that may or may not be related to swallowing and is a more dominant feature than dysphagia.
Ch. 46 Diffuse Oesophageal Spasm, p. 1025.

A **4.17**   Regarding inflammatory disease of the stomach

A. True   In more than 95%, of gastric ulcers they are benign with 70% due to *H. pylori* infection and the remainder due to non-steroidal anti-inflammatory agents and alcohol abuse.
Ch. 46 Inflammatory Disease, p. 1040.

B. True   Benign ulcers are much less common in the fundus and along the proximal half of the greater curvature. Lesions should be suspicious for malignancy.
Ch. 46 Inflammatory Disease, p. 1041.

C. True   This is more common in advancing age and the disease is caused by a decreased production of intrinsic factor with malabsorption of vitamin B_{12}.
Ch. 46 Inflammatory Disease, p. 1045.

D. False   When the upper gastrointestinal tract is affected by Crohn's disease, both the stomach and the duodenum are involved.
Ch. 46 Inflammatory Disease, p. 1045.

E. True   It is a rare entity but well known in the radiology literature because of its dramatic and characteristic appearance.
Ch. 46 Menetrier's Disease, p. 1046.

Q 4.18   Regarding the duodenum

A. In crush injuries, the most frequent site of rupture is at the junction of the first and second parts of the duodenum.

B. On barium studies, superior mesenteric artery compression syndrome is characterized by a sharp cut-off of the third part in the right anterior oblique position.

C. Incidental diverticula of the duodenum on barium studies, are seen in approximately 20% of examinations.

D. Abdominal aortic aneurysms are a recognized cause of duodenal obstruction from mechanical compression.

E. Bouveret's syndrome is characterized by gastric outlet obstruction due to a gallstone impacted in the duodenal cap.

Q 4.19   Regarding imaging of the small intestine

A. Mesenteric abscesses and mesenteric lymphadenopathy are recognized CT findings in Crohn's disease.

B. A 'coiled spring' appearance is a sign of coeliac disease on a barium follow-through.

C. Isolated focal dilatation of a small bowel loop is a sign of lymphoma.

D. Primary carcinoma is more common in the ileum than the jejunum.

E. Deep ulceration occurs in 80% of cases of radiation enteritis.

(Answers overleaf)

A **4.18**   Regarding the duodenum

A. False   The most frequent site is at the junction of the second and third parts of the duodenum.
Ch. 48 Traumatic Rupture, p. 1072.

B. True   It commonly affects the third part of the duodenum, and barium examination shows strong to-and-fro peristalsis with duodenal dilatation.
Ch. 48 Superior Mesenteric Artery Compression Syndrome, p. 1072.

C. False   These diverticula, which are lined with intestinal epithelium, are frequently an incidental finding but present in only 2–5% of examinations.
Ch. 48 Diverticula, p. 1066.

D. True   Abdominal aortic aneurysms may compress a third part of the duodenum and can occasionally cause obstruction.
Ch. 48 Compression from Aortic Aneurysm, p. 1072.

E. True   The mortality is high and it is, therefore, important to recognize this complication of gallstone disease.
Ch. 48 Bouveret's Syndrome, p. 1073.

A **4.19**   Regarding imaging of the small intestine

A. True
Ch. 49 Crohn's Disease, p. 1078.

B. True   Non-obstructive intussusception commonly occurs in this condition, which most characteristically causes small bowel dilation.
Ch. 49 Coeliac Disease, p. 1082.

C. True   This is occasionally seen owing presumably to loss of intestinal muscle tone as a result of lymphomatous invasion of muscle layers and neural plexus. Also known as focal aneurysmal dilatation.
Ch. 49 Lymphoma, p. 1085.

D. False   The reverse is true. Ileal carcinoma is rare.
Ch. 49 Primary Carcinoma, p. 1085.

E. False   Deep ulceration is uncommon in radiation enteritis. Ulcers when present are typically too shallow to be appreciated radiologically.
Ch. 49 Chronic Radiation Enteritis, p. 1089.

Q **4.20** **Thickened valvulae conniventes on small-bowel enemas are a characteristic feature of**

A. Carcinoid tumour.
B. Zollinger-Ellison syndrome.
C. Coeliac disease.
D. Mastocytosis.
E. Behçet's disease.

Q **4.21** **Regarding the anatomy of the large bowel**

A. Both the ascending and descending colon are predominantly extraperitoneal.
B. The proximal descending colon is supplied by the superior mesenteric artery.
C. Absence of haustration in the proximal colon is always abnormal.
D. A presacral space of 15 mm or greater can be a normal finding.
E. The start of the ascending colon is demarcated by the ileocaecal valve.

(Answers overleaf)

A **4.20** **Thickened valvulae conniventes on small-bowel enemas are a characteristic feature of**

A. True
Ch. 49 Table 49.3, p. 1095.

B. True
Ch. 49 Table 49.3, p. 1095.

C. True Characteristic radiological sign of coeliac disease with dilation of the small bowel. The valvulae conniventes are straightened, moderately thickened and separated.
Ch. 49 Coeliac Disease, p. 1082.

D. True
Ch. 49 Table 49.3, p. 1095.

E. False In Behçet's disease, there is more frequently ulceration in the ileo-caecal region with an appearance resembling ileocaecal tuberculosis or Crohn's disease.
Ch. 49 Behçet's Disease, p. 1095.

A **4.21** **Regarding the anatomy of the large bowel**

A. True The transverse and sigmoid colons both have a mesentery, whereas, the ascending and descending colon are partly extraperitoneal.
Ch. 50 Anatomy, p. 1099.

B. False The colon distal to the splenic flexure is supplied by the inferior mesenteric artery.
Ch. 50 Anatomy, p. 1099.

C. True There is often no haustration visible from mid transverse colon to the rectum during a barium enema, however, haustra should always be visible in the ascending colon.
Ch. 50 Anatomy, p. 1099.

D. True In the obese and elderly, up to 20 mm is within normal limits.
Ch. 50 Anatomy, p. 1099.

E. True The ileocaecal valve demarcates the junction between the caecum and the ascending colon.
Ch. 50 Anatomy, p. 1101.

Q **4.22**   **Regarding large bowel polyps**

A.   More than 50% of adenomatous polyps are found in the recto-sigmoid region.

B.   Metaplastic polyps greater than 1 cm across have an incidence of malignancy of less than 1%.

C.   On double contrast barium enema, a ring of barium having a sharp inner edge and an unsharp outer margin are characteristic of a polyp.

D.   Familial adenomatous polyposis patients have an increased risk of desmoid tumours.

E.   Size is the most important radiographic criterion of malignancy.

Q **4.23**   **Regarding abnormalities of the peritoneum, mesenteries and omentum**

A.   Gas within a loculated mesenteric fluid collection is pathognomic of a peritoneal abscess.

B.   Peritoneal mesothelioma is associated with asbestos exposure.

C.   Ascites with septations is a recognized feature of pseudomyxoma-peritonei.

D.   Fibrosing mesenteritis is a mimic of carcinoid tumours on CT.

E.   Lipomas are the commonest primary benign solid tumour in the mesentery.

(Answers overleaf)

A **4.22** Regarding large bowel polyps

A. True

 Ch. 50 Adenomatous Polyps, p. 1109.

B. False These lesions are common in the rectum and appear as sessile nodules less than 1cm across and have no malignant potential.
Ch. 50 Metaplastic Polyps, p. 1109.

C. True

 Ch. 50 Meniscus Sign, p. 1109.

D. True Gardner's syndrome is now considered as part of the spectrum of familial adenomatous polyposis. Desmoid formation is often precipitated by surgery, and is a major cause of morbidity and mortality owing to recurrent local invasion and small-bowel obstruction.
Ch. 50 Familial Adenomatous Polyposis, p. 1113.

E. True

 Ch. 50 Assessment and Management of Ppolyps, p. 1111.

A **4.23** Regarding abnormalities of the peritoneum, mesenteries and omentum

A. False This is highly suggestive of an abscess, however, a necrotic non-infected tumour and a mass that communicates with the bowel may also contain air.
Ch. 51 Abnormalities of the Peritoneum, p. 1146.

B. True It also has an extremely poor prognosis.
Ch. 51 Peperitoneal Mesothelioma, p. 1149.

C. True These features are characteristic, however, it may be difficult to distinguish from simple ascites. This is commonly due to intraperitoneal spread of a mucinous adenocarcinoma or an ovarian or appendiceal mucinous adenoma.
Ch. 51 Intraperitoneal Seeding, p. 1148.

D. True In retractile or fibrosing mesenteritis, there is also an infiltrative soft-tissue mass with associated radiating linear strands of soft-tissue attenuation. MRI might help in the differentiation by showing low signal intensity on T1 and T2 images in fibrosing mesenteritis.
Ch. 51 Mesenteric Panniculitis, p. 1154.

E. False It is the second most common primary solid tumour after fibromatosis. Fibromatosis may be isolated or occur in association with Gardner's syndrome and arises after surgery or trauma.
Ch. 51 Primary Neoplasms, p. 1157.

Q **4.24** Regarding gastrointestinal bleeding and angiography

A. Vasodilators should be used regularly in arteriography to improve the diagnostic accuracy.

B. Angiodysplasia when demonstrated on arteriography, is frequently the source of haemorrhage.

C. A hypervascular lesion with a corkscrew pattern of vessels and venous occlusions are characteristics of adenocarcinomas of the gastrointestinal tract.

D. Stent insertion into the superior mesenteric artery is a recognized treatment for patients with mesenteric ischaemia.

E. Bowel infarction is not a risk following embolization due to the rich collateral supplies found throughout the upper GI tract.

Q **4.25** Regarding delayed passage of meconium

A. On a water soluble contrast medium enema, a rectum:sigmoid ratio greater than 1 is suggestive of Hirschsprung's disease.

B. Meconium plug syndrome is associated with cystic fibrosis.

C. Ninety per cent of infants with meconium ileus have cystic fibrosis and have a similar long-term outcome in comparison with other cystic fibrosis patients who do not present with meconium ileus.

D. Volvulus is a recognized feature in meconium ileus.

E. The 'soap bubble' appearance in the right iliac fossa on AXR is pathognomomic of meconium ileus.

(Answers overleaf)

A **4.24** Regarding gastrointestinal bleeding and angiography

A. False Although there has been much attempt to improve images using these substances, there is controversy as to its effects. The operator should aim to acquire good selective arteriography using adequate amounts of contrast medium delivered at the right rate.
Ch. 52 Role of Vasoactive Drugs, p. 1174.

B. False Demonstration of angiodysplasia on arteriography does not prove that it is the source of haemorrhage unless it is actively bleeding.
Ch. 52 Angiodysplasia, p. 1175.

C. False Adenocarcinomas are usually hypovascular with areas of subtle neovascularity and vascular irregularity and can easily be overlooked at angiography. Corkscrew patterns of vessels and venous drainage occlusion are common with carcinoid tumours.
Ch. 52 Adenocarcinoma, p. 1178.

D. True Angioplasty with or without stent insertion has been shown to be helpful in selected patients with coeliac axis, SMA or IMA stenosis.
Ch. 52 Percutaneous Angioplasty and Mesenteric Ischaemia, p. 1178.

E. False Although bowel infarction is rare after embolization, there is still a risk especially if multiple simultaneous embolizations are performed and if there is pre-existing arterial disease or if surgery has compromised the collateral circulation.
Ch. 52 Interventional Techniques, p. 1172.

A **4.25** Regarding delayed passage of meconium

A. False This is the norm and reversed with Hirschprung's as the rectum would be narrowed and a cone-shape transition zone is seen in the more proximal dilated aganglionic bowel.
Ch. 54 Hirschsprung's Disease, p. 1208.

B. False This condition is not associated with cystic fibrosis. The exact cause of this syndrome remains unknown, but immaturity of the myenteric plexus has been postulated.
Ch. 54 Functional Immaturity of the Colon, p. 1209.

C. True
Ch. 54 Meconium Ileus, p. 1210.

D. True Volvulus of a heavy, meconium-laden loop of bowel is common.
Ch. 54 Meconium Ileus, p. 1212.

E. False Although characteristic, it is a non-specific feature. Distal ileal atresia may give a similar appearance.
Ch. 54 Meconium Ileus, p. 1212.

The liver, biliary tract, pancreas, endocrine system and lymphoma

Q 5.1 Regarding normal visceral anatomy and physiology

- **A.** The caudate lobe separates porta hepatis from inferior vena cava.
- **B.** The pressure difference between the hepatic sinusoids and inferior vena cava is normally between 12 and 15 mm Hg.
- **C.** Inferior mesenteric vein drains into right gastroepipioic vein in 50% of cases.
- **D.** The caudate lobe receives vascular supply from both right and left portal veins.
- **E.** Riedel's lobe drains directly into the IVC.

Q 5.2 Regarding normal hepatic variants

- **A.** The gallbladder is displaced posteriorly if there is agenesis of the right lobe of liver.
- **B.** When the caudate lobe is enlarged there is increased distance between the portal vein and inferior vena cava.
- **C.** A replaced left hepatic artery arises from the right gastric artery.
- **D.** Duplication of the portal vein occurs in 10% of the normal population.
- **E.** Absence of the inferior vena cava is associated with a right-sided liver.

Q 5.3 Concerning normal imaging findings in the liver

- **A.** The walls of the hepatic veins are distinguishable from the adjacent parenchyma on ultrasound.
- **B.** The normal portal venous trace on Doppler examination is continuously antegrade.
- **C.** Normal portal venous flow varies with respiration and the cardiac cycle.
- **D.** Optimal portal phase imaging in contrast-enhanced CT of the liver is achieved 30-40 seconds after injection.
- **E.** Liver attenuation at computed tomography is usually 8–10 HU greater than the spleen.

(Answers overleaf)

A **5.1** **Regarding normal visceral anatomy and physiology**

A. True
> *Ch. 55 The Liver, p, 1237*

B. False The corrected sinusoidal pressure is normally between 4 and 8 mm Hg.
> *Ch. 55 The Liver, p. 1237.*

C. False The IMV normally drains into the splenic vein.
> *Ch. 55 The Liver, p. 1238.*

D. True
> *Ch. 55 The Liver, p. 1239.*

E. False The caudate lobe drains directly into the IVC.
> *Ch. 55 The Liver, p. 1239.*

A **5.2** **Regarding normal hepatic variants**

A. True It assumes a retrohepatic location and the left lobe rotates to fill the hepatic fossa.
> *Ch. 55 The Liver, p. 1239.*

B. True The papillary process of caudate insinuates between these vessels.
> *Ch. 55 The Liver, p. 1239.*

C. False The left hepatic artery arises from the left gastric artery.
> *Ch. 55 The Liver, p. 1240.*

D. False Variations in portal venous anatomy are infrequent.
> *Ch. 55 The Liver, p. 1240.*

E. True In this circumstance the hepatic veins drain directly into a cardiac atrium while the azygous vein replaces the IVC.
> *Ch. 55 The Liver, p. 1240.*

A **5.3** **Concerning normal imaging findings in the liver**

A. False
> *Ch. 55 The Liver, p. 1241.*

B. True
> *Ch. 55 The Liver, p. 1241.*

C. True There is slight variant with breathing and cardiac systole.
> *Ch. 55 The Liver, p. 1241.*

D. False Portal phase imaging is used for detection of relatively hypovascular lesions (which include the majority of metastases). Optimal data acquisition occurs between 70 and 90 seconds after injection.
> *Ch. 55 The Liver, p. 1241.*

E. True
> *Ch. 55 The Liver, p. 1242.*

Q 5.4   Concerning magnetic resonance imaging of the liver

A. Iron oxide particles shorten T2.

B. Particles that target the reticulo-endothelial system are generally larger than those that target hepatocytes.

C. The intensity of normal liver parenchyma on T1 weighted MRI is the same or slightly higher than that of adjacent muscles

D. Many malignant liver lesions have T1 and T2 values that mirror those of the spleen.

E. The spleen should be darker than the liver on T1 weighted images and brighter than the liver on T2 weighted images.

Q 5.5   Regarding liver scintigraphy

A. ^{99m}Tc sulphur colloid is superior to ^{99m}Tc-labelled red blood cells for the detection of haemangioma.

B. Following injection of sulphur colloid 80-90% of the dose is taken up by hepatocytes in the liver.

C. During imaging with sulphur colloid data may begin to be acquired 5–10 minutes after injection.

D. When there is portal hypertension optimal concentration of sulphur colloid takes longer and imaging should not begin before 20 minutes following the injection.

E. In a normal liver-spleen scintigram a small amount of activity is seen in the reticulo-endothelial cells of the skeleton.

Q 5.6   Concerning imaging findings in cirrhosis

A. The commonest finding in advanced cirrhosis is atrophy of segments V and VII of the right lobe.

B. Pure hepatic fibrosis results in loss of the margins of the portal vein branches on ultrasound examination.

C. In end-stage cirrhosis the hepatic veins become attenuated and difficult to visualize.

D. Hepatic arterial flow is usually increased in advanced cirrhosis.

E. In cirrhosis there is enlargement of the hepatic arteries, which may simulate enlarged bile ducts on ultrasound.

(Answers overleaf)

A **5.4** **Concerning magnetic resonance imaging of the liver**

A. True Accumulation of iron oxide particles causes a reduction in signal due to susceptibility-induced dephasing of protons
Ch. 55 The Liver, p. 1243.

B. True Larger particles (50–100 nm) exploit the ability of Kupffer and endothelial cells to take up starch-coated particles of iron oxide.
Ch. 55 The Liver, p. 1243.

C. True This holds for virtually all sequence combinations except for certain inversion recovery techniques.
Ch. 55 The Liver, p. 1243.

D. True
Ch. 55 The Liver, p. 1243.

E. True
Ch. 55 The Liver, p. 1243.

A **5.5** **Regarding liver scintigraphy**

A. False
Ch. 55 The Liver, p. 1243.

B. False From 80 to 90% of the dose is taken up by the Kupffer cells of the liver and 5–10% is taken up by the spleen. A small proportion is also absorbed by the bone marrow.
Ch. 55 The Liver, p. 1243.

C. True
Ch. 55 The Liver, p. 1244.

D. True
Ch. 55 The Liver, p. 1244.

E. False
Ch. 55 The Liver, p. 1244.

A **5.6** **Concerning imaging findings in cirrhosis**

A. False The posterior segments (VI and VII) of the right lobe.
Ch. 55 The Liver, p. 1248.

B. True Owing to increased reflectivity of hepatic parenchyma.
Ch. 55 The Liver, p. 1248.

C. True
Ch. 55 The Liver, p. 1248.

D. True This occurs as the portal contribution to hepatocyte perfusion decreases.
Ch. 55 The Liver, p. 1248.

E. True
Ch. 55 The Liver, p. 1248.

Q 5.7 Concerning imaging findings in diffuse liver disease

A. The majority of cases of acute viral hepatitis have normal parenchyma on ultrasound.

B. Gallbladder wall thickening is a common finding in acute hepatitis.

C. Haemochromatosis results in an increased risk of developing malignancy in general and hepato-cellular carcinoma in particular.

D. There is less risk of liver damage from iron overload from transfusions than from haemochromatosis.

E. Copper accumulation in Wilson's disease causes a detectable increase in hepatic attenuation on CT examination.

Q 5.8 Causes of calcification in the liver include

A. *Pneumocystis carinii* infection.

B. Giant haemangioma.

C. Hepatoblastoma.

D. Fibrolamellar hepatoma.

E. Wilson's disease.

Q 5.9 Causes of portal vein gas include

A. Necrotizing entercolitis.

B. Interstinal volvulus.

C. Crohn's disease.

D. Hyperventilation.

E. Colonic carcinoma.

(Answers overleaf)

A **5.7** **Concerning imaging findings in diffuse liver disease**

A. True Occasionally there is a generalized decrease in reflectivity.
Ch. 55 The Liver, p. 1249.

B. True
Ch. 55 The Liver, p. 1249.

C. True
Ch. 55 The Liver, p. 1249.

D. True
Ch. 55 The Liver, p. 1249.

E. True This occurs in some cases.
Ch. 55 The Liver, p. 1250.

A **5.8** **Causes of calcification in the liver include**

A. True Benign parenchymal calcification is a relatively common end result of previous infection with this organism.
Ch. 55 The Liver, p. 1250.

B. True
Ch. 55 The Liver, p. 1250.

C. True There may be chunky calcification in this childhood neoplasm.
Ch. 55 The Liver, p. 1250.

D. True
Ch. 55 The Liver, p. 1250.

E. False
Ch. 55 The Liver, p. 1250.

A **5.9** **Causes of portal vein gas include**

A. True
Ch. 55 The Liver, p. 1251.

B. True
Ch. 55 The Liver, p. 1251.

C. True
Ch. 55 The Liver, p. 1251.

D. False
Ch. 55 The Liver, p. 1251.

E. True
Ch. 55 The Liver, p. 1251.

Q 5.10   Regarding hepatic cysts

A. Simple cysts return greater T2-weighted signal than the spleen on MRI.
B. Choledochal cysts show increased activity on HIDA scans.
C. Cysts may be indistinguishable from haemangiomas on T2-weighted MRI.
D. Attenuation of 20–30 HU suggests the presence of a simple cyst on CT.
E. The walls of a simple cyst show mild enhancement with intravenous contrast medium.

Q 5.11   Concerning hepatic cystic lesions

A. Hydatid cysts may be indistinguishable from simple cysts on ultrasound.
B. MRI is sensitive at identifying calcification in hydatid cyst walls.
C. Rim enhancement of abscesses is often not apparent once antibiotic treatment has started.
D. Liver metastases from ovarian tumours simulate simple cysts.
E. Early abscesses simulate solid tumours on virtually all imaging modalities.

Q 5.12   Regarding liver haemangiomas

A. They are multiple in 40%.
B. They have high signal on T2-weighted MRI that is less than the spleen.
C. Haemangiomas become more prominent on T2-weighted MRI when the TE is increased from 90 to 160 ms.
D. In adult haemangiomas there is usually detectable flow on colour Doppler ultrasound.
E. Haemangiomas are photopenic on sulphur colloid studies.

(Answers overleaf)

A **5.10** Regarding hepatic cysts

A. **True**

Ch. 55 The Liver, p. 1252.

B. **True**

Ch. 55 The Liver, p. 1252.

C. **True**

Ch. 55 The Liver, p. 1252.

D. **False** Attenuation of 0–10 HU is typical of a simple cyst on CT
Ch. 55 The Liver, p. 1252.

E. **False**

Ch. 55 The Liver, p. 1252.

A **5.11** Concerning hepatic cystic lesions

A. **True**

Ch. 55 The Liver, p. 1253.

B. **False**

Ch. 55 The Liver, p. 1253.

C. **True**

Ch. 55 The Liver, p. 1253.

D. **True**

Ch. 55 The Liver, p. 1254.

E. **True**

Ch. 55 The Liver, p. 1254.

A **5.12** Regarding liver haemangiomas

A. **False** They are mutiple in up to 10% of cases.
Ch. 55 The Liver, p. 1254.

B. **False** Homogeneously high signal on T2 weighting is seen in haemangiomas. This is in excess of the spleen and similar to that of fluid.
Ch. 55 The Liver, p. 1254.

C. **True**

Ch. 55 The Liver, p. 1254.

D. **False**

Ch. 55 The Liver, p. 1254.

E. **True** They do not contain Kupffer cells but they show an increase in uptake on blood pool studies.
Ch. 55 The Liver, p. 1255.

Q **5.13**   Regarding focal liver lesions

A. Paediatric haemangiomas are hyporeflective on ultrasound.
B. Core biopsy of haemangiomas is no longer used owing to the risk of serious haemorrhage.
C. Focal nodular hyperplasia is more common in men aged 20–50.
D. Multiple adenomas occur in glycogen storage disease type I
E. Focal confluent fibrosis affects the anterior segments of the right lobe of liver.

Q **5.14**   Concerning focal nodular hyperplasia

A. It presents with pain and hepatomegaly.
B. It arises from a congenital vascular malformation.
C. Contains Kupffer cells.
D. Contains hepatocytes.
E. Contains normal portal triads.

Q **5.15**   Regarding hepatic adenoma

A. Kupffer cells are present in 50% of cases.
B. The presence of haemorrhage thrombosis and necrosis favours the diagnosis of focal nodular hyperplasia over adenoma.
C. Adenomas may contain fat.
D. Most adenomas are hypervascular on angiography.
E. Adenomas are hyperreflective well-defined masses that mimic haemangiomas on ultrasound.

(Answers overleaf)

A **5.13** Regarding focal liver lesions

A. True As are some adult cavernous haemangiomas.
Ch. 55 The Liver, p. 1256

B. False In adult core needle biopsy rather than aspiration is occasionally useful. It is less likely to provoke serious haemorrhage than previously thought particularly if the needle route is via intervening normal liver.
Ch. 55 The Liver, p. 1256.

C. False Women between the ages are more likely to be affected.
Ch. 55 The Liver, p. 1256.

D. True
Ch. 55 The Liver, p. 1257.

E. True
Ch. 55 The Liver, p. 1259.

A **5.14** Concerning focal nodular hyperplasia

A. True
Ch. 55 The Liver, p. 1257.

B. True
Ch. 55 The Liver, p. 1257.

C. True
Ch. 55 The Liver, p. 1257.

D. True
Ch. 55 The Liver, p. 1257.

E. False
Ch. 55 The Liver, p. 1257.

A **5.15** Regarding hepatic adenoma

A. False Kupffer cell activity is usually absent but it may be seen in 20% of cases.
Ch. 55 The Liver, p. 1258.

B. False
Ch. 55 The Liver, p. 1258.

C. True Substantial amounts of fat lower the attenuation of adenomas on CT.
Ch. 55 The Liver, p. 1258.

D. True
Ch. 55 The Liver, p. 1258.

E. True Especially if they contain a lot of fat.
Ch. 55 The Liver, p. 1258.

Q 5.16 Regarding focal liver abnormalities

A. Focal confluent fibrosis occurs in established cirrhosis.
B. The segment involved by focal confluent fibrosis is usually atrophic.
C. Focal confluent fibrosis has increased signal on T2-weighted MRI.
D. Atypical regenerative nodules have reduced signal on T2-weighted MRI images.
E. Atypical regenerative nodules have increased signal on T1-weighted MRI images.

Q 5.17 Concerning primary hepatocellular carcinoma

A. It occurs with a normal a-fetoprotein level.
B. Contains areas of fat.
C. Vascular invasion is rare.
D. High-velocity Doppler signal occurs within the lesion.
E. Calcification is more likely to occur in focal nodular hyperplasia than primary hepato-cellular carcinoma.

Q 5.18 Concerning fibrolamellar hepatoma

A. It is predisposed to by chronic hepatitis B infection.
B. It is usually multiple.
C. Calcification is commoner in fibrolamellar hepatoma than primary hepato-cellular carcinoma.
D. There is delayed enhancement of the central scar.
E. Unlike focal nodular hyperplasia, the central scar in fibrolamellar hepatoma has low signal on T1-and T2-weighting.

(Answers overleaf)

A **5.16** **Regarding focal liver abnormalities**

A. **True**
Ch. 55 The Liver, p. 1259

B. **Irue**
Ch. 55 The Liver, p. 1259.

C. **True**
Ch. 55 The Liver, p. 1259.

D. **True** Owing to their iron content.
Ch. 55 The Liver, p. 1259.

E. **True** Owing to fat or glycogen accumulation rather than copper as previously thought.
Ch. 55 The Liver, p. 1259.

A **5.17** **Concerning primary hepatocellular carcinoma**

A. **True**
Ch. 55 The Liver, p. 1260.

B. **True**
Ch. 55 The Liver, p. 1260.

C. **False** It is a typical feature which tends to occur in large lesions causing portal vein invasion and thrombosis.
Ch. 55 The Liver, p. 1260.

D. **True** This occurs in the majority of cases as a result or arterio-portal shunting.
Ch. 55 The Liver, p. 1260.

E. **False**
Ch. 55 The Liver, p. 1261.

A **5.18** **Concerning fibrolamellar hepatoma**

A. **False** It arises spontaneously with no known predisposing factors.
Ch. 55 The Liver, p. 1263.

B. **False**
Ch. 55 The Liver, p. 1263.

C. **True**
Ch. 55 The Liver, p. 1263.

D. **True**
Ch. 55 The Liver, p. 1263.

E. **True**
Ch. 55 The Liver, p. 1263.

Q **5.19** Concerning liver metastases

A. Right colon primary tumours are more likely to metastasize to the right lobe of liver.

B. FDG-PET is useful at detecting metastatic disease in the presence of cirrhosis.

C. On CT the majority of metastases have low attenuation on unenhanced images, which remain so on portal phase images.

D. On MRI the signal of metastases roughly parallels that of the spleen.

E. On colloid radionuclide imaging the majority of metastases appear as areas of increased activity.

Q **5.20** **Metastatic tumours that may demonstrate increased vascularity compared to normal liver parenchyma include**

A. Breast.

B. Cervix.

C. Kidney.

D. Thyroid.

E. Melanoma.

Q **5.21** **Regarding Budd-Chiari syndrome**

A. In Budd-Chiari syndrome the caudate lobe is relatively spared because it drains into IVC above the hepatic venous confluence.

B. Core biopsy is frequently required in Budd-Chiari syndrome.

C. Inability to demonstrate any hepatic venous flow is diagnostic of Budd-Chiari syndrome.

D. On unenhanced CT images the enlarged congested peripheral liver has lower attenuation than normal.

E. The differential diagnosis of Budd-Chiari syndrome on contrast enhanced CT is diffuse tumour invasion.

(Answers overleaf)

A **5.19** **Concerning liver metastases**

A. True This extraordinary finding is evidence of blood flow separation in the portal vein.
Ch. 55 The Liver, p. 1264.

B. False
Ch. 55 The Liver, p. 1264.

C. True
Ch. 55 The Liver, p. 1265.

D. True
Ch. 55 The Liver, p. 1265.

E. False They appear as areas of reduced activity owing to a lack of Kupffer cells.
Ch. 55 The Liver, p. 1265.

A **5.20** **Metastatic tumours that may demonstrate increased vascularity compared to normal liver parenchyma include**

A. True
Ch. 55 The Liver, p. 1264.

B. False
Ch. 55 The Liver, p. 1264.

C. True
Ch. 55 The Liver, p. 1264.

D. True
Ch. 55 The Liver, p. 1264.

E. True
Ch. 55 The Liver, p. 1264.

A **5.21** **Regarding Budd-Chiari syndrome**

A. False It drains into the IVC inferior to the normal hepatic venous confluence.
Ch. 55 The Liver, p. 1265.

B. True
Ch. 55 The Liver, p. 1266.

C. False This finding needs to be interpreted with caution in the presence of cirrhosis.
Ch. 55 The Liver, p. 1266.

D. True Where as the caudate is often preserved with normal attenuation on unenhanced image and a normal enhancement pattern.
Ch. 55 The Liver, p. 1266.

E. True
Ch. 55 The Liver, p. 1266.

Q **5.22** Regarding portal hypertension

A. The absence of splenomegaly does not exclude portal hypertension.

B. A portal vein diameter in excess than 10 mm is highly suggestive of portal venous hypertension.

C. Portal venous flow of less than 10 cm per second on Doppler is likely to reflect significant portal venous hypertension.

D. Gastric and bowel wall oedema is a sign of portal hypertension on CT.

E. The mesenteric veins are distended on Doppler examination.

Q **5.23** Causes of portal venous thrombosis include

A. Acute cholecystitis.

B. Necrotizing enterocolitis.

C. Trauma.

D. Pancreatitis.

E. β-blockers.

Q **5.24** Regarding congenital anomalies of the biliary tree

A. Agenesis of the gallbladder occurs more frequently than double gallbladder.

B. In double gallbladder there are usually 2 cystic ducts.

C. Biliary leaks post cholecystectomy occur when the ducts of Magendie are severed.

D. The gallbladder is intrahepatic in the first month of intra-uterine life.

E. An anomalous cystic duct enters the right posterior sectoral duct more commonly than the segment 5 duct.

(Answers overleaf)

A **5.22**   Regarding portal hypertension

A. True

> *Ch. 55 The Liver, p. 1267.*

B. False   The normal portal vein diameter does not exclude the diagnosis, however, a diameter in excess of 15 mm is highly suggestive of portal venous hypertension.
> *Ch. 55 The Liver, p. 1267.*

C. True

> *Ch. 55 The Liver, p. 1267.*

D. True

> *Ch. 55 The Liver, p. 1267.*

E. True

> *Ch. 55 The Liver, p. 1267.*

A **5.23**   Causes of portal venous thrombosis include

A. True

> *Ch. 55 The Liver, p. 1268.*

B. True

> *Ch. 55 The Liver, p. 1268.*

C. True

> *Ch. 55 The Liver, p. 1268.*

D. True

> *Ch. 55 The Liver, p. 1268.*

E. False

> *Ch. 55 The Liver, p. 1268.*

A **5.24**   Regarding congenital anomalies of the biliary tree

A. False   Absence or agenesis of the gallbladder is extremely rare. It is associated with extra vaginal fistula, imperforate anus and the absence of one or more bones.
> *Ch. 56 The Biliary Tract, p. 1277.*

B. False

> *Ch. 56 The Biliary Tract, p. 1278.*

C. False   Leaks from the ducts of Luschka account for a third of biliary leaks that occur after laproscopic cholecystectomy.
> *Ch. 56 The Biliary Tract, p. 1278.*

D. True

> *Ch. 56 The Biliary Tract, p. 1279.*

E. True

> *Ch. 56 The Biliary Tract, p. 1279.*

Q **5.25**   Concerning hepatobiliary anatomy

A. Separate pancreatic and biliary duct orifices occur in 10% of patients.
B. The superior mesenteric artery gives rise to partial hepatic arterial flow in about 20% of patients.
C. In 25% of individuals a portion of the hepatic arterial supply arises from the left gastric artery.
D. The left portal vein gives rise to a branch which supplies segment 4.
E. Double portal vein is usually caused by fenestration at the confluence of SMV and splenic vein.

Q **5.26**   Causes of acoustic shadowing during gallbladder ultrasound include

A. Pigment calculi.
B. Valves of Houston.
C. Polyps.
D. Biliary sludge.
E. Cholesterol stones.

(Answers overleaf)

177

A **5.25** Concerning hepatobiliary anatomy

A. False From 30 to 40%.
Ch. 56 The Biliary Tract, p. 1280.

B. True
Ch. 56 The Biliary Tract, p. 1280.

C. True
Ch. 56 The Biliary Tract, p. 1280.

D. True If the right portal vein is occluded this recurrent branch may be mistaken for that vessel giving the erroneous impression that the portal system is normal.
Ch. 56 The Biliary Tract, p. 1280.

E. False
Ch. 56 The Biliary Tract, p. 1280.

A **5.26** Causes of acoustic shadowing during gallbladder ultrasound include

A. True
Ch. 56 The Biliary Tract, p. 1284.

B. False The valves of Heister may cause distal acoustic shadowing.
Ch. 56 The Biliary Tract, p. 1284.

C. False
Ch. 56 The Biliary Tract, p. 1284.

D. False Layered bile in which the lower or more dependent layer is diffusely and homogeneous echogenic has been termed biliary sludge. It disappears when the patients who have been fasting resume eating, although in some it is seen to predispose to the development of gallstones in the future. Biliary sludge has been chemically characterized as calcium bilirubinate.
Ch. 56 The Biliary Tract, p. 1284.

E. True
Ch. 56 The Biliary Tract, p. 1284.

Q **5.27** **Regarding biliary imaging**

- **A.** An ejection fraction of 20% is found in a normal gallbladder.
- **B.** The calibre of the right or left hepatic duct is usually 1–3 mm.
- **C.** CT cholangiography is dependent on hepatocellular function whereas magnetic resonance chole-pancreatography is not.
- **D.** During HIDA imaging the patient is in the prone position.
- **E.** During HIDA scanning most gallbladders are visualized within 60 minutes.

Q **5.28** **Causes of non-opacification of the gallbladder during hida scanning include**

- **A.** Acute cholecystitis.
- **B.** The patient has not fasted.
- **C.** Opiates.
- **D.** Alcohol abuse.
- **E.** Phrygian cap deformity.

Q **5.29** **Regarding primary sclerosing cholangitis**

- **A.** It is associated with ulcerative colitis.
- **B.** Scintigraphy with ^{99m}Tc-labelled HIDA reveals multiple focal areas of reduced uptake.
- **C.** The appearance on ERCP is mimicked by biliary cystadenoma.
- **D.** Involvement of the intrahepatic ducts occurs in only 20% of cases.
- **E.** There is an increased risk of bile duct cancer.

(Answers overleaf)

179

A **5.27** Regarding biliary imaging

A. True

Ch. 56 The Biliary Tract, p. 1285.

B. True

Ch. 56 The Biliary Tract, p. 1285.

C. True

Ch. 56 The Biliary Tract, p. 1285.

D. False The patient is supine with the gamma camera in place anteriorly and sequential images are obtained continuously for the first hour at approximately 1-minute intervals.

Ch. 56 The Biliary Tract, p. 1286.

E. True

Ch. 56 The Biliary Tract, p. 1286.

A **5.28** Causes of non-opacification of the gallbladder during HIDA scanning include

A. True

Ch. 56 The Biliary Tract, p. 1286.

B. True

Ch. 56 The Biliary Tract, p. 1286.

C. True

Ch. 56 The Biliary Tract, p. 1286.

D. True

Ch. 56 The Biliary Tract, p. 1286.

E. False

Ch. 56 The Biliary Tract, p. 1286.

A **5.29** Regarding primary sclerosing cholangitis

A. True Although it is an association of ulcerative colitis there is no cause–effect relationship.

Ch. 57 The Liver, Biliary Tract, Pancreas, Endocrine System and Lymphoma, p. 1302.

B. False

Ch. 57 The Liver, Biliary Tract, Pancreas, Endocrine System and Lymphoma, p. 1302.

C. False The diffuse form of cholangiocarcinoma can mimic sclerosing cholangitis.

Ch. 57 The Liver, Biliary Tract, Pancreas, Endocrine System and Lymphoma, p. 1302.

D. False The intrahepatic ducts are nearly always involved.

Ch. 57 The Liver, Biliary Tract, Pancreas, Endocrine System and Lymphoma, p. 1302.

E. True

Ch. 57 The Liver, Biliary Tract, Pancreas, Endocrine System and Lymphoma, p. 1302.

Q 5.30   Regarding the radiology of liver transplantation

A. Portal vein thrombosis is an absolute contraindication to liver transplantation.

B. The commonest vascular complication of liver transplantation is hepatic artery thrombosis.

C. Changes to the biliary tree seen on ERCP after hepatic artery thrombosis simulate sclerosing cholangitis.

D. Hepatic artery stenosis can be treated by angioplasty.

E. Hepatic artery pseudoaneurysms post-transplantation are best treated with embolization.

Q 5.31   Regarding imaging of the pancreas

A. The normal pancreatic duct measures up to 4 mm.

B. Peripancreatic fluid collections resolve spontaneously in more than half of cases.

C. Dilation of peri-pancreatic veins is a sign of vascular invasion by carcinoma.

D. A pancreatic mass comprising multiple small cysts less than 2 cm across is more likely to be benign than malignant.

E. Fluid lying between the splenic vein and main body of pancreas is a sign of post-traumatic pancreatic injury.

(Answers overleaf)

181

A 5.30   Regarding the radiology of liver transplantation

A. False   Portal vein thrombectomy and/or reconstruction can successfully circumvent this problem.
Ch. 57 The Liver, Biliary Tract, Pancreas, Endocrine System and Lymphoma, p. 1304.

B. True   This occurs in approximately 5% of adult transplant patients.
Ch. 57 The Liver, Biliary Tract, Pancreas, Endocrine System and Lymphoma, p. 1307.

C. True   Multiple intrahepatic strictures may develop and are associated with recurrent fever and sepsis.
Ch. 57 The Liver, Biliary Tract, Pancreas, Endocrine System and Lymphoma, p. 1338.

D. True   This may prevent progression to complete hepatic artery occlusion. However, some patients experience ischaemic biliary complication despite successful angioplasty.
Ch. 57 The Liver, Biliary Tract, Pancreas, Endocrine System and Lymphoma, p. 1338.

E. False   These are usually infected and surgical excision and reconstruction are the preferred therapy.
Ch. 57 The Liver, Biliary Tract, Pancreas, Endocrine System and Lymphoma, p. 1338.

A 5.31   Regarding imaging of the pancreas

A. False   Greater than 3 mm is abnormal.
Ch. 59 The Pancreas, p. 1354.

B. True   Fluid collections differ from pseudocysts in that they have no detectable wall or capsule and are confined by the anatomical compartment within which they arise.
Ch. 59 The Pancreas, p. 1358.

C. True   When the superior mesenteric vein is involved by tumour, the peri-pancreatic veins become dilated and more visible on CT.
Ch. 59 The Pancreas, p. 1359.

D. True   Serous cystic tumours are generally benign. They are composed of numerous tiny cysts – more than six in number and less than 2 cm in diameter. Malignancy mucinous cystic neoplasms are more common but associated with larger cysts, fewer in number and amorphous calcification.
Ch. 59 The Pancreas, p. 1360.

E. True   Thickening of the anterior adrenal fascia, fluid in the lesser sac, increased attenuation of peri-pancreatic fat and fluid lying between splenic vein and pancreas are all signs of serious pancreatic injury. The fluid as described may be associated with laceration of the pancreatic duct.
Ch. 59 The Pancreas, p. 1361.

Q 6.1 Concerning radionuclide imaging in the genitourinary tract

A. Divided renal function is measured by calculating ^{99m}Tc-DTPA uptake at 2 minutes.

B. Differential renal blood flow is measured during the first-pass phase of ^{99m}Tc-DTPA.

C. Renovascular hypertension is assessed using the captopril stress test.

D. Vesico-ureteric reflux is measured by instilling ^{99m}Tc-DTPA into the bladder.

E. Residual urine volume is calculated with quantitative bladder emptying following ^{99m}Tc-DTPA administration.

Q 6.2 Regarding dynamic renal imaging

A. ^{99m}Tc-DTPA is handled by glomerular filtration and tubular excretion.

B. ^{99m}Tc-MAG3 is excreted only by glomerular filtration.

C. When a rapid bolus injection of ^{99m}Tc-DTPA is employed this optimizes the measurement of first pass renal blood flow.

D. Intravenous diuretic is administered before ^{99m}Tc-DTPA when investigating outflow obstruction.

E. Vesico-ureteric reflux is associated with a saw-tooth activity pattern in the renal pelvis.

Q 6.3 Regarding static renal radionuclide imaging with ^{99m}tc-dmsa

A. ^{99m}Tc-DMSA is fixed within the kidney parenchyma with no significant excretion.

B. Seven hundred to nine hundred MBq of ^{99m}Tc-DMSA are injected.

C. Obstruction artificially increases apparent functional cortical mass.

D. DMSA is retained mainly in the proximal tubules.

E. Images are normally obtained after 30 minutes.

(Answers overleaf)

A **6.1** Concerning radionuclide imaging in the genitourinary tract

A. True
Ch. 65 Table 65.1, p. 1498.

B. True
Ch. 65 Table 65.1, p. 1498.

C. True
Ch. 65 Table 65.1, p. 1498.

D. False The agent is ^{99m}Tc-pertechnetate. IV ^{99m}Tc-DTPA is used during a dynamic indirect voiding study.
Ch. 65 Radionuclide Imaging in the Genitourinary Tract, p. 1498.

E. True
Ch. 65 Radionuclide Imaging in the Genitourinary Tract, p. 1498.

A **6.2** Regarding dynamic renal imaging

A. False It is handled by glomerular filtration in the same way as inulin.
Ch. 65 Radionuclide Imaging in the Genitourinary Tract, p. 1498

B. False It is exreted by glomerular filtration and tubular excretion and it has the advantage of higher renal concentration than DTPA.
Ch. 65 Radionuclide Imaging in the Genitourinary Tract, p. 1498

C. True
Ch. 65 Radionuclide Imaging in the Genitourinary Tract, p. 1498

D. True IV furosemide (frusemide) has traditionally been injected 20 minutes after the radionuclide, however it has become increasingly popular to inject it before the DTPA in order to obtain high urine flow.
Ch. 65 Radionuclide Imaging in the Genitourinary Tract, p. 1499.

E. True Owing to radionuclide washing up and down the ureter into the renal pelvis.
Ch. 65 Radionuclide Imaging in the Genitourinary Tract, p. 1500.

A **6.3** Regarding static renal radionuclide imaging with ^{99M}tc-dmsa

A. False Approximately 15% is excreted during the first 3 hours.
Ch. 65 Radionuclide Imaging in the Genitourinary Tract, p. 1501.

B. False Approximately 80 MBq.
Ch. 65 Radionuclide Imaging in the Genitourinary Tract, p. 1501.

C. True Because the excreted 15% may stay within the upper collecting system.
Ch. 65 Radionuclide Imaging in the Genitourinary Tract, p. 1501.

D. True
Ch. 65 Radionuclide Imaging in the Genitourinary Tract, p. 1501.

E. False After 3 hours.
Ch. 65 Radionuclide Imaging in the Genitourinary Tract, p. 1501.

Q **6.4** **Concerning renovascular disease**

A. Selective renal arteriography requires pump injection of contrast medium for adequate opacification.
B. Fibromuscular dysplasia most commonly affects the renal ostium.
C. CT angiography is less nephrotoxic than selective renal angiography.
D. During time of flight MR angiography thrombus mimics flowing blood.
E. Gadolinium DTPA injection doubles the signal to noise ration in distal renal arteries.

Q **6.5** **Concerning renal angiography**

A. IVU and renal arteriography are mandatory prior to live renal donation.
B. Single renal artery aneurysms are usually atheromatous.
C. Arteriovenous fistula after renal core biopsy is best treated by embolization with polyvinyl alcohol particles.
D. Renal arteries may arise from the iliac arteries.
E. Multiple renal arteries are associated with ectopic kidney.

Q **6.6** **Renal artery aneurysms are associated with**

A. Polyarteritis nodosa.
B. Gouty nephropathy.
C. Goodpasture's syndrome.
D. Neurofibromatosis.
E. Fibromuscular dysplasia.

(Answers overleaf)

A **6.4** Concerning renovascular disease

A. False Hand injections are adequate.
Ch. 67 Renovascular Disease, p. 1514.

B. False
Ch. 67 Renovascular Disease, p. 1514.

C. False The amount of contrast medium used is much greater using the CT technique, however, selective renal angiography has a risk of arterial damage and subsequent renal impairment.
Ch. 67 Renovascular Disease, p. 1514.

D. True High signal from thrombus may mimic flowing blood
Ch. 67 Renovascular Disease, p. 1515.

E. True
Ch. 67 Renovascular Disease, p. 1515.

A **6.5** Concerning renal angiography

A. False Spiral CT and MRA are adequate in this regard.
Ch. 67 Renovascular Disease, p. 1517.

B. True
Ch. 67 Renovascular Disease, p. 1519.

C. False Coils are the embolic material of choice for preserving the greatest amount of renal parenchyma.
Ch. 67 Renovascular Disease, p. 1520.

D. True
Ch. 67 Renovascular Disease, p. 1517.

E. True
Ch. 67 Renovascular Disease, p. 1517.

A **6.6** Renal artery aneurysms are associated with

A. True
Ch. 67 Renovascular Disease, p. 1519.

B. False
Ch. 67 Renovascular Disease, p. 1519.

C. False
Ch. 67 Renovascular Disease, p. 1519.

D. True
Ch. 67 Renovascular Disease, p. 1519.

E. True
Ch. 67 Renovascular Disease, p. 1519.

Q **6.7**   **Spontaneous renal haemorrhage is associated with**

    A. Polyarteritis nodosa.
    B. Simple cortical cysts.
    C. Angiomyolipoma.
    D. Renal cell carcinoma.
    E. Xanthogranulomatous pyelonephritis.

Q **6.8**   **Regarding renovascular pathology**

    A. The cortical rim sign occurs when the renal artery is occluded.
    B. The presence of central medullary enhancement rules out a diagnosis of renal artery occlusion.
    C. Renal vein thrombosis is associated with membranous glomerulonephritis.
    D. An increasingly dense nephrogram at IVU occurs in renal vein thrombosis.
    E. Curvilinear calcification is associated with chronic renal vein thrombosis.

Q **6.9**   **Concerning renal artery stenosis**

    A. It is suspected if there is sudden onset hypertension.
    B. Stenosis is more likely to progress to occlusion in children.
    C. Medial fibroplasia responds better to angioplasty than subadventitial fibroplasia.
    D. Post-stenotic dilation is a good indicator of the severity of the stenosis.
    E. Involvement of distal renal arterial branches by atheroma is associated with improved outcome after angioplasty.

(Answers overleaf)

A **6.7** Spontaneous renal haemorrhage is associated with

A. True   Intrarenal aneurysms in this condition bleed rarely
Ch. 67 Renovascular Disease, p. 1518.

B. True   Spontaneous haemorrhage is not uncommon. After the haematoma resolves follow-up CT is required to ensure that there is no aggressive underlying cause.
Ch. 67 Renovascular Disease, p. 1520.

C. True   Especially if larger than 4 cm. Pregnancy is a risk factor.
Ch. 67 Renovascular Disease, p. 1518.

D. True
Ch. 67 Renovascular Disease, p. 1520.

E. False
Ch. 67 Renovascular Disease, p. 1520.

A **6.8** Regarding renovascular pathology

A. True   Owing to enhancement via cortical collaterals.
Ch. 67 Renovascular Disease, p. 1523.

B. False   Central medullary enhancement may occur when the renal artery is occluded because cortical or ureteric collaterals may supply blood to the medulla.
Ch. 67 Renovascular Disease, p. 1523.

C. True
Ch. 67 Renovascular Disease, p. 1523.

D. True   More commonly a faint or absent nephrogram occurs in renal vein thrombosis.
Ch. 67 Renovascular Disease, p. 1523.

E. True
Ch. 67 Renovascular Disease, p. 1524.

A **6.9** Concerning renal artery stenosis

A. True
Ch. 67 Renovascular Disease, p. 1524.

B. False   Atheromatous renal artery stenosis in adults is much more likely to be progressive than the non-atheromatous type in children.
Ch. 67 Renovascular Disease, p. 1524.

C. True   The medial fibroplasia subtype of fibromuscular dysplasia dilates easily at lower pressures and there are excellent long-term results.
Ch. 67 Renovascular Disease, p. 1525.

D. False
Ch. 67 Renovascular Disease, p. 1525.

E. False
Ch. 67 Renovascular Disease, p. 1525.

Q 6.10   Regarding middle aortic syndrome

A.   It is associated with dextrocardia.
B.   An abdominal bruit may be audible.
C.   The angiographic findings are similar to Takaysu's disease.
D.   There is an association with William's syndrome.
E.   Neurofibromatosis may result in a middle aortic syndrome.

Q 6.11   Features suggesting the presence of significant renal artery stenosis include

A.   Peak systolic velocity in renal artery of more than 100 cm per second.
B.   Renal artery to aorta velocity ration of 0.35.
C.   Prolonged intrarenal parenchymal transit time on ACE inhibitor radionuclide renography.
D.   Failure to identify intrarenal branches on contrast-enhanced MRA.
E.   Elevated ipsilateral renal vein renin level.

Q 6.12   Regarding excretion urography (IVU)

A.   A faint nephrogram 6 hours after injection of contrast medium may be seen in normal patients.
B.   Kidney length is normally greater than four and a half lumbar vertebrae and their intervening disc spaces.
C.   The left kidney is normally longer than the right by up to 2 cm.
D.   Compound calices occur most commonly around the middle of the kidney.
E.   Narrowing of an upper pole infundibulum by vascular impression may be associated with dilation of the calyx.

(Answers overleaf)

A **6.10** **Regarding middle aortic syndrome**

A. False

Ch. 67 Renovascular Disease, p. 1527.

B. True Owing to abdominal aortic coarctation or other visceral arterial stenosis.
Ch. 67 Renovascular Disease, p. 1527.

C. True It has been suggested that middle aortic syndrome and inactive Takayasu's aortoarteritis are indistinguishable entities.
Ch. 67 Renovascular Disease, p. 1527.

D. True

Ch. 67 Renovascular Disease, p. 1527.

E. True In this condition renal artery stenosis and abdominal aortic stenosis may co-exist.
Ch. 67 Renovascular Disease, p. 1527.

A **6.11** **Features suggesting the presence of significant renal artery stenosis include**

A. True

Ch. 67 Renovascular Disease, p. 1527.

B. False Three and a half or greater.
Ch. 67 Renovascular Disease, p. 1527.

C. True

Ch. 67 Renovascular Disease, p. 1527.

D. False

Ch. 67 Renovascular Disease, p. 1529.

E. True This is a good predictor of successful blood pressure response to angioplasty in hypertension.
Ch. 67 Renovascular Disease, p. 1532.

A **6.12** **Regarding excretion urography (IVU)**

A. True Faint opacification in normal patients may be seen even at 24 hours
Ch. 68 Renal Parenchymal Disease, p. 1538.

B. False Three and a half vertebrae and intervening disc spaces.
Ch. 68 Renal Parenchymal Disease, p. 1539.

C. True

Ch. 68 Renal Parenchymal Disease, p. 1539.

D. False These are commonest at the poles.
Ch. 68 Renal Parenchymal Disease, p. 1539.

E. True This simulates obstruction.
Ch. 68 Renal Parenchymal Disease, p. 1539.

Q **6.13**　**Radiological features supporting a diagnosis of glomerulonephritis include**

    A.　Four centimetre difference in renal length.
    B.　Rim calcification on plain radiography.
    C.　Bilateral renal enlargement on ultrasound.
    D.　Changes of papillary necrosis on IVU.
    E.　Delayed persistent nephrogram on IVU.

Q **6.14**　**Causes of renal enlargement on ultrasound**

    A.　Renal vein thrombosis.
    B.　Leukaemia.
    C.　Multiple myeloma.
    D.　Primary amyloidosis.
    E.　Acute papillary necrosis.

(Answers overleaf)

A **6.13** **Radiological features supporting a diagnosis of glomerulonephritis include**

A. **False** Glomerulonephritis is a bilateral, symmetrical nephropathy.
Ch. 68 Renal Parenchymal Disease, p. 1543.

B. **False**
Ch. 68 Renal Parenchymal Disease, p. 1543.

C. **True**
Ch. 68 Renal Parenchymal Disease, p. 1543.

D. **False**
Ch. 68 Renal Parenchymal Disease, p. 1542.

E. **True**
Ch. 68 Renal Parenchymal Disease, p. 1543.

A **6.14** **Causes of renal enlargement on ultrasound**

A. **True**
Ch. 68 Renal Parenchymal Disease, p. 1544.

B. **True** Non-Hodgkin's lymphoma also.
Ch. 68 Renal Parenchymal Disease, p. 1544.

C. **True** Owing to amyloid deposition.
Ch. 68 Renal Parenchymal Disease, p. 1544.

D. **True** In 30% of cases or primary amyloidosis the kidneys are involved leading to renal enlargement and stretching of the calices.
Ch. 68 Renal Parenchymal Disease, p. 1544.

E. **True**
Ch. 68 Renal Parenchymal Disease, p. 1544.

Q 6.15   Concerning papillary necrosis

A. It is associated with sickle cell trait.
B. Presents with haematuria and renal colic.
C. Raised white cell count in the urine suggests an alternative diagnosis.
D. There is usually symmetrical involvement of the kidneys.
E. Rapid deterioration in renal function is a complication.

Q 6.16   Regarding renal tuberculosis

A. Bilateral abnormalities are usually seen on IVU.
B. Ulceration of renal papillae occurs late.
C. Calcification occurs within caseous pyelonephritis.
D. Renal cavitation may simulate hydronephrosis.
E. Vesico-ureteric reflux is an association.

(Answers overleaf)

A **6.15**   Concerning papillary necrosis

A. True   In one study 50% of parents with sickle cell trait had minor changes on excretion urography.
Ch. 68 Renal Parenchymal Disease, p. 1544.

B. True   Owing to obstruction of the ureter by a sloughed papilla.
Ch. 68 Renal Parenchymal Disease, p. 1544.

C. False   Sterile pyuria is a well-recognized feature.
Ch. 68 Renal Parenchymal Disease, p. 1544.

D. True   Asymmetry suggests co-existent obstruction, chronic infection or even renal artery stenosis.
Ch. 68 Renal Parenchymal Disease, p. 1545.

E. True   The combination of infection and obstruction in a diabetic patient can lead to papillary necrosis with rapid destruction of renal substance.
Ch. 68 Renal Parenchymal Disease, p. 1546.

A **6.16**   Regarding renal tuberculosis

A. False   It is usually radiologically unilateral, and asymmetrical when bilateral.
Ch. 68 Renal Parenchymal Disease, p. 1548.

B. False   This is one of the earliest signs. TB should always be considered in the differential diagnosis of papillary necrosis.
Ch. 68 Renal Parenchymal Disease, p. 1547.

C. True   This has a characteristic cloudy appearance that progresses to produce homogeneous collecting system calcification. Eventually a lobulated calcified mass is seen: 'Tuberculous autonephrectomy'.
Ch. 68 Renal Parenchymal Disease, p. 1548.

D. True   Absence of infundibular and pelvic dilation are clues to the presence of cavitation as opposed to hydronephrosis.
Ch. 68 Renal Parenchymal Disease, p. 1549.

E. True   In chronic TB affecting bladder and ureter, bladder function is altered and there is free reflux back through the VUJ into a dilated, fixed upper tract.
Ch. 68 Renal Parenchymal Disease, p. 1549.

Q **6.17**   Regarding tuberculosis of the urinary tract

    A. Renal calcification occurs in 90% or cases.

    B. Ureteric calcification does not occur.

    C. Calcification in the vas deferens looks similar to the pattern seen in diabetes.

    D. Hydrocalicosis is a feature.

    E. Concentration of contrast medium by an affected kidney is often poor relative to the degree of obstruction.

Q **6.18**   Concerning infection in the urinary tract

    A. Involvement of the bladder in schistosomiasis leads to rigid non-function in the majority of cases.

    B. Schistosomiasis causes fibrotic strictures of the bladder neck and ureters.

    C. Gas in the renal collecting system and bladder occurs with infection by *Candidia albicans*.

    D. *Proteus mirabilis* infection is associated with the development of xanthogranulomatous pyelonephritis.

    E. Gas within the renal parenchyma caused by infection indicates a worse prognosis than gas within the pelvi-calyceal system.

(Answers overleaf)

A **6.17** **Regarding tuberculosis of the urinary tract**

A. False About 30%.
Ch. 68 Renal Parenchymal Disease, p. 1548.

B. False This is the second commonest site of calcification.
Ch. 68 Renal Parenchymal Disease, p. 1548.

C. False In TB calcification of the vas deferens has a chunky beaded appearance unlike the fine tramline pattern seen in diabetes.
Ch. 68 Renal Parenchymal Disease, p. 1549.

D. True Caused by infundibular stricture.
Ch. 68 Renal Parenchymal Disease, p. 1549.

E. True
Ch. 68 Renal Parenchymal Disease, p. 1549.

A **6.18** **Concerning infection in the urinary tract**

A. False The calcification is submucosal and a heavily calcified bladder may empty normally.
Ch. 68 Renal Parenchymal Disease, p. 1551.

B. True This leads to hydronephrosis.
Ch. 68 Renal Parenchymal Disease, p. 1551.

C. True This is a gas-forming organism.
Ch. 68 Renal Parenchymal Disease, p. 1551.

D. True Usually in the presence of calculi.
Ch. 68 Renal Parenchymal Disease, p. 1551.

E. True Emphysematous pyelonephritis is often fatal.
Ch. 68 Renal Parenchymal Disease, p. 1552.

Q **6.19**   **Filling defects within the renal collecting system are caused by**

   A.   Schistosomiasis.
   B.   *Candida albicans* infection.
   C.   Cholesteatoma.
   D.   *E. coli* infection.
   E.   Pyeloureteritis cystica.

Q **6.20**   **Regarding cystic renal masses**

   A.   Peripelvic cysts are lymphatic in origin.
   B.   Congenital multi-cystic renal dysplasia enlarges progressively into adulthood.
   C.   Wilm's tumour may develop within the wall of a cystic partially differentiated nephroblastoma.
   D.   Renal hydatid cysts rupture into the collecting system.
   E.   Most patients with adult polycystic kidney disease have a berry aneurysm demonstrable at angiography or autopsy.

(Answers overleaf)

A **6.19**   **Filling defects within the renal collecting system are caused by**

A. True   Owing to oedema or polypoid granulomas seen in the renal pelvis or bladder.
Ch. 68 Renal Parenchymal Disease, p. 1551.

B. True   A shaggy fungus ball may be seen in the renal pelvis or bladder.
Ch. 68 Renal Parenchymal Disease, p. 1551.

C. True   This is a mass of desquamated keratin, which lies free in the lumen of the collecting system. A whorled pattern on IVU is typical.
Ch. 68 Renal Parenchymal Disease, p. 1553.

D. True   Malacoplakia is a rare granulomatous response to infection with this organism which results in multiple small filling defects in renal pelvis and ureter.
Ch. 68 Renal Parenchymal Disease, p. 1553.

E. True   This is considered to be associated with infection and the differential includes papillomas, calculi and multiple vascular impressions.
Ch. 68 Renal Parenchymal Disease, p. 1553.

A **6.20**   **Regarding cystic renal masses**

A. True
Ch. 69 Renal Masses, p. 1561.

B. False   Spontaneous reduction in size occurs and this condition is undetectable with ultrasound in the adult.
Ch. 69 Renal Masses, p. 1562.

C. True
Ch. 69 Renal Masses, p. 1562.

D. True   This gives rise to acute flank pain, voiding of scolices in the urine and possibly haematuria.
Ch. 69 Renal Masses, p. 1562.

E. False   Up to 40% at angiography, much less at autopsy.
Ch. 69 Renal Masses, p. 1562.

Q **6.21** **Concerning inflammatory disease in the renal tract**

    A. Infection in the perinephric space is more often a consequence of a ruptured hydronephrosis than ruptured renal abscess.

    B. Acute focal pyelonephritis causes a hyporeflective mass on ultrasound.

    C. Focal pyelonephritis is associated with areas of increased density on CT.

    D. Xanthogranulomatous pyelonephritis differs from actinomycetes infection in that it does not cause sinus tracks to the skin.

    E. The bladder is more frequently involved by malacoplakia than the kidneys.

Q **6.22** **Regarding renal masses**

    A. Pulmonary involvement by malacoplakia simulates metastases from renal carcinoma.

    B. Angiomyolipomas are distinguished from renal carcinomas by the presence of hyper-reflectivity on ultrasound.

    C. Renal sinus lipomatosis is associated with calculi in most cases.

    D. Oncocytomas metastasize.

    E. Rim and spoke-wheel appearance on angiography is pathognomonic of oncocytoma.

Q **6.23** **Concerning renal cancer**

    A. Most patient with Von-Hippel Lindau syndrome eventually develop renal cell carcinoma.

    B. Perinephric stranding on CT implies tumour extension outside the kidney.

    C. Enhancement of thrombus within renal vein is diagnostic of tumour thrombus.

    D. The sensitivity of CT staging is higher for stage III than stage IV disease.

    E. Wilm's tumour usually presents in adolescence.

(Answers overleaf)

A **6.21** Concerning inflammatory disease in the renal tract

A. **True**
Ch. 69 Renal Masses, p. 1562.

B. **True**
Ch. 69 Renal Masses, p. 1563.

C. **True** Owing to focal haemorrhage.
Ch. 69 Renal Masses, p. 1563.

D. **False** Both conditions are associated with sinuses to skin.
Ch. 69 Renal Masses, p. 1563.

E. **True**
Ch. 69 Renal Masses, p. 1563.

A **6.22** Regarding renal masses

A. **True**
Ch. 69 Renal Masses, p. 1564.

B. **False** A significant proportion of renal cell carcinomas are hyper-reflective on ultrasound.
Ch. 69 Renal Masses, p. 1565.

C. **False** It is an overbalance of renal sinus fat unassociated with calculus or inflammatory disease.
Ch. 69 Renal Masses, p. 1566.

D. **True**
Ch. 69 Renal Masses, p. 1566.

E. **False**
Ch. 69 Renal Masses, p. 1566.

A **6.23** Concerning renal cancer

A. **False** About one-third develop renal cell carcinoma.
Ch. 69 Renal Masses, p. 1567.

B. **False** Oedema, fibrosis and vascular engorgement can all cause this sign.
Ch. 69 Renal Masses, p. 1570.

C. **True**
Ch. 69 Renal Masses, p. 1570.

D. **False** Stage III disease includes renal vein, nodal and local vessel involvement. Sensitivity of disease spread is higher for spread to adjacent organs outside Gerota's fascia and distant metastases.
Ch. 69 Renal Masses, p. 1570.

E. **False** Most present before 7 years of age

Ch. 69 Renal Masses, p. 1570.

Q **6.24**   Regarding Wilm's tumour

A.   Histologically this is an oncocytoma.
B.   The majority of Wilm's tumours have calcification visible on CT.
C.   Fifty per cent are bilateral.
D.   Tumour invasion and obstruction of the renal vein is a recognized finding.
E.   Large focal hypoechoic area on ultrasound are seen.

Q **6.25**   Concerning renal neoplasms

A.   Renal sarcomas present with abdominal pain.
B.   Primary renal lymphoma and secondary lymphoma involving the kidneys are equally common.
C.   Secondary renal lymphoma usually shows as a focal mass on IVU.
D.   Renal lymphoma is usually hyperechoic on ultrasound.
E.   Metastases to the kidney almost always have an exophytic appearance.

(Answers overleaf)

A **6.24**   **Regarding Wilm's tumour**

A. False   It is a nephroblastoma, which is very occasionally seen in adults with identical histology but poorer prognosis.
Ch. 69 Renal Masses, p. 1571.

B. False   Up to 10% on plain radiograph and a little more commonly on CT.
Ch. 69 Renal Masses, p. 1571.

C. False   Up to 10%.
Ch. 69 Renal Masses, p. 1571.

D. True
Ch. 69 Renal Masses, p. 1572.

E. True   These may increase in size indicating necrosis and/or haemorrhage and as a result of treatment with chemotherapy/radiotherapy.
Ch. 69 Renal Masses, p. 1571.

A **6.25**   **Concerning renal neoplasms**

A. True   These present late as a large mass and metastases are common at the time of diagnosis.
Ch. 69 Renal Masses, p. 1572.

B. False   Primary renal lymphoma is very rare as there is no lymphatic tissue within the kidneys. Secondary involvement is usually haematogenous but contiguous involvement from retroperitoneal lymphadenopathy may occur.
Ch. 69 Renal Masses, p. 1572.

C. False   The appearance on IVU is usually that of diffuse renal enlargement rather than single or multiple masses.
Ch. 69 Renal Masses, p. 1572.

D. False   It is usually hypoechoic or even anechoic with no distal acoustic enhancement.
Ch. 69 Renal Masses, p. 1572.

E. False   An exophytic renal neoplasm is more likely to be a primary than a secondary tumour. The latter are more infiltrative in appearance.
Ch. 69 Renal Masses, p. 1572.

Q **6.26** Concerning renal urothelial tumours

A. Transitional cell carcinoma of the renal pelvis usually presents as a palpable abdominal mass.

B. Most urothelial tumours present as an infiltrative mass rather than a filling defect in the pelvi-calyceal system.

C. Urothelial tumours are usually hypoechoic on ultrasound

D. Transitional cell carcinoma invades the renal vein in 30–40% of cases.

E. Squamous cell carcinoma is associated with renal calculi.

Q **6.27** Risk factors for the development of urinary calculi include

A. Excessive tea drinking.

B. Elevated urinary pH.

C. High consumption of cocoa.

D. High consumption of peanuts.

E. Low urine volumes.

(Answers overleaf)

A **6.26** **Concerning renal urothelial tumours**

A. False Most present with haematuria before a palpable mass is present.
Ch. 69 Renal Masses, p. 1573.

B. False
Ch. 69 Renal Masses, p. 1573.

C. True
Ch. 69 Renal Masses, p. 1573.

D. False This is rare with transitional cell tumours.
Ch. 69 Renal Masses, p. 1573.

E. True Stones are present in 57% of patients with this aggressive tumour.
Ch. 69 Renal Masses, p. 1573.

A **6.27** **Risk factors for the development of urinary calculi include**

A. True Tea has a high oxalate content.
Ch. 70 Calculus Disease and Urothelial Lesions, p. 1578.

B. True
Ch. 70 Calculus Disease and Urothelial Lesions, p. 1578.

C. True Chocolate addiction leads to high oxalate intake from cocoa as well as increased calcium intake from its milk content.
Ch. 70 Calculus Disease and Urothelial Lesions, p. 1578.

D. True Peanuts, rhubarb and spinach lead to high urinary oxalate levels.
Ch. 70 Calculus Disease and Urothelial Lesions, p. 1578.

E. True Concentrated urine predisposes to crystalluria and stone formation.
Ch. 70 Calculus Disease and Urothelial Lesions, p. 1578.

Q **6.28**   Concerning urinary calculi and infection

A. Fewer than 5% of UK stones are infective in origin.

B. Infection causes a rise in urinary citrate, which predisposes to stones.

C. Urease is produced by *Escherichia coli*.

D. Most staghorn calculi are infection stones.

F The recurrence rate of staghorn calculi after complete clearance at open surgery is less than 5%.

Q **6.29**   Anatomical factors predisposing to renal calculi include

A. Horseshoe kidney.

B. Caliceal cysts.

C. Medullary sponge kidney.

D. Tall stature.

E. Ureterocele.

(Answers overleaf)

A **6.28**   Concerning urinary calculi and infection

A. **False**   One UK study of 1000 stones found evidence of an infective aetiology in nearly 30% using quantitative analysis for the detection of magnesium ammonium phosphate – a crystal formed when infection is present.
Ch. 70 Calculus Disease and Urothelial Lesions, p. 1578.

B. **False**   The urinary citrate is reduced by infection. This reduces the solubility of calcium salts predisposing to stones.
Ch. 70 Calculus Disease and Urothelial Lesions, p. 1578.

C. **True**   Proteus, E. coli, Klebsiella and some pseudomonas produce urease. Magnesium ammonium phosphate (struvite or triple phosphate) stones are formed by splitting urea.
Ch. 70 Calculus Disease and Urothelial Lesions, p. 1578.

D. **True**   They may start with a glycoprotein matrix, upon which triple phosphate deposition occurs.
Ch. 70 Calculus Disease and Urothelial Lesions, p. 1579.

E. **False**   It may be a high as 30%.
Ch. 70 Calculus Disease and Urothelial Lesions, p. 1579.

A **6.29**   Anatomical factors predisposing to renal calculi include

A. **True**
Ch. 70 Calculus Disease and Urothelial Lesions, p. 1579.

B. **True**
Ch. 70 Calculus Disease and Urothelial Lesions, p. 1579.

C. **True**
Ch. 70 Calculus Disease and Urothelial Lesions, p. 1579.

D. **False**
Ch. 70 Calculus Disease and Urothelial Lesions, p. 1579.

E. **True**
Ch. 70 Calculus Disease and Urothelial Lesions, p. 1579.

Q **6.30** **Regarding the appearance of urinary calculi on plain abdominal radiographs**

    A. Oxalate stones are usually denser than adjacent transverse processes.
    B. Cystine stones are usually less dense than adjacent transverse processes.
    C. Ring calcification is seen in sloughed papillae.
    D. Pure uric acid calculi are radiolucent
    E. A high kV technique optimizes detection of urinary calculi.

Q **6.31** **Concerning the detection of urinary calculi**

    A. The IVU control film need extend down only as far as the ischial tuberocities.
    B. CT demonstrates uric acid calculi as areas of marked hyperdensity.
    C. Contrast-enhanced helical CT is now preferable to IVU for the detection of ureteric calculi.
    D. Ureteric obstruction by calculus requires tomography for adequate evaluation during an intravenous urogram.
    E. Perirenal streaking persists on CT after the calculus has passed.

Q **6.32** **Regarding nephrocalcinosis**

    A. Cortical calcification may occur in nephrotic syndrome induced by glomerlonephritis.
    B. Nephrocalcinosis is associated with secondary hyperparathyroidism.
    C. The pattern of renal calcification in renal tubular acidosis can be reliably distinguished form that caused by hyperparathyroidism.
    D. Hyperoxaluria secondary to bowel disorders does not cause nephrocalcinosis.
    E. Hemi-hypertrophy is an association.

(Answers overleaf)

A **6.30** **Regarding the appearance of urinary calculi on plain abdominal radiographs**

A. True

Ch. 70 Calculus Disease and Urothelial Lesions, p. 1580.

B. True

Ch. 70 Calculus Disease and Urothelial Lesions, p. 1580.

C. True

Ch. 70 Calculus Disease and Urothelial Lesions, p. 1580.

D. True

Ch. 70 Calculus Disease and Urothelial Lesions, p. 1580.

E. False

Ch. 70 Calculus Disease and Urothelial Lesions, p. 1580.

A **6.31** **Concerning the detection of urinary calculi**

A. False Bladder calculi will be missed if it doesn't extend down as far as the symphysis pubis.
Ch. 70 Calculus Disease and Urothelial Lesions, p. 1581.

B. True

Ch. 70 Calculus Disease and Urothelial Lesions, p. 1581.

C. False Non-contrast CT is useful in the emergency setting.
Ch. 70 Calculus Disease and Urothelial Lesions, p. 1581.

D. False A limited IVU comprising control and full-length 15-minute image is adequate in this clinical setting.
Ch. 70 Calculus Disease and Urothelial Lesions, p. 1581.

E. True

Ch. 70 Calculus Disease and Urothelial Lesions, p. 1581.

A **6.32** **Regarding nephrocalcinosis**

A. True

Ch. 70 Calculus Disease and Urothelial Lesions, p. 1582.

B. True

Ch. 70 Calculus Disease and Urothelial Lesions, p. 1583.

C. False No pattern of calcification is diagnostic.
Ch. 70 Calculus Disease and Urothelial Lesions, p. 1582.

D. False Both primary and secondary hyperoxaluria are associated with nephrocalcinosis.
Ch. 70 Calculus Disease and Urothelial Lesions, p. 1583.

E. True Medullary sponge kidney is associated with hemi-hypertrophy.
Ch. 70 Calculus Disease and Urothelial Lesions, p. 1584.

Q **6.33** **Focal renal calcificaion on plain radiography is associated with**

    A. Small-bowel resection.
    B. Renal-artery aneurysm.
    C. Squamous-cell carcinoma of the renal pelvis.
    D. Schistosomiasis.
    E. Histiocytosis X.

Q **6.34** **Concerning extrarenal urothelial neoplasms**

    A. There is an increased risk of bladder cancer in hairdressers.
    B. Schistosomiasis is particularly associated with squamous carcinoma of the bladder.
    C. There is an association with Balkan nephropathy.
    D. Fifty per cent of patients with a renal pelvic tumour will develop a bladder tumour within 15 months.
    E. The commonest bladder carcinoma is papillary carcinoma.

(Answers overleaf)

A **6.33**   **Focal renal calcificaion on plain radiography is associated with**

A. True   If this is extensive it is associated with excessive oxalate absorption and
hyperoxaluria.
Ch. 70 Calculus Disease and Urothelial Lesions, p. 1584.

B. True   This may affect hilar or intrarenal branches and demonstrate rim calcification.
Ch. 70 Calculus Disease and Urothelial Lesions, p. 1584.

C. True
Ch. 70 Calculus Disease and Urothelial Lesions, p. 1584.

D. True   Very rarely submucosal pelvicaliceal calcification is seen. More commonly,
stones are associated.
Ch. 70 Calculus Disease and Urothelial Lesions, p. 1584.

E. False
Ch. 70 Calculus Disease and Urothelial Lesions, p. 1584.

A **6.34**   **Concerning extrarenal urothelial neoplasms**

A. True   Printers, tailors, leather workers and those involved in rubber and the chemical
dye industry are at an increased risk of bladder cancer.
Ch. 70 Calculus Disease and Urothelial Lesions, p. 1585.

B. True
Ch. 70 Calculus Disease and Urothelial Lesions, p. 1586.

C. True   Ninety per cent of the associated papillary tumours seen in this condition affect
the upper tracts.
Ch. 70 Calculus Disease and Urothelial Lesions, p. 1586.

D. True
Ch. 70 Calculus Disease and Urothelial Lesions, p. 1586.

E. True   This accounts for nearly 80% of transitional cell tumours of the bladder.
Ch. 70 Calculus Disease and Urothelial Lesions, p. 1586.

Q **6.35** **Concerning urothelial cancer**

    A. Ten per cent of bladder tumours present only with urgency or frequency.
    B. Papillary bladder tumours are less invasive than squamous-cell tumours.
    C. Co-existent bladder and upper-tract tumours are very rare (less than 0.1%).
    D. A single retrograde image taken during surgery is sufficient to rule out a tumour in 95% of cases.
    E. Crossed calices simulate a renal pelvis filling defect.

Q **6.36** **Transitional cell carcinoma of the pelvi-ureteric system is simulated by**

    A. Tuberculosis.
    B. Pyeloureteritis cystica.
    C. Cholesteatoma.
    D. Vascular impression.
    E. Uric-acid calculi.

(Answers overleaf)

A **6.35** **Concerning urothelial cancer**

A. True
Ch. 70 Calculus Disease and Urothelial Lesions, p. 1586.

B. True
Ch. 70 Calculus Disease and Urothelial Lesions, p. 1587.

C. False Synchronous tumours are not rare hence the need for meticulous upper-tract assessment in all patients with bladder cancer. IVU is mandatory and some will require retrograde pyelography for adequate assessment.
Ch. 70 Calculus Disease and Urothelial Lesions, p. 1588.

D. False Retrograde urography needs to be done in the radiology department employing meticulous technique. This includes oblique views and images taken as the catheter is being withdrawn.
Ch. 70 Calculus Disease and Urothelial Lesions, p. 1588.

E. True
Ch. 70 Calculus Disease and Urothelial Lesions, p. 1589.

A **6.36** **Transitional cell carcinoma of the pelvi-ureteric system is simulated by**

A. True
Ch. 70 Calculus Disease and Urothelial Lesions, p. 1589.

B. True
Ch. 70 Calculus Disease and Urothelial Lesions, p. 1589.

C. True
Ch. 70 Calculus Disease and Urothelial Lesions, p. 1589.

D. True Usually eliminated by prone, oblique or compression images.
Ch. 70 Calculus Disease and Urothelial Lesions, p. 1589.

E. True These can be identified on ultrasound and/or CT.
Ch. 70 Calculus Disease and Urothelial Lesions, p. 1589.

Q **6.37**   **Causes of functional obstruction in the absence of demonstrable anatomical narrowing include**

    A. Detrusor – bladder-neck dyssynergia.
    B. Pyelonephritis cystica.
    C. Primary megaureter.
    D. Pelviureteric junction obstruction.
    E. Detrusor – external sphincter dyssynergia.

Q **6.38**   **Regarding hydronephrosis**

    A. The pathological definition requires back-pressure changes in the renal parenchyma to be present.
    B. The presence of hydronephrosis is conclusive proof of obstruction.
    C. Mild hydronephrosis proves that the degree of obstruction is mild.
    D. The absence of hydronephrosis is a reliable indicator that obstruction is not present.
    E. Abdominal compression during IVU simulates hydronephrosis.

Q **6.39**   **Concerning the physiology of urinary obstruction**

    A. Renal pelvic pressure is normally between 20 and 30 mm Hg.
    B. Pressures within the ureter are generally higher than in the renal pelvis.
    C. When obstruction is present pressure in the renal pelvis may reach 70 mm Hg.
    D. There is an increase in renal blood flow when obstruction is present.
    E. Pressure inside the renal pelvis returns to normal when chronic obstruction is present.

(Answers overleaf)

A **6.37** **Causes of functional obstruction in the absence of demonstrable anatomical narrowing include**

A. True
Ch. 71 Urinary Obstruction, p. 1594.

B. False
Ch. 71 Urinary Obstruction, p. 1594.

C. True
Ch. 71 Urinary Obstruction, p. 1594.

D. True
Ch. 71 Urinary Obstruction, p. 1594.

E. True
Ch. 71 Urinary Obstruction, p. 1594.

A **6.38** **Regarding hydronephrosis**

A. True
Ch. 71 Urinary Obstruction, p. 1594.

B. False Vesico-ureteric reflux may cause severe hydronephrosis in the absence of obstruction.
Ch. 71 Urinary Obstruction, p. 1594.

C. False
Ch. 71 Urinary Obstruction, p. 1594.

D. False
Ch. 71 Urinary Obstruction, p. 1594.

E. True This manoeuvre often causes mild calyceal blunting, which is the earliest change seen in hydronephrosis.
Ch. 71 Urinary Obstruction, p. 1594.

A **6.39** **Concerning the physiology of urinary obstruction**

A. False Normally below 12 mm Hg.
Ch. 71 Urinary Obstruction, p. 1594.

B. True Owing to peristalsis.
Ch. 71 Urinary Obstruction, p. 1594.

C. True This may occur in acute severe obstruction.
Ch. 71 Urinary Obstruction, p. 1594.

D. True This occurs early and is transient. Later renal blood flow reduces by up to 30%.
Ch. 71 Urinary Obstruction, p. 1594.

E. True
Ch. 71 Urinary Obstruction, p. 1595.

Q 6.40   Concerning urinary obstruction

A. Acute obstruction needs to be relieved immediately in order to avoid measurable deterioration in renal function.

B. The gold-standard test for quantifying obstruction is the Doppler ultrasound resistivity index.

C. An increase in the number of 'ureteric jets' is seen on the affected side due to peristalsis.

D. Magnetic resonance imaging is the best imaging modality for diagnosing urinary obstruction.

E. The diagnosis of obstruction requires the correlation of anatomical and functional information.

Q 6.41   Changes on the IVU during acute obstruction include

A. Increasingly dense nephrogram on the contralateral side.

B. Renal enlargement.

C. Delayed opacification of the collecting system.

D. Spontaneous pyelosinus extravasation.

E. Severe pelvicaliectasis.

Q 6.42   Concerning the IVU in acute obstruction in the diagnosis of an ureteric stone

A. If no contrast medium has appeared in the collecting system at 30 minutes, the next should be taken after a further hour.

B. In an obstructive nephrogram, contrast material accumulates in the renal interstitium.

C. The striated nephrogram occurs as a result of contrast failing to opacify tubules.

D. An obstructive nephrogram may not become manifest if there is co-existent infection.

E. From 80 to 90% of obstructing calculi pass spontaneously.

(Answers overleaf)

A **6.40** **Concerning urinary obstruction**

A. **False** In animal experiments the kidney may withstand total obstruction for up to 1 week without suffering irreversible damage.
Ch. 71 Urinary Obstruction, p. 1595.

B. **False**
Ch. 71 Urinary Obstruction, p. 1595.

C. **False**
Ch. 71 Urinary Obstruction, p. 1595.

D. **False**
Ch. 71 Urinary Obstruction, p. 1595.

E. **True**
Ch. 71 Urinary Obstruction, p. 1595.

A **6.41** **Changes on the IVU during acute obstruction include**

A. **False**
Ch. 71 Urinary Obstruction, p. 1595.

B. **True** This is usually mild.
Ch. 71 Urinary Obstruction, p. 1595.

C. **True**
Ch. 71 Urinary Obstruction, p. 1595.

D. **True** Caused by fornix tears in up to 24% of patients.
Ch. 71 Urinary Obstruction, p. 1595.

E. **False** This is a late finding.
Ch. 71 Urinary Obstruction, p. 1595.

A **6.42** **Concerning the IVU in acute obstruction in the diagnosis of an ureteric stone**

A. **False** This is too early! The 'rule of eight' applies: no contrast at 15 mins – the next image at 2 hours. No contrast at 30 mins – next image at 4 hours.
Ch. 71 Urinary Obstruction, p. 1597.

B. **False** It remains in the tubules.
Ch. 71 Urinary Obstruction, p. 1596.

C. **False** Opacification of bundles of proximal tubules within the medullary rays is responsible for this phenomenon.
Ch. 71 Urinary Obstruction, p. 1596.

D. **True**
Ch. 71 Urinary Obstruction, p. 1596.

E. **True**
Ch. 71 Urinary Obstruction, p. 1596.

Q 6.43 Concerning the renal tract on IVU

A. The degree of pelvicaliceal dilation reflects the degree of obstruction.
B. A standing column of contrast medium may be seen in normal individuals.
C. The normal female ureter is wider on average than the male ureter.
D. Gall bladder opacification may occur in the normal patient after IVU.
E. Extravasation of contrast medium during IVU of an obstructed system requires urgent drainage.

Q 6.44 The following are imaging findings in chronic urinary obstruction

A. Large kidney size.
B. Small kidney size.
C. Normal nephrographic density.
D. Longitudinal striations in ureteric mucosa.
E. Negative pyelogram.

Q 6.45 Concerning ultrasound in urinary obstruction

A. Separation of central medullary sinus fat echoes by areas of hydroreflectivity occurs in normal individuals.
B. A urine-debris level is a sign of pyonephrosis.
C. Acute urinary obstruction is ruled out by normal renal appearances on ultrasound.
D. Elevation of the resistivity index occurs only after hydronephrosis has developed.
E. MRI is preferable to ultrasound in the evaluation of transplant kidneys for suspected acute obstruction.

(Answers overleaf)

A **6.43** Concerning the renal tract on IVU

A. False
  Ch. 71 Urinary Obstruction, p. 1597.

B. True This may occur but will not be seen on more than one or two radiographs in the normal patient.
  Ch. 71 Urinary Obstruction, p. 1597.

C. True The male ureter (with compression applied) is usually less than 7 mm. The female ureter averages a couple of millimetres wider.
  Ch. 71 Urinary Obstruction, p. 1597.

D. False Heterotopic excretion occurs in obstruction of the renal tract.
  Ch. 71 Urinary Obstruction, p. 1597.

E. False It is almost always benign and self-limiting.
  Ch. 71 Urinary Obstruction, p. 1598.

A **6.44** The following are imaging findings in chronic urinary obstruction

A. True If obstruction is partial.
  Ch. 71 Urinary Obstruction, p. 1599.

B. True If obstruction is complete.
  Ch. 71 Urinary Obstruction, p. 1599.

C. True
  Ch. 71 Urinary Obstruction, p. 1599.

D. True
  Ch. 71 Urinary Obstruction, p. 1599.

E. True
  Ch. 71 Urinary Obstruction, p. 1599.

A **6.45** Concerning ultrasound in urinary obstruction

A. True In 20% of normal people.
  Ch. 71 Urinary Obstruction, p. 1601.

B. True
  Ch. 71 Urinary Obstruction, p. 1601.

C. False It takes approximately 24 hours for demonstrable caliectasis to develop.
  Ch. 71 Urinary Obstruction, p. 1601.

D. False This feature may precede hydronephrosis.
  Ch. 71 Urinary Obstruction, p. 1601.

E. False
  Ch. 71 Urinary Obstruction, p. 1601.

Q **6.46**   **The following are signs of urinary obstruction on CT**

    A. Peri-vesical stranding.
    B. Peri-ureteric stranding.
    C. Delayed nephrogram.
    D. Medullary pyramids more densely opacified than cortex.
    E. Delayed pyelogram.

Q **6.47**   **Ureteric obstruction is associated with**

    A. Desmoid tumour.
    B. Peri-aneurysmal fibrosis.
    C. Tuberculosis.
    D. Pelvic lipomatosis.
    E. Peri-ureteric fibrovenous entrapment.

Q **6.48**   **Cause of congenital ureteric obstruction include**

    A. Cholesteatoma.
    B. Circumcaval ureter.
    C. Bladder diverticulum.
    D. Epidermolysis bullosa.
    E. Primary megaureter.

(Answers overleaf)

A **6.46**   **The following are signs of urinary obstruction on CT**

A. False   Perinephric stranding.
Ch. 71 Urinary Obstruction, p. 1601.

B. True
Ch. 71 Urinary Obstruction, p. 1603.

C. True
Ch. 71 Urinary Obstruction, p. 1603.

D. True
Ch. 71 Urinary Obstruction, p. 1603.

E. True
Ch. 71 Urinary Obstruction, p. 1604.

A **6.47**   **Ureteric obstruction is associated with**

A. True   Retroperitoneal desmoids can cause ureteric obstruction.
Ch. 71 Urinary Obstruction, p. 1609.

B. True   Typically this occurs in association with peri-aortic fibrosis, but obstruction may occur at an aneurysmal common iliac artery.
Ch. 71 Urinary Obstruction, p. 1609.

C. True   Granulomatous retroperitoneal infection or inflammation can be causative.
Ch. 71 Urinary Obstruction, p. 1609.

D. True
Ch. 71 Urinary Obstruction, p. 1609.

E. True   Previously called 'ovarian vein syndrome'.
Ch. 71 Urinary Obstruction, p. 1609.

A **6.48**   **Cause of congenital ureteric obstruction include**

A. False   This is an acquired intra-luminal lesion, which may obstruct the PUJ.
Ch. 71 Urinary Obstruction, p. 1608.

B. True
Ch. 71 Urinary Obstruction, p. 1608.

C. False
Ch. 71 Urinary Obstruction, p. 1608.

D. False   Ureteric obstruction in this condition is acquired not congenital.
Ch. 71 Urinary Obstruction, p. 1609.

E. True
Ch. 71 Urinary Obstruction, p. 1608.

Q **6.49** **Consider the following statements regarding obstruction in the urinary tract**

    A. Differential renal function can be calculated during ^{99m}Tc-DTPA diuresis renography.
    B. Antegrade pyelography in an obstructed system has a high associated risk of infection.
    C. The Whitaker test is almost invariably conclusive.
    D. MRI is more sensitive than CT at diagnosing the cause of obstruction.
    E. The commonest site for an impacted stone is at the PUJ.

Q **6.50** **Regarding dilation of the urinary tract**

    A. Massive hydronephrosis and hydroureter imply that obstruction must be present.
    B. After obstruction is relieved, the ureter may remain dilated permanently.
    C. Congenital megacalices are a consequence of multiple stenosed infundibula.
    D. Renal cortical thickness is normal when congenital megacalices are present.
    E. Most patients with primary megaureter have significant vesico-ureteric reflux.

Q **6.51** **Infection with the following organisms causes ureteric obstruction**

    A. *Actinomycetes israelii.*
    B. *Schistosoma haematobium.*
    C. *Mycobacterium tuberculosis.*
    D. Cytomegalovirus.
    E. *Clonorchis sinensis.*

(Answers overleaf)

A **6.49** Consider the following statements regarding obstruction in the urinary tract

A. True Differential renal function is also measurable using $^{99\,m}$Tc-DMSA in a separate procedure.
Ch. 71 Urinary Obstruction, p. 1604.

B. False
Ch. 71 Urinary Obstruction, p. 1604.

C. False It is often helpful diagnosing surgically corrective obstruction but equivocal results are not uncommon.
Ch. 71 Urinary Obstruction, p. 1510.

D. False
Ch. 71 Urinary Obstruction, p. 1606.

E. False
Ch. 71 Urinary Obstruction, p. 1607.

A **6.50** Regarding dilation of the urinary tract

A. False Longstanding vesico-ureteric reflux will cause this appearance.
Ch. 71 Urinary Obstruction, p. 1606.

B. True
Ch. 71 Urinary Obstruction, p. 1606.

C. False This is non-obstructive and felt to be a consequence of renal medullary hypoplasia.
Ch. 71 Urinary Obstruction, p. 1607.

D. True This distinguishes the condition from post-obstructive atrophy.
Ch. 71 Urinary Obstruction, p. 1607.

E. False A small minority have reflux.
Ch. 71 Urinary Obstruction, p. 1607.

A **6.51** Infection with the following organisms causes ureteric obstruction

A. False
Ch. 71 Urinary Obstruction, p. 1610.

B. True
Ch. 71 Urinary Obstruction, p. 1610.

C. True
Ch. 71 Urinary Obstruction, p. 1610.

D. False
Ch. 71 Urinary Obstruction, p. 1610.

E. False
Ch. 71 Urinary Obstruction, p. 1610.

Q 6.52 Urethral obstruction in children is caused by

A. Anterior urethral valve.
B. Leiomyoma.
C. Epidermolysis bullosa.
D. Hirschprung's disease.
E. Down's syndrome.

Q 6.53 Concerning the anatomy of the normal bladder

A. Obturator internus lies infero-laterally.
B. In infants the internal sphincter often lies above the level of the symphysis pubis.
C. Normal distended bladder wall thickness is 6–8 mm.
D. The trigone is covered in rugose mucosa in the undistended bladder.
E. A normal-sized prostate does not indent the bladder base.

Q 6.54 Concerning imaging of the bladder

A. A contrast-urine level on CT is seen only when there is pathological stasis.
B. Catheterization is the routine method of choice for measuring bladder residual volume.
C. Chemical shift artefact causes spurious bladder wall thickening on MRI.
D. Bladder wall resolution is improved when an endorectal coil is used instead of a body coil.
E. Mucosal enhancement precedes muscular wall enhancement after intravenous gadolinium administration.

(Answers overleaf)

A **6.52** **Urethral obstruction in children is caused by**

A. True
Ch. 71 Urinary Obstruction, p. 1612.

B. True
Ch. 71 Urinary Obstruction, p. 1612.

C. True
Ch. 71 Urinary Obstruction, p. 1612.

D. True
Ch. 71 Urinary Obstruction, p. 1612.

E. False This is associated with a narrowed posterior urethra but obstruction is not a feature.
Ch. 71 Urinary Obstruction, p. 1738.

A **6.53** **Concerning the anatomy of the normal bladder**

A. True Along with levator ani.
Ch. 71 Urinary Obstruction, p. 1615.

B. True
Ch. 71 Urinary Obstruction, p. 1615.

C. False Less than 5 mm.
Ch. 71 Urinary Obstruction, p. 1615.

D. False The trigone is smooth.
Ch. 71 Urinary Obstruction, p. 1615.

E. False
Ch. 71 Urinary Obstruction, p. 1615.

A **6.54** **Concerning imaging of the bladder**

A. False
Ch. 72 Radiological Evaluation of the Urinary Bladder, p. 1616.

B. False Ultrasound is an accurate non-invasive way of measuring bladder volume.
Ch. 72 Radiological Evaluation of the Urinary Bladder, p. 1616.

C. True
Ch. 72 Radiological Evaluation of the Urinary Bladder, p. 1617.

D. True
Ch. 72 Radiological Evaluation of the Urinary Bladder, p. 1616.

E. True
Ch. 72 Radiological Evaluation of the Urinary Bladder, p. 1617.

Q **6.55**   Regarding imaging findings of bladder pathology

A. The normal width of the symphysis pubis exceeds 15 mm.
B. Fungus balls are usually caused by actinomycetes species.
C. A gas-filled, laminated, hyperdense, rounded masses seen on CT suggests cystitis cystica.
D. The commonest cause of ruptured bladder on CT is blunt abdominal trauma.
E. Bladder calculi formed predominantly from uric acid are very rare.

Q **6.56**   Regarding bladder rupture

A. Extraperitoneal rupture is more common than intraperitoneal rupture.
B. Pelvic fractures are more strongly associated with intraperitoneal then extraperitoneal rupture.
C. Most causes of bladder rupture follow a motor vehicle accident.
D. In intraperitoneal rupture contrast accumulates around the dome of the bladder.
E. Subserosal rupture is rare.

Q **6.57**   Concerning bladder pathology

A. Surgery is required more for intraperitoneal than extraperitoneal bladder rupture.
B. Most bladder tumours are epithelial in origin.
C. CT cystscopy requires bladder catheterization.
D. An IVU is mandatory for staging bladder carcinoma.
E. A staging cystogram is used when cystoscopy for bladder carcinoma is negative.

(Answers overleaf)

A **6.55**   **Regarding imaging findings of bladder pathology**

A. False   Normal width at all ages is less than 10 mm.
Ch. 72 Radiological Evaluation of the Urinary Bladder, p. 1618.

B. False   Usually Candida albicans.
Ch. 72 Radiological Evaluation of the Urinary Bladder, p. 1619.

C. False   This is the description of a fungus ball.
Ch. 72 Radiological Evaluation of the Urinary Bladder, p. 1619.

D. True

Ch. 72 Radiological Evaluation of the Urinary Bladder, p. 1619.

E. False   One study found that nearly 50% of bladder calculi are composed of uric acid.
Ch. 72 Radiological Evaluation of the Urinary Bladder, p. 1619.

A **6.56**   **Regarding bladder rupture**

A. True

Ch. 72 Radiological Evaluation of the Urinary Bladder, p. 1619.

B. False

Ch. 72 Radiological Evaluation of the Urinary Bladder, p. 1619.

C. True   Approximately 90%.
Ch. 72 Radiological Evaluation of the Urinary Bladder, p. 1619.

D. True   It gathers here and also extends laterally, outlining bowel.
Ch. 72 Radiological Evaluation of the Urinary Bladder, p. 1621.

E. True   This is seen as an elliptical extravasation adjacent to the bladder.
Ch. 72 Radiological Evaluation of the Urinary Bladder, p. 1621.

A **6.57**   **Concerning bladder pathology**

A. True

Ch. 72 Radiological Evaluation of the Urinary Bladder, p. 1621.

B. True   Over 90%.
Ch. 72 Radiological Evaluation of the Urinary Bladder, p. 1621.

C. False

Ch. 72 Radiological Evaluation of the Urinary Bladder, p. 1623.

D. False

Ch. 72 Radiological Evaluation of the Urinary Bladder, p. 1623.

E. False

Ch. 72 Radiological Evaluation of the Urinary Bladder, p. 1623.

Q 6.58　Regarding imaging of the bladder carcinoma on CT

   A. CT is used to distinguish T1 from T2 tumours.
   B. CT can distinguish T3a from T3b tumours.
   C. High doses of intravenous contrast medium facilitate the detection of small mucosal tumours.
   D. Nodes greater than 10 mm short axis are considered malignant.
   E. Loss of the seminal vesicle fat angle occurs in constipated patients.

Q 6.59　Concerning MRI of bladder carcinoma

   A. Papillary tumours have higher signal than urine on T1-weighted sequences.
   B. T2-weighted sequences diminish the contrast between urine and tumour.
   C. T1-weighted post-gadolinium sequences are more sensitive at detecting carcinoma than unenhanced T2-weighted sequences.
   D. Bladder tumours show earlier enhancement after intravenous gadolinium than inflammatory non-neoplastic lesions.
   E. The staging accuracy of MRI is vastly superior to CT.

Q 6.60　Concerning the anatomy of the prostate

   A. Denonvillier's fascia separates posterior surface of prostate from rectum.
   B. The pubovesical ligament is attached to the prostate capsule.
   C. The central zone accounts for 90% of the bulk of the gland.
   D. The volume of the central zone decreases with age.
   E. The transitional zone develops benign prostatic hypertrophy.

(Answers overleaf)

A **6.58** **Regarding imaging of the bladder carcinoma on CT**

A. False
> *Ch. 72 Radiological Evaluation of the Urinary Bladder, p. 1624.*

B. True
> *Ch. 72 Radiological Evaluation of the Urinary Bladder, p. 1624.*

C. False   High-density intravesical contrast medium obscures small tumours.
> *Ch. 72 Radiological Evaluation of the Urinary Bladder, p. 1624.*

D. True
> *Ch. 72 Radiological Evaluation of the Urinary Bladder, p. 1625.*

E. True   Rectal distension obliterates this sign.
> *Ch. 72 Radiological Evaluation of the Urinary Bladder, p. 1625.*

A **6.59** **Concerning MRI of bladder carcinoma**

A. True
> *Ch. 72 Radiological Evaluation of the Urinary Bladder, p. 1625.*

B. True
> *Ch. 72 Radiological Evaluation of the Urinary Bladder, p. 1625.*

C. True
> *Ch. 72 Radiological Evaluation of the Urinary Bladder, p. 1626.*

D. True
> *Ch. 72 Radiological Evaluation of the Urinary Bladder, p. 1626.*

E. False
> *Ch. 72 Radiological Evaluation of the Urinary Bladder, p. 1627.*

A **6.60** **Concerning the anatomy of the prostate**

A. True
> *Ch. 72 Radiological Evaluation of the Urinary Bladder, p. 1629.*

B. True
> *Ch. 72 Radiological Evaluation of the Urinary Bladder, p. 1629.*

C. False
> *Ch. 72 Radiological Evaluation of the Urinary Bladder, p. 1629.*

D. True
> *Ch. 72 Radiological Evaluation of the Urinary Bladder, p. 1629.*

E. True
> *Ch. 72 Radiological Evaluation of the Urinary Bladder, p. 1629.*

Q **6.61** Regarding prostatic anatomy

A. The anterior fibromuscular band separates prostate gland from the peri-prostatic spaces.

B. The central zone accounts for 40% of carcinomas.

C. The prostatic urethra contacts the peripheral zone at the verumontanum.

D. The base of the prostate extends from bladder floor to symphysis pubis

E. The apex of prostate extends from bladder neck to obturator internus.

Q **6.62** Regarding transrectal ultrasound of normal prostate

A. Zonal anatomy is usually visible.

B. The transition zone is hypo-reflective.

C. Corpora amylacea are demonstrated.

D. The prostatic urethra is seen in 90% of cases.

E. The vas deferens is not visualized unless it is pathologically enlarged.

Q **6.63** Concerning prostatic imaging

A. The peripheral zone is more reflective than the transition zone on transrectal ultrasound.

B. Dynamic helical CT can demonstrate zonal anatomy.

C. On spin-echo T1-weighted MRI, the zonal anatomy cannot be differentiated.

D. On T2-weighted MRI sequences, the peripheral zone has a higher signal intensity than the transition zone.

E. The transition zone has a low signal, which becomes heterogeneous with the development of benign prostatic hyperplasia.

(Answers overleaf)

A **6.61** **Regarding prostatic anatomy**

A. True

Ch. 72 Radiological Evaluation of the Urinary Bladder, p. 1629.

B. False The peripheral zone is the site of a considerable majority.

Ch. 72 Radiological Evaluation of the Urinary Bladder, p. 1629.

C. True

Ch. 72 Radiological Evaluation of the Urinary Bladder, p. 1629.

D. False

Ch. 72 Radiological Evaluation of the Urinary Bladder, p. 1629.

E. False

Ch. 72 Radiological Evaluation of the Urinary Bladder, p. 1629.

A **6.62** **Regarding transrectal ultrasound of normal prostate**

A. True

Ch. 72 Radiological Evaluation of the Urinary Bladder, p. 1630.

B. True

Ch. 72 Radiological Evaluation of the Urinary Bladder, p. 1630.

C. True These may be seen as dense echogenic foci between peripheral and transition zones.

Ch. 72 Radiological Evaluation of the Urinary Bladder, p. 1630.

D. False The normal prostatic urethra is rarely seen.

Ch. 72 Radiological Evaluation of the Urinary Bladder, p. 1630.

E. False The normal vas deferens may be seen.

Ch. 72 Radiological Evaluation of the Urinary Bladder, p. 1630.

A **6.63** **Concerning prostatic imaging**

A. True

Ch. 72 Radiological Evaluation of the Urinary Bladder, p. 1630.

B. True

Ch. 72 Radiological Evaluation of the Urinary Bladder, p. 1631.

C. True

Ch. 72 Radiological Evaluation of the Urinary Bladder, p. 1631.

D. True

Ch. 72 Radiological Evaluation of the Urinary Bladder, p. 1632.

E. True

Ch. 72 Radiological Evaluation of the Urinary Bladder, p. 1632.

Q **6.64** **Regarding prostatic pathology**

 A. Mullerian cysts usually lie in the midline.
 B. Acquired prostatic cysts usually lie in the transition zone.
 C. Prostatic abscess usually begins in the peripheral zone.
 D. Granulomatous prostatitis is usually infective in origin.
 E. The prostatic urethra is shortened and widened on micturating cystourethrography in acute prostatitis.

Q **6.65** **Concerning the imaging of prostatic pathology**

 A. Calcification caused by tuberculous infection can be reliably distinguished from calcified prostatic calculi.
 B. The CT attenuation value allows diffuse prostatitis to be distinguished from normal prostate.
 C. Prostatic ductal calcification is a pre-cancerous finding.
 D. Prostate enlargement on CT is diagnosed when the prostate gland is seen on axial slices at least 3 cm or more above the pubic symphysis.
 E. Prostate enlargement is associated with 'fish-hook' ureters.

Q **6.66** **Regarding prostate cancer**

 A. From 60 to 80% of cancers begin in the peripheral zone.
 B. Over 90% of cancers are adenocarcinomas.
 C. Release of prostatic fibrinolysin may lead to rectal haemorrhage.
 D. Prostate cancer is usually under-staged by digital rectal examination.
 E. Transabdominal ultrasound now has the spatial resolution necessary to demonstrate the majority of prostatic carcinomas.

(Answers overleaf)

231

A **6.64** Regarding prostatic pathology

A. True
> *Ch. 72 Radiological Evaluation of the Urinary Bladder, p. 1633.*

B. True
> *Ch. 72 Radiological Evaluation of the Urinary Bladder, p. 1633.*

C. True It may spread to other areas and rupture into urethra, rectum, perineum or even peritoneum.
> *Ch. 72 Radiological Evaluation of the Urinary Bladder, p. 1633.*

D. False M. Tuberculosis, Brucella abortus and other organism are rare cause of granulomatous prostatitis.
> *Ch. 72 Radiological Evaluation of the Urinary Bladder, p. 1633.*

E. False Narrowed and lengthened.
> *Ch. 72 Radiological Evaluation of the Urinary Bladder, p. 1634.*

A **6.65** Concerning the imaging of prostatic pathology

A. False
> *Ch. 72 Radiological Evaluation of the Urinary Bladder, p. 1634.*

B. False On the other hand, prostatic abscess may be visible as a reduced density focus with rim enhancement.
> *Ch. 72 Radiological Evaluation of the Urinary Bladder, p. 1634.*

C. False
> *Ch. 72 Radiological Evaluation of the Urinary Bladder, p. 1634.*

D. False One centimetre or more .
> *Ch. 72 Radiological Evaluation of the Urinary Bladder, p. 1635.*

E. True Owing to elevation of the bladder base.
> *Ch. 72 Radiological Evaluation of the Urinary Bladder, p. 1636.*

A **6.66** Regarding prostate cancer

A. True
> *Ch. 72 Radiological Evaluation of the Urinary Bladder, p. 1636.*

B. True
> *Ch. 72 Radiological Evaluation of the Urinary Bladder, p. 1636.*

C. True
> *Ch. 72 Radiological Evaluation of the Urinary Bladder, p. 1636.*

D. True
> *Ch. 72 Radiological Evaluation of the Urinary Bladder, p. 1636.*

E. False
> *Ch. 72 Radiological Evaluation of the Urinary Bladder, p. 1636.*

Q **6.67**   **Consider the following statements regarding the radiological evaluation of prostatic carcinoma**

  A.   A hypoechoic focus in the peripheral zone is pathognomonic of carcinoma.
  B.   Transrectal ultrasound is an effective screening examination for prostatic cancer.
  C.   T2 tumours are usually indefinable on CT.
  D.   Low signal intensity of the seminal vesicles on T2-weighted imaging suggest invasion by carcinoma.
  E.   Locally increased signal intensity of the levator ani muscle on T2-weighting suggests invasion by carcinoma.

Q **6.68**   **Regarding imaging of prostate tumour spread**

  A.   Transrectal ultrasound is useful for the detection of lymph node metastases.
  B.   CT can detect microinvasion of normal sized nodes.
  C.   CT is the best screening test for bony metastases.
  D.   Bone scintigraphy is more sensitive than CT at detecting small metastatic lesions.
  E.   Para-aortic node involvement by prostatic cancer is usually accompanied by pelvic lymphadenopathy.

Q **6.69**   **Causes of low signal intensity within the peripheral zone of prostate on t2-weighted MRI include**

  A.   Radiation fibrosis.
  B.   Post-orchidectomy.
  C.   Benign prostatic hyperplasia.
  D.   Post-biopsy haemorrhage.
  E.   Dystrophic change.

(Answers overleaf)

A **6.67** Consider the following statements regarding the radiological evaluation of prostatic carcinoma

A. False A variety of benign disorders can cause this appearance.
Ch. 72 Radiological Evaluation of the Urinary Bladder, p. 1637.

B. False Digital rectal examination and serum PSA estimation are more sensitive and less expensive.
Ch. 72 Radiological Evaluation of the Urinary Bladder, p. 1637.

C. False
Ch. 72 Radiological Evaluation of the Urinary Bladder, p. 1637.

D. True
Ch. 72 Radiological Evaluation of the Urinary Bladder, p. 1637.

E. True
Ch. 72 Radiological Evaluation of the Urinary Bladder, p. 1637.

A **6.68** Regarding imaging of prostate tumour spread

A. False
Ch. 72 Radiological Evaluation of the Urinary Bladder, p. 1638.

B. False
Ch. 72 Radiological Evaluation of the Urinary Bladder, p. 1639.

C. False
Ch. 72 Radiological Evaluation of the Urinary Bladder, p. 1639.

D. True
Ch. 72 Radiological Evaluation of the Urinary Bladder, p. 1639.

E. True
Ch. 72 Radiological Evaluation of the Urinary Bladder, p. 1639.

A **6.69** Causes of low signal intensity within the peripheral zone of prostate on t2-weighted MRI include

A. True
Ch. 72 Radiological Evaluation of the Urinary Bladder, p. 1639.

B. True
Ch. 72 Radiological Evaluation of the Urinary Bladder, p. 1639.

C. False
Ch. 72 Radiological Evaluation of the Urinary Bladder, p. 1639.

D. True
Ch. 72 Radiological Evaluation of the Urinary Bladder, p. 1639.

E. True
Ch. 72 Radiological Evaluation of the Urinary Bladder, p. 1639.

Q 6.70 Concerning the embryology of the urinary tract

A. The pronephros develops into the kidney.
B. The mesonephric duct migrates caudally to enter the prostatic urethra.
C. The metanephros is initially located above the diaphragm.
D. Unilateral renal agenesis is usually diagnosed antenatally.
E. Bilateral renal agenesis is associated with urinary tract infections in the infant.

Q 6.71 Features used to detect extracapsular extension of prostate cancer on t2-weighted images include

A. Focal capsular retraction.
B. Ductal calcification.
C. Obliteration of the recto-prostatic angle.
D. Asymmetry of the neurovascular bundle.
E. Low signal in the seminal vesicles.

Q 6.72 Concerning the anatomy of the normal urethra

A. The prostatic urethra starts at the external sphincter and ends at the superior aspect of the urogenital diaphragm.
B. The posterior wall of the membranous urethra contains the verumotanum.
C. The verumontanum contains the two orifices of the ejaculatory ducts.
D. The membranous urethra is lined by transitional epithelium.
E. The bulbar urethra extends from the inferior urogenital diaphragm to the suspensory penile ligament.

(Answers overleaf)

A **6.70**   **Concerning the embryology of the urinary tract**

A. False   It is reabsorbed by the 4th week.
Ch. 76 Imaging of the Kidneys and Urinary Tract in Children, p. 1719.

B. True
Ch. 76 Imaging of the Kidneys and Urinary Tract in Children, p. 1719.

C. False   It starts off in the lumbo-sacral region.
Ch. 76 Imaging of the Kidneys and Urinary Tract in Children, p. 1720.

D. False   It is usually an acquired pathology caused by involution of a multi-cystic kidney.
Ch. 76 Imaging of the Kidneys and Urinary Tract in Children, p. 1720.

E. False   It is incompatible with life.
Ch. 76 Imaging of the Kidneys and Urinary Tract in Children, p. 1720.

A **6.71**   **Features used to detect extracapsular extension of prostate cancer on t2-weighted images include**

A. True
Ch. 72 Radiological Evaluation of the Urinary Bladder, Prostate and Urethra, p. 1641.

B. False
Ch. 72 Radiological Evaluation of the Urinary Bladder, Prostate and Urethra, p. 1641.

C. True
Ch. 72 Radiological Evaluation of the Urinary Bladder, Prostate and Urethra, p. 1641.

D. True
Ch. 72 Radiological Evaluation of the Urinary Bladder, Prostate and Urethra, p. 1641.

E. True
Ch. 72 Radiological Evaluation of the Urinary Bladder, Prostate and Urethra, p. 1641.

A **6.72**   **Concerning the anatomy of the normal urethra**

A. False   It starts at the vesical orifice (internal sphincter) and ends at the external sphincter, which is located at the superior aspect of the urogenital diaphragm.
Ch. 72 Radiological Evaluation of the Urinary Bladder, Prostate and Urethra, p. 1644.

B. False   The verumontanum is located on the posterior aspect of the prostatic urethra.
Ch. 72 Radiological Evaluation of the Urinary Bladder, Prostate and Urethra, p. 1644.

C. True
Ch. 72 Radiological Evaluation of the Urinary Bladder, Prostate and Urethra, p. 1644.

D. False   It is lined by stratified columnar epithelium. The prostatic urethra is lined by transitional epithelium, which is continuous with bladder epithelium.
Ch. 72 Radiological Evaluation of the Urinary Bladder, Prostate and Urethra, p. 1644.

E. True
Ch. 72 Radiological Evaluation of the Urinary Bladder, Prostate and Urethra, p. 1644.

Q **6.73**   Regarding the technique of retrograde urethrography

A.   A nutcracker clamp is used.
B.   Two balloons are used in the female urethra.
C.   A 5 ml syringe filled with contrast medium is sufficient for most patients.
D.   Lipiodol should be used if a false passage is suspected.
E.   Prostatic urethra is better imaged by retrograde urethrography than by antegrade voiding studies.

Q **6.74**   Concerning imaging of the urethra

A.   The female urethra has a target-like appearance on T1-weighted images.
B.   Posterior urethral valves are best detected on retrograde urethrography.
C.   Urethral diverticulum is seen most commonly in the mid-urethra.
D.   Filling defects are seen on urethrography when acute infection is present.
E.   The urethritis of Reiter's syndrome can be differentiated from gonococcal urethritis by the presence of strictures.

(Answers overleaf)

A **6.73** Regarding the technique of retrograde urethrography

A. False
Ch. 72 Radiological Evaluation of the Urinary Bladder, Prostate and Urethra, p. 1645.

B. True One to occlude the bladder end and the other to occlude the external orifice.
Ch. 72 Radiological Evaluation of the Urinary Bladder, Prostate and Urethra, p. 1645.

C. False A 30 ml syringe is normally used.
Ch. 72 Radiological Evaluation of the Urinary Bladder, Prostate and Urethra, p. 1645.

D. False
Ch. 72 Radiological Evaluation of the Urinary Bladder, Prostate and Urethra, p. 1645.

E. False There is better distension with the antegrade technique.
Ch. 72 Radiological Evaluation of the Urinary Bladder, Prostate and Urethra, p. 1645.

A **6.74** Concerning imaging of the urethra

A. False This is the appearance on T2 weighted images where the high signal smooth muscle layer is sandwiched between low signal striated muscle and stratified epithelial layers.
Ch. 72 Radiological Evaluation of the Urinary Bladder, Prostate and Urethra, p. 1645.

B. False Antegrade studies or ultrasound depict this lesion best.
Ch. 72 Radiological Evaluation of the Urinary Bladder, Prostate and Urethra, p. 1645.

C. True Complications include stone formation, infection and carcinoma.
Ch. 72 Radiological Evaluation of the Urinary Bladder, Prostate and Urethra, p. 1646.

D. True Owing to the presence of sloughed mucosa.
Ch. 72 Radiological Evaluation of the Urinary Bladder, Prostate and Urethra, p. 1646.

E. False Proximal dilation, false passages, pseudo-diverticula, fistulas and reflux into Cowper's gland ducts, prostatic ducts and seminal vesicles can occur in both conditions.
Ch. 72 Radiological Evaluation of the Urinary Bladder, Prostate and Urethra, p. 1646.

Q 6.75   Regarding the urethra in trauma

A.   Traumatic urethral injuries most commonly involve the bulbar urethra.
B.   From 5 to 15% of pelvic fractures are associated with urethral injury.
C.   During retrograde urethrography contrast medium entering the retropubic space means that the penile urethra has been damaged.
D.   Complete tears are less common than partial tears.
E.   Strictures are more likely to occur after complete tears.

Q 6.76   Causes of filling defects on urethrography

A.   Amyloidosis.
B.   Condylomata acuminata.
C.   Sarcoidosis.
D.   Caplan's nodules.
E.   Melanoma.

(Answers overleaf)

A **6.75**   Regarding the urethra in trauma

A. False   Membranous urethra is most commonly traumatized because it is relatively fixed in the urogenital diaphragm.
Ch. 72 Radiological Evaluation of the Urinary Bladder, Prostate and Urethra, p. 1647.

B. True
Ch. 72 Radiological Evaluation of the Urinary Bladder, Prostate and Urethra, p. 1647.

C. False   This sign means that the urethra above the urogenital diaphragm has been torn.
Ch. 72 Radiological Evaluation of the Urinary Bladder, Prostate and Urethra, p. 1647.

D. False   Complete tears are twice as common.
Ch. 72 Radiological Evaluation of the Urinary Bladder, Prostate and Urethra, p. 1647.

E. True
Ch. 72 Radiological Evaluation of the Urinary Bladder, Prostate and Urethra, p. 1647.

A **6.76**   Causes of filling defects on urethrography

A. True
Ch. 72 Radiological Evaluation of the Urinary Bladder, Prostate and Urethra, p. 1648.

B. True
Ch. 72 Radiological Evaluation of the Urinary Bladder, Prostate and Urethra, p. 1648.

C. True
Ch. 72 Radiological Evaluation of the Urinary Bladder, Prostate and Urethra, p. 1648.

D. False
Ch. 72 Radiological Evaluation of the Urinary Bladder, Prostate and Urethra, p. 1648.

E. True
Ch. 72 Radiological Evaluation of the Urinary Bladder, Prostate and Urethra, p. 1648.

Q **6.77** **Concerning renal trauma**

A. Microscopic haematuria without hypotension is very unlikely to be associated with major renal injury.

B. Normal urinalysis excludes significant renal injury.

C. Most traumatic injuries are visible on ultrasound.

D. A striated nephrogram on CT is a sign of renal trauma.

E. Subcapsular haematomas on CT are seen in over 20% of adult renal injuries.

Q **6.78** **Regarding imaging findings in major renal injury**

A. Peripheral renal enhancement is seen in renal artery avulsion.

B. Renal angiography is required to diagnose renal artery occlusion.

C. Right renal artery occlusion is associated with retrograde blood flow from IVC into right renal vein.

D. Significant renal vein injury is more common than significant injury to the renal artery.

E. Renal fragmentation is an absolute indication for nephrectomy.

(Answers overleaf)

241

A **6.77**   **Concerning renal trauma**

A. True   Only 3 of 1558 blunt trauma patients without haematuria or hypotension had significant renal injury in one study.
Ch. 73 Injuries to the Genitourinary Tract, p. 1654.

B. False   This finding may be seen when the renal artery has been avulsed and has been reported in one-quarter of patients with major renal artery trauma.
Ch. 73 Injuries to the Genitourinary Tract, p. 1654.

C. False   The majority of renal injuries have normal ultrasound appearances (low negative predictive value).
Ch. 73 Injuries to the Genitourinary Tract, p. 1654.

D. True   This is seen when the kidney is irregularly perfused because it is oedematous.
Ch. 73 Injuries to the Genitourinary Tract, p. 1655.

E. False   These are rare in the adult as the renal capsule is not easily separated from the cortex.
Ch. 73 Injuries to the Genitourinary Tract, p. 1655.

A **6.78**   **Regarding imaging findings in major renal injury**

A. True   Owing to retroperitoneal collaterals.
Ch. 73 Injuries to the Genitourinary Tract, p. 1657.

B. False   This diagnosis can be made on CT.
Ch. 73 Injuries to the Genitourinary Tract, p. 1657.

C. True   This mimics contrast medium in the collecting system only after injection into the femoral vein.
Ch. 73 Injuries to the Genitourinary Tract, p. 1657.

D. False
Ch. 73 Injuries to the Genitourinary Tract, p. 1657.

E. False   In the haemodynamically stable patient an expectant approach can sometimes result in remarkable restoration of renal contour and function.
Ch. 73 Injuries to the Genitourinary Tract, p. 1657.

Q **6.79** **Regarding traumatic injury to the collecting system**

    A. Ureteral injury usually occurs at the vesico-ureteric junction.
    B. Ureteral penetrating injuries are best diagnosed using IVU.
    C. Traumatic bladder injury is associated with pelvic fractures in 60–80% of cases.
    D. Cystography should be performed in all patients with gross haematuria associated with fractures.
    E. Cystography in an adult requires instillation of 100–200 ml of contrast medium to effectively examine its contour.

Q **6.80** **Regarding bladder rupture**

    A. Intraperitoneal rupture results from blunt trauma to a full bladder.
    B. CT of the pelvis after intravenous contrast and clamping of the bladder reliably excludes bladder injury.
    C. Extraperitoneal bladder rupture accounts for most bladder ruptures.
    D. Contrast medium extravasation into the scrotum occurs after disruption of the urogenital diaphragm.
    E. Most cases of extraperitoneal bladder rupture require surgical repair.

(Answers overleaf)

A **6.79** **Regarding traumatic injury to the collecting system**

A. False This is usually at the pelvi-ureteric junction.
Ch. 73 Injuries to the Genitourinary Tract, p. 1662,

B. False This technique is very insensitive at demonstrating penetrating injury to the ureter.
Ch. 73 Injuries to the Genitourinary Tract, p. 1662.

C. True
Ch. 73 Injuries to the Genitourinary Tract, p. 1662.

D. True
Ch. 73 Injuries to the Genitourinary Tract, p. 1662.

E. False From 350 to 400 ml is required for adequate distension but if bladder rupture is likely it should be instilled in 100 ml 'stages'.
Ch. 73 Injuries to the Genitourinary Tract, p. 1663.

A **6.80** **Regarding bladder rupture**

A. True
Ch. 73 Injuries to the Genitourinary Tract, p. 1663.

B. False Bladder clamping is an unreliable method of achieving sufficient distension to diagnose bladder injury.
Ch. 73 Injuries to the Genitourinary Tract, p. 1663.

C. True From 80 to 90%.
Ch. 73 Injuries to the Genitourinary Tract, p. 1663.

D. True
Ch. 73 Injuries to the Genitourinary Tract, p. 1664.

E. False Most are treated conservatively with transurethral or suprapubic catheterization.
Ch. 73 Injuries to the Genitourinary Tract, p. 1664.

Q 6.81 **Contrast medium extravasation from extraperitoneal bladder rupture may be seen in the following areas**

    A. Pouch of Douglas.
    B. Prevesical space of Retzius.
    C. Upper thigh.
    D. Presacral space.
    E. Lateral paravesical space.

Q 6.82 **Concerning imaging and biopsy of the failing kidney**

    A. Normal renal cortical thickness in an adult is 2–2.5 cm.
    B. Renal biopsy from upper pole of kidney is the preferred method of obtaining diagnostic samples.
    C. Renal biopsy samples should ideally contain 50% cortex and 50% medulla.
    D. Symptomatic perinephric haematoma occurs after renal biopsy in approximately 20% of subjects.
    E. Increased resistivity index in the failing kidney strongly suggests a diagnosis of renal vein thrombosis.

Q 6.83 **Regarding renal cystic disease**

    A. High density in a cyst in a patient with adult polycystic kidney disease is usually caused by adenocarcinoma.
    B. Calculi are seen in 20–40% of patients with adult polycystic kidney.
    C. Cystic renal disease complicating tuberous sclerosis can be distinguished from autosomal dominant (adult) polycystic kidney disease on MRI of the kidneys.
    D. Cysts acquired as a result of chronic renal impairment can usually be distinguished from adult polycystic kidney disease on ultrasound.
    E. From 10 to 15% of patients receiving dialysis have autosomal dominant polycystic renal disease.

(Answers overleaf)

245

A **6.81** **Contrast medium extravasation from extraperitoneal bladder rupture may be seen in the following areas**

A. False

Ch. 73 Injuries to the Genitourinary Tract, p. 1663.

B. True

Ch. 73 Injuries to the Genitourinary Tract, p. 1663.

C. True

Ch. 73 Injuries to the Genitourinary Tract, p. 1663.

D. True

Ch. 73 Injuries to the Genitourinary Tract, p. 1663.

E. True Contrast material can extend retroperitoneally to the level of the kidney simulating renal injury.
Ch. 73 Injuries to the Genitourinary Tract, p. 1663.

A **6.82** **Concerning imaging and biopsy of the failing kidney**

A. True

Ch. 74 Renal Failure and Transplantation, p. 1674.

B. False The lower pole is easier to biopsy more safely.
Ch. 74 Renal Failure and Transplantation, p. 1674.

C. False One hundred per cent cortex is desirable. Medulla should be avoided.
Ch. 74 Renal Failure and Transplantation, p. 1674.

D. False Less than 10%.
Ch. 74 Renal Failure and Transplantation, p. 1674.

E. False This is a non-specific finding seen in chronic renal failure of many different causes.
Ch. 74 Renal Failure and Transplantation, p. 1674.

A **6.83** **Regarding renal cystic disease**

A. False Usually simple haemorrhage.
Ch. 74 Renal Failure and Transplantation, p. 1675.

B. True

Ch. 74 Renal Failure and Transplantation, p. 1675.

C. False They are indistinguishable.
Ch. 74 Renal Failure and Transplantation, p. 1675.

D. True The kidneys are small or normal in size and the cyst are smaller and less numerous.
Ch. 74 Renal Failure and Transplantation, p. 1675.

E. True

Ch. 74 Renal Failure and Transplantation, p. 1674.

Q **6.84** Concerning contrast medium nephrotoxicity

A. Dehydration is a predisposing factor.
B. High-osmolality contrast medium is safer.
C. Myeloma is a risk factor.
D. Diabetic nephropathy is a risk factor.
E. Pre-treatment with steriods reduces the risk.

Q **6.85** The following pathologies and nephrographic appearances are associated

A. Acute tubular necrosis and immediate homogeneous nephrogram.
B. Acute glomerulonephritis and increasingly dense nephrogram.
C. Acute intratubular block by uric acid crystals and striated nephrogram.
D. Contrast medium nephropathy and persistent homogeneous nephrogram 24 hours after intravenous contrast medium.
E. Renal vein thrombosis and striated nephrogram.

Q **6.86** Concerning acquired cystic disease of the kidneys

A. The prevalence increases with longer durations of dialysis.
B. Most cysts are asymptomatic.
C. Massive retroperitoneal haemorrhage is associated.
D. There is a three- to sixfold increase in the risk of renal adenocarcinoma.
E. Following renal transplantation, the risk of developing haemorrhage or renal carcinoma diminishes.

(Answers overleaf)

A **6.84** **Concerning contrast medium nephrotoxicity**

A. **True**
> *Ch. 74 Renal Failure and Transplantation, p. 1676.*

B. **False**
> *Ch. 74 Renal Failure and Transplantation, p. 1676.*

C. **True**
> *Ch. 74 Renal Failure and Transplantation, p. 1676.*

D. **True**
> *Ch. 74 Renal Failure and Transplantation, p. 1676.*

E. **False** There is some evidence that N-acetyloysteine is protective.
> *Ch. 74 Renal Failure and Transplantation, p. 1676.*

A **6.85** **The following pathologies and nephrographic appearances are associated**

A. **True** It may persist for 24 hours or longer.
> *Ch. 74 Renal Failure and Transplantation, p. 1677.*

B. **True**
> *Ch. 74 Renal Failure and Transplantation, p. 1677.*

C. **True** This is also associated with an increasingly dense nephrogram.
> *Ch. 74 Renal Failure and Transplantation, p. 1677.*

D. **True**
> *Ch. 74 Renal Failure and Transplantation, p. 1677.*

E. **True**
> *Ch. 74 Renal Failure and Transplantation, p. 1677.*

A **6.86** **Concerning acquired cystic disease of the kidneys**

A. **True**
> *Ch. 74 Renal Failure and Transplantation, p. 1677.*

B. **True** Occasionally pain from cyst rupture and haematuria may occur.
> *Ch. 74 Renal Failure and Transplantation, p. 1677.*

C. **True** This is rare.
> *Ch. 74 Renal Failure and Transplantation, p. 1677.*

D. **True**
> *Ch. 74 Renal Failure and Transplantation, p. 1677.*

E. **False**
> *Ch. 74 Renal Failure and Transplantation, p. 1677.*

Q **6.87**   **The following conditions preclude kidney donation**

    A. Pelvicalyceal duplication.
    B. Horseshoe kidney.
    C. Papillary necrosis.
    D. Bilateral reflux nephropathy.
    E. Large solitary renal cyst.

Q **6.88**   **Concerning imaging in renal transplantation**

    A. The donor right kidney is usually placed in the recipient's left iliac fossa and vice versa.
    B. Transplant renal artery stenosis may occur as early as 6 weeks post-transplantation.
    C. An ipsilateral approach is usually adequate when performing transplant angiography.
    D. Ciclosporin A toxicity is reliably distinguished from other causes of renal impairment on MRI.
    E. Most lymphoceles resolve spontaneously.

(Answers overleaf)

A **6.87** The following conditions preclude kidney donation

A. False

Ch. 74 Renal Failure and Transplantation, p. 1678.

B. True

Ch. 74 Renal Failure and Transplantation, p. 1678.

C. True

Ch. 74 Renal Failure and Transplantation, p. 1678.

D. True

Ch. 74 Renal Failure and Transplantation, p. 1678.

E. False

Ch. 74 Renal Failure and Transplantation, p. 1678.

A **6.88** Concerning imaging in renal transplantation

A. True Owing to the easier vascular anastomoses with this arrangement. The normal anatomy is vein anterior pelvic posterior and artery in the middle. This is reversed using the technique above.
Ch. 74 Renal Failure and Transplantation, p. 1679.

B. True

Ch. 74 Renal Failure and Transplantation, p. 1681.

C. True

Ch. 74 Renal Failure and Transplantation, p. 1682.

D. False The distinction between acute rejection, acute tubular necrosis and ciclosporin A toxicity is best made with biopsy. All imaging modalities have difficulty distinguishing these conditions.
Ch. 74 Renal Failure and Transplantation, p. 1684.

E. True

Ch. 74 Renal Failure and Transplantation, p. 1685.

Q **6.89** Concerning renal anomalies in children

A. Bilateral renal agenesis is associated with marked oligohydramnios.
B. Ectopic kidney may present as a mass adjacent to the thyroid in the neck.
C. In horseshoe kidney, the pelves and ureters usually pass posteriorly behind the fused lower poles.
D. There is an increased incidence of vesico-ureteric reflux into the crossed kidney in crossed fused renal ectopia.
E. A pancake kidney lies flat between right lobe of liver and chest wall.

Q **6.90** Indications for micturating cysto-urethrography include

A. All boys under 1 year of age who have had a urinary-tract infection.
B. Ureteric dilation in infants.
C. Renal failure of undetermined cause.
D. Infant screening in whom an older sibling has vesico-ureteric reflux.
E. Potter's syndrome.

Q **6.91** Concerning micturating cysto-urethrography technique in children

A. A 14–18 Fr catheter is usually used.
B. A balloon catheter is preferable to a feeding tube.
C. Images of the urethra are best achieved with the catheter in situ.
D. Iohexol 350 mg per ml is used.
E. Oblique voiding views of the male urethra are mandatory.

(Answers overleaf)

A **6.89**   Concerning renal anomalies in children

A. True   There is a high incidence of pulmonary hypoplasia in addition.
        Ch. 76 Imaging of the Kidneys and Urinary Tract in Children, p. 1720.

B. False   It may pass through diaphragm to lie behind the heart.
        Ch. 76 Imaging of the Kidneys and Urinary Tract in Children, p. 1721.

C. False
        Ch. 76 Imaging of the Kidneys and Urinary Tract in Children, p. 1721.

D. True
        Ch. 76 Imaging of the Kidneys and Urinary Tract in Children, p. 1722.

E. False   Pancake kidney occurs when both kidneys fail to migrate from the pelvis and
        fuse in situ.
        Ch. 76 Imaging of the Kidneys and Urinary Tract in Children, p. 1722.

A **6.90**   Indications for micturating cysto-urethrography include

A. True
        Ch. 76 Imaging of the Kidneys and Urinary Tract in Children, p. 1723.

B. True
        Ch. 76 Imaging of the Kidneys and Urinary Tract in Children, p. 1723.

C. True
        Ch. 76 Imaging of the Kidneys and Urinary Tract in Children, p. 1723.

D. True
        Ch. 76 Imaging of the Kidneys and Urinary Tract in Children, p. 1723.

E. False
        Ch. 76 Imaging of the Kidneys and Urinary Tract in Children, p. 1723.

A **6.91**   Concerning micturating cysto-urethrography technique in children

A. False   A 6 Fr tube suits most circumstances.
        Ch. 76 Imaging of the Kidneys and Urinary Tract in Children, p. 1723.

B. False   A balloon may obstruct adequate visualization of the urethra.
        Ch. 76 Imaging of the Kidneys and Urinary Tract in Children, p. 1724.

C. False   The catheter is removed to allow anterior urethral pathology such as
        syringocele to be imaged.
        Ch. 76 Imaging of the Kidneys and Urinary Tract in Children, p. 1724.

D. False   One hundred and forty milligrams per ml is a suitable concentration.
        Ch. 76 Imaging of the Kidneys and Urinary Tract in Children, p. 1724.

E. True
        Ch. 76 Imaging of the Kidneys and Urinary Tract in Children, p. 1724.

Q **6.92** Causes of bilateral prenatal hydronephrosis

    A. Bilateral vesico-ureteric reflux.
    B. Neurogenic bladder.
    C. Marfan syndrome.
    D. Posterior urethral valves.
    E. Multicystic kidney on one side and cystic dysplastic kidney on the other.

Q **6.93** Causes of bilateral hyper-reflective kidneys in the neonate

    A. Laurence Moon Biedl syndrome.
    B. Congenital cytomegalovirus infection.
    C. Maternal warfarin ingestion.
    D. Xanthogranulomatous pyelonephritis.
    E. Nephroblastomatosis.

Q **6.94** Regarding benign renal tumours in children

    A. Nephroblastomatosis is associated with an increased risk of nephroblastoma (Wilm's tumour).
    B. Diffuse nephroblastomatosis looks like lymphoma on renal ultrasound.
    C. Mesoblastic nephroma does not metastasize.
    D. Multi-locular cystic nephroma is treated with nephrectomy because of its malignant potential.
    E. Angiomyolipoma may invade renal vein and inferior vena cava.

(Answers overleaf)

A **6.92**   **Causes of bilateral prenatal hydronephrosis**

A. True
> *Ch. 76 Imaging of the Kidneys and Urinary Tract in Children, p. 1730.*

B. True
> *Ch. 76 Imaging of the Kidneys and Urinary Tract in Children, p. 1730.*

C. False
> *Ch. 76 Imaging of the Kidneys and Urinary Tract in Children, p. 1730.*

D. True
> *Ch. 76 Imaging of the Kidneys and Urinary Tract in Children, p. 1730.*

E. True
> *Ch. 76 Imaging of the Kidneys and Urinary Tract in Children, p. 1730.*

A **6.93**   **Causes of bilateral hyper-reflective kidneys in the neonate**

A. True
> *Ch. 76 Imaging of the Kidneys and Urinary Tract in Children, p. 1733.*

B. True
> *Ch. 76 Imaging of the Kidneys and Urinary Tract in Children, p. 1733.*

C. False
> *Ch. 76 Imaging of the Kidneys and Urinary Tract in Children, p. 1733.*

D. False   This occurs later in childhood.
> *Ch. 76 Imaging of the Kidneys and Urinary Tract in Children, p. 1733.*

E. True
> *Ch. 76 Imaging of the Kidneys and Urinary Tract in Children, p. 1733.*

A **6.94**   **Regarding benign renal tumours in children**

A. True
> *Ch. 76 Imaging of the Kidneys and Urinary Tract in Children, p. 1757.*

B. True
> *Ch. 76 Imaging of the Kidneys and Urinary Tract in Children, p. 1757.*

C. True
> *Ch. 76 Imaging of the Kidneys and Urinary Tract in Children, p. 1757.*

D. True
> *Ch. 76 Imaging of the Kidneys and Urinary Tract in Children, p. 1757.*

E. True
> *Ch. 76 Imaging of the Kidneys and Urinary Tract in Children, p. 1758.*

Q **6.95**   Cause of increased renal medullary reflectivity in children include

A. Silicosis.

B. Klinefelter syndrome.

C. Renal tubular acidosis.

D. *Candida albicans* infection.

F Autosomal recessive polycystic kidney disease.

(Answers overleaf)

255

A **6.95**   **Cause of increased renal medullary reflectivity in children include**

A. **False**

Ch. 76 Imaging of the Kidneys and Urinary Tract in Children, p. 1763.

B. **False**

Ch. 76 Imaging of the Kidneys and Urinary Tract in Children, p. 1763.

C. **True**

Ch. 76 Imaging of the Kidneys and Urinary Tract in Children, p. 1763.

D. **True**

Ch. 76 Imaging of the Kidneys and Urinary Tract in Children, p. 1763.

E. **True**

Ch. 76 Imaging of the Kidneys and Urinary Tract in Children, p. 1763.

7 The skeletal system

Q 7.1 Regarding general radiology for skeletal trauma

A. Most fractures are apparent clinically.

B. Soft tissue injuries are not well demonstrated.

C. Two orthogonal views are required to fully characterize lesions.

D. Skeletal scintigraphy utilizes a phosphate analogue to assess osteoclastic activity.

E. CT is more sensitive and specific for detection of fractures of the face.

Q 7.2 Regarding MRI in trauma

A. MRI is not sensitive to acute changes in bone marrow.

B. The patient has to be moved during the different sequences.

C. On T1-weighted fat suppressed images fluid will appear of high signal intensity.

D. T2-weighted fat suppression usually makes intramedullary lesions more conspicuous.

E. MRI is acceptable for assessing damage to articular cartilage.

(Answers overleaf)

A **7.1** Regarding general radiology for skeletal trauma

A. True
> *Ch. 78 Skeletal Trauma, p. 1777.*

B. False
> *Ch. 78 Skeletal Trauma, p. 1777.*

C. True
> *Ch. 78 Skeletal Trauma, p. 1777.*

D. False Uptake on a radiopharmeceutical (usually a phosphate analogue) is related to *osteoblastic* activity; the radioactive tracer is attached to the phosphate compound and incorporated into the new bone as it is built, thus lesions with a high rate of bone turnover will demonstrate increased tracer activity.
> *Ch. 78 Skeletal Trauma, p. 1777.*

E. True
> *Ch. 78 Skeletal Trauma, p. 1778.*

A **7.2** Regarding MRI in trauma

A. False
> *Ch. 78 Skeletal Trauma, p. 1778.*

B. False Multiplanar orthogonal and non-orthogonol views can easily be obtained.
> *Ch. 78 Skeletal Trauma, p. 1778.*

C. False Fluid appears dark on T1-weighted images whether they are fat suppressed or non-fat suppressed.
> *Ch. 78 Skeletal Trauma, p. 1778.*

D. True
> *Ch. 78 Skeletal Trauma, p. 1778.*

E. True
> *Ch. 78 Skeletal Trauma, p. 1778.*

Q 7.3   Regarding fractures

A. A fracture in osteoporotic bone is defined as a *pathological fracture*.
B. Metastatic disease is the most common underlying process in which pathological fractures occur.
C. Pathological fractures are rare in Paget's disease and renal osteodystrophy.
D. Transversely orientated fractures are typical in abnormal bone.
E. Pseudofractures are a recognized feature of Paget's disease.

Q 7.4   Regarding the aetiology of fractures

A. Stress fractures are often difficult to diagnose at the initial presentation.
B. The pubic ramus is a common location for stress fractures.
C. A *fatigue fracture* is a stress fracture that occurs in otherwise normal bone.
D. An *insufficiency fracture* is a stress fracture that occurs in osteopenic bone.
E. A stress fracture can occur anywhere where chronic repetitive stress is placed on bone.

(Answers overleaf)

A **7.3** **Regarding fractures**

A. True A pathological fracture occurs in weakened bone and, therefore, requires substantially less force. Pathological fractures may occur in bones with underlying metabolic problems, e.g. osteoporosis, osteomalacia, etc. and in certain circumstances across tumours whether primary or secondary.
Ch. 78 Skeletal Trauma, p. 1778.

B. True Metastatic disease is the most common underlying process in which pathological fractures occur. It must be remembered that pathological fractures may occur through benign tumours such as enchondroma or solitary bone cyst.
Ch. 78 Skeletal Trauma, p. 1778.

C. False In diffuse bony diseases such as Paget's disease, renal osteodystrophy or osteogenesis impefecta there is increased risk of pathological fracture.
Ch. 78 Skeletal Trauma, p. 1778.

D. True
Ch. 78 Skeletal Trauma, p. 1778.

E. True In the context of patients with osteomalacia – fibrous dysplasia and Paget's disease small transversely orientated cortical fractures – so-called 'pseudo-fractures' can be demonstrated.
Ch. 78 Skeletal Trauma, p. 1778.

A **7.4** **Regarding the aetiology of fractures**

A. True Stress fractures occur due to chronic repetitive trauma ultimately resulting in structural failure of bone. Such injuries may be difficult to diagnose at initial presentation and may only be demonstrated radiographically by subtle periosteal reaction or a transverse band of linear sclerosis which may develop after 1–2 weeks after the onset of injury.
Ch. 78 Skeletal Trauma, p. 1778.

B. True Other common locations include the femoral neck, tibia and fibular shafts and the tuberosity of the calcaneum.
Ch. 78 Skeletal Trauma, p. 1778.

C. True
Ch. 78 Skeletal Trauma, p. 1778.

D. True
Ch. 78 Skeletal Trauma, p. 1778.

E. True
Ch. 78 Skeletal Trauma, p. 1778.

Q 7.5 Regarding neuropathic joint disease

A. Destruction of the joint is a recognized feature.

B. The neuropathic joint demonstrates increased density and heterotopic new bone formation.

C. The neuropathic joint usually demonstrates joint marginal lucencies.

D. Frank dislocation is rare.

E. Debris around a neuropathic joint raises the possibility of infection especially in diabetics.

Q 7.6 Concerning injuries to the pelvis

A. If a pelvic fracture is suspected a routine PA view is indicated.

B. Judet's views are valuable for assessing the anterior and posterior walls of the acetabulum.

C. Lateral compressive forces usually result in fractures of the iliac crest and pubic bone.

D. The Malgaigne complex is usually produced by vertical sheer forces.

E. Stable pelvic fractures are unlikely to produce urethral injuries.

(Answers overleaf)

A 7.5 Regarding neuropathic joint disease

A. True
> *Ch. 78 Skeletal Trauma, p. 1778.*

B. True
> *Ch. 78 Skeletal Trauma, p. 1778.*

C. False The neuropathic joint demonstrates marked sclerosis.
> *Ch. 78 Skeletal Trauma, p. 1778.*

D. False Dislocation is a typical finding of a neuropathic joint.
> *Ch. 78 Skeletal Trauma, p. 1778.*

E. False Debris is a typical finding of a neuropathic joint per se.
> *Ch. 78 Skeletal Trauma, p. 1778.*

A 7.6 Concerning injuries to the pelvis

A. False Routine views are AP and maybe augmented by a variety of oblique views.
> *Ch. 78 Skeletal Trauma, p. 1780.*

B. True
> *Ch. 78 Skeletal Trauma, p. 1780.*

C. True These fractures maybe associated with a sacral fracture. Their displacement is uncommon with these injuries.
> *Ch. 78 Skeletal Trauma, p. 1781.*

D. True Vertical sheer forces often result in a particular pattern of injury (Malgaigne complex) in which the fracture of the medial ilium or sacrum is seen in conjunction with fractures of the superior and inferior rami on the ipsilateral side. Superior displacement of the affected hemipelvis and hip usually results.
> *Ch. 78 Skeletal Trauma, p. 1782.*

E. False Urethral injury is associated typically with stable pelvic fractures, though unstable fractures may also produce urethral injury. The injury is usually produced by straddling an object (e.g. bicycle).
> *Ch. 78 Skeletal Trauma, p. 1782.*

Q **7.7** The following muscles and bony sites are associated with avulsion injuries

A. Avulsion of the anterior inferior iliac spine and the sartorius muscle.

B. Avulsion of the anterior superior iliac spine and the straight head of rectus femoris.

C. The hamstring muscles and the ischial tuberosity.

D. Avulsion of the obturator internus muscle and the inferior ischial ramus.

E. Avulsion of the iliopsoas and the lesser of the femur trochanter.

Q **7.8** Match the following fracture classification with its description

A. Open fracture: a fracture which communicates with the outside environment.

B. A complete fracture: this is a fracture extending across the bone to involve both cortices.

C. A comminuted fracture: a fracture that divides into more than two separate fragments.

D. A segmental fracture: an injury that divides the bone into three usually transverse fragments.

E. A butterfly fragment: a large triangular fragment of bone associated with an incomplete fracture.

(Answers overleaf)

A **7.7** The following muscles and bony sites are associated with avulsion injuries

A. False Avulsion of the anterior superior iliac spine is related to sartorius injury.
Ch. 78 Skeletal Trauma, p. 1782.

B. False Avulsion of the anterior inferior iliac spine and the reflected head of rectus femoris.
Ch. 78 Skeletal Trauma, p. 1783.

C. True
Ch. 78 Skeletal Trauma, p. 1783.

D. False
Ch. 78 Skeletal Trauma, p. 1783.

E. True
Ch. 78 Skeletal Trauma, p. 1783.

A **7.8** Match the following fracture classification with its description

A. True
Ch. 78 Skeletal Trauma, p. 1784.

B. True
Ch. 78 Skeletal Trauma, p. 1784.

C. True
Ch. 78 Skeletal Trauma, p. 1784.

D. True
Ch. 78 Skeletal Trauma, p. 1785.

E. False
Ch. 78 Skeletal Trauma, p. 1785.

Q **7.9**   **The following radiographic views are recommended for the shoulder joint**

A. AP radiographs in internal and external rotation of the arm.
B. A Grashey view.
C. An axial view.
D. A 'Y' view.
E. The 'Kitty Clark' view.

Q **7.10**   **Regarding shoulder dislocation**

A. Forced adduction and internal rotation produce an anterior dislocation.
B. Sixty per cent of shoulder dislocations show anterior dislocation of the humeral head.
C. In most cases of anterior dislocation the humeral head lies anterior to the acromion process.
D. In approximately 2% of patients there is an impaction fracture of the posterior humeral head on the inferior glenoid.
E. If the anterior inferior glenoid rim is fractured it is referred to as a Bankhart lesion.

(Answers overleaf)

265

A **7.9** The following radiographic views are recommended for the shoulder joint

A, True The routine radiographic evaluation of the shoulder should include AP views in both internal and external rotation – although many authors suggest this is not common practice. The typical view is an oblique coronal where the scapular blade is parallel to the film plate – the so called AP view (which is actually oblique!).
Ch. 78 Skeletal Trauma, p. 1788.

B. True This is an augmented AP view, which is truly tangential to the glenohumeral joint.
Ch. 78 Skeletal Trauma, p. 1788.

C. True This view requires abduction of the arm and can be difficult in patients with pain – it is often the case that if this view can be performed there is little identifiable pathology in the shoulder joint.
Ch. 78 Skeletal Trauma, p. 1789.

D. True This is the transcapular view, which projects along the long axis of the scapula approximately 20° off true lateral.
Ch. 78 Skeletal Trauma, p. 1786.

E. False There is no Kitty Clark view, though there is an excellent book that is to be found in most casualty X-ray departments giving most of the standard and non-standard views of the shoulder joint.
Ch. 78 Skeletal Trauma, p. 1789.

A **7.10** Regarding shoulder dislocation

A. False A frequent mechanism of anterior dislocation involves forced abduction and external rotation of the arm.
Ch. 78 Skeletal Trauma, p. 1789.

B. False The vast majority (90%) are anterior dislocations of the humeral head.
Ch. 78 Skeletal Trauma, p. 1789.

C. False In most instances the humeral head lies beneath the coracoid process and is referred to as a subcoracoid dislocation.
Ch. 78 Skeletal Trauma, p. 1789.

D. False About 20% of the time the anterior shoulder dislocation results in impaction fracture of the posterior superior humeral head when it strikes the inferior glenoid after coming to rest in the sub coracoid position. This indentation is termed the Hill-Sachs fracture and is best seen on the internal rotational axillary views.
Ch. 78 Skeletal Trauma, p. 1789.

E. True A Bankhart lesion is a fracture of the anterior inferior glenoid labrum.
Ch. 78 Skeletal Trauma, p. 1789.

Q 7.11   Concerning posterior dislocation of the shoulder

    A.   These account for approximately 20% of shoulder dislocations.

    B.   The diagnosis of posterior dislocation is more straightforward than anterior dislocation.

    C.   Typically the humerus is fixed in internal rotation.

    D.   The 'lightbulb' sign is a characteristic radiological feature.

    E.   Widening of the joint space greater than 6 mm may be detected on the Grashey view.

Q 7.12   Concerning rotator cuff disease

    A.   Trauma is the commonest cause of rotator cuff tear in a younger patient.

    B.   The commonest muscle to be involved is the infraspinatus.

    C.   On T2-weighted MR images there is usually an area of high signal intensity within 2 cm of the supraspinatus attachment to the greater tuberosity.

    D.   Full-thickness tears may be confused with the 'magic angle' phenomenon on T2-weighted images.

    E.   Most tears in the supraspinatus tendon occur at the insertion onto the greater tubercle.

(Answers overleaf)

A **7.11** Concerning posterior dislocation of the shoulder

A. False They account for approximately 5% of cases and in half of these they usually are related to seizures or electrocution; in these cases bilateral dislocation may occur.
Ch. 78 Skeletal Trauma, p. 1789.

B. False Diagnosis of posterior dislocation on the routine AP shoulder radiograph is often difficult.
Ch. 78 Skeletal Trauma, p. 1789.

C. True In this position of internal rotation the humeral head appears to resemble a 'lightbulb' – the 'lightbulb' sign.
Ch. 78 Skeletal Trauma, p. 1789.

D. True
Ch. 78 Skeletal Trauma, p. 1789.

E. True
Ch. 78 Skeletal Trauma, p. 1790.

A **7.12** Concerning rotator cuff disease

A. True
Ch. 78 Skeletal Trauma, p. 1790.

B. False The supraspinatus.
Ch. 78 Skeletal Trauma, p. 1790.

C. True
Ch. 78 Skeletal Trauma, p. 1790.

D. False The magic angle phenomenon is best demonstrated on T1 – and proton density – weighted images and is a positional artefact of tendon.
Ch. 78 Skeletal Trauma, p. 1790.

E. False
Ch. 78 Skeletal Trauma, p. 1790.

Q 7.13 Concerning shoulder trauma

A. Most scapular injuries occur in the neck or the body.
B. Most clavicular fractures occur within the medial 3rd.
C. Stress views are unnecessary to diagnose grade 3 acromioclavicular separation.
D. CT is the preferred method of imaging for sternoclavicular dislocation.
E. Anterior dislocation of the clavicle is the most common form of dislocation.

Q 7.14 Concerning trauma to the upper limb

A. Fractures of the mid shaft of the humerus are commonest in the elderly.
B. Fractures of the mid humeral shaft are usually due to severe trauma in non-pathological bone.
C. An angulated fracture of the mid shaft of the humerus may damage the radial artery.
D. Most radial head fractures are orientated vertically.
E. Displacement of the posterior fatpad is pathognomonic for a fracture of the radial head.

(Answers overleaf)

A **7.13** Concerning shoulder trauma

A. True Most scapular fractures are located in the scapular neck or body. Ipsilateral upper rib and clavicle fractures, pulmonary contusion, and pleural effusion are often seen in association with a scapular fracture.
Ch. 78 Skeletal Trauma, p. 1791.

B. False Middle 3rd.
Ch. 78 Skeletal Trauma, p. 1798.

C. True Grade 3 acromioclavicular injuries involve disruption of the acromioclavicular ligaments and the coracoclavicular ligaments the criteria on plain radiograph for a grade 3 injury is upward subluxation in the non-weight-bearing view.
Ch. 78 Skeletal Trauma, p. 1791.

D. True
Ch. 78 Skeletal Trauma, p. 1792.

E. True The less common posterior displacement is more dangerous is because it could injure the great vessels at the thoracic inlet.
Ch. 78 Skeletal Trauma, p. 1792.

A **7.14** Concerning trauma to the upper limb

A. False Fractures of the proximal humerus are most common in the elderly; the surgical neck of the humerus is the most typical location.
Ch. 78 Skeletal Trauma, p. 1793.

B. True
Ch. 78 Skeletal Trauma, p. 1793.

C. False The radial artery is not formed in the upper.
Ch. 78 Skeletal Trauma, p. 1793.

D. True Falls on the outstretched hand in an adult may result in radial head fracture, which is usually orientated vertically. All may cause radial head fracture, which tends to be impacted and slightly angulated.
Ch. 78 Skeletal Trauma, p. 1793.

E. False The anterior and posterior fatpad signs can be demonstrated when there is an elbow effusion. Given the correct clinical setting this is very supportive of a fracture, though certainly not pathognomonic.
Ch. 78 Skeletal Trauma, p. 1795.

Q 7.15 Concerning trauma of the upper limb

A. Fractures of the capitellum usually result from valgus impaction forces.
B. Olecranon fractures are usually due to either a direct blow or an avulsion injury due to vigorous contraction of the triceps muscle.
C. Anterior dislocation of the ulna is extremely rare.
D. Traumatic avulsion of the ulnar collateral ligament is associated with impaction fractures to the radiocapitellar joint.
E. Collateral ligament injury around the elbow joint is best appreciated on coronal MRI images.

Q 7.16 Concerning fractures of the forearm

A. A nightstick injury refers usually to a midshaft radial fracture.
B. A fracture of one bone usually necessitates fracture or displacement of the other.
C. A Monteggia fracture is a fracture of the proximal ulna with dislocation of the radial head.
D. A Galeazzi fracture is a fracture of the distal ulna with distal radial dislocation.
E. A Colles' fracture is the same as a reverse Galeazzi fracture.

Q 7.17 Match the age with the wrist fracture

A. Fracture of distal radius: children.
B. Fractures of the distal radius: adults over 40.
C. Fractures of the scaphoid bone: teenagers and young adults.
D. Carpal fractures: greater than 45 years old.
E. Pisiform fracture: under 12 years old.

(Answers overleaf)

A **7.15**   Concerning trauma of the upper limb

A. **True**
> *Ch. 78 Skeletal Trauma, p. 1795.*

B. **True**
> *Ch. 78 Skeletal Trauma, p. 1795.*

C. **True**   Most dislocations are posterior in relation to the radius and ulna.
> *Ch. 78 Skeletal Trauma, p. 1795.*

D. **True**   These are best appreciated on MRI.
> *Ch. 78 Skeletal Trauma, p. 1795.*

E. **True**
> *Ch. 78 Skeletal Trauma, p. 1796.*

A **7.16**   Concerning fractures of the forearm

A. **False**   A nightstick injury is due to a direct blow on the forearm and usually results in a midshaft ulnar fracture.
> *Ch. 78 Skeletal Trauma, p. 1796.*

B. **True**
> *Ch. 78 Skeletal Trauma, p. 1796.*

C. **True**
> *Ch. 78 Skeletal Trauma, p. 1796.*

D. **False**   A Galeazzi fracture is a dorsally angulated distal radial fracture seen in conjunction with the dorsal dislocation of the distal ulnar. Both the Monteggia and Galeazzi fracture classically occur when the patient falls onto the flexed arm.
> *Ch. 78 Skeletal Trauma, p. 1796.*

E. **False**
> *Ch. 78 Skeletal Trauma, p. 1798.*

A **7.17**   Match the age with the wrist fracture

A. **True**
> *Ch. 78 Skeletal Trauma, p. 1797.*

B. **True**
> *Ch. 78 Skeletal Trauma, p. 1797.*

C. **True**
> *Ch. 78 Skeletal Trauma, p. 1797.*

D. **False**
> *Ch. 78 Skeletal Trauma, p. 1797.*

E. **False**
> *Ch. 78 Skeletal Trauma, p. 1797.*

Q **7.18**   Match the following wrist fracture with its eponymous term

A. Colles' fracture: fracture of the distal radius with dorsal angulation.

B. Smith's fracture: a volarly angulated distal radial fragment.

C. Barton's fracture: a displaced fracture of the volar lip of the distal radius without involvement of the dorsal lip.

D. Hutchinson's fracture: a fracture of the ulnar styloid process

E. Jones' fracture: fracture of the base of the 5th metacarpal.

Q **7.19**   Regarding fractures around the wrist joint

A. The pronator quadratus sign suggests an acute distal forearm fracture.

B. The scaphoid bone only accounts for approximately 40% of carpal fractures.

C. Most scaphoid fractures occur in the distal 3rd.

D. If there is doubt concerning a fracture of the scaphoid a radiograph obtained 7–10 days is now not regarded as necessary.

E. Early osteonecrosis of the distal pole of the scaphoid is best detected by PET.

(Answers overleaf)

A **7.18** **Match the following wrist fracture with its eponymous term**

A. True   The term Colles' fracture is often inappropriately used to refer to any fracture of the distal radius resulting from a fall on the outstretched hand. It is important that the radiologist avoids the use of eponymous names as they can be somewhat misleading. In almost every situation, a description of the injury will avoid potential confusion. Unfortunately, some clinicians still use these terms.
Ch. 78 Skeletal Trauma, p. 1797.

B. True
Ch. 78 Skeletal Trauma, p. 1799.

C. True
Ch. 78 Skeletal Trauma, p. 1799.

D. False   It is an isolated fracture of the distal radial styloid process.
Ch. 78 Skeletal Trauma, p. 1799.

E. False   This is an ankle injury (metatarsal).
Ch. 78 Skeletal Trauma, p. 1799.

A **7.19** **Regarding fractures around the wrist joint**

A. True   An indirect sign of an acute forearm fracture is displacement of the pronator quadratus fat plane.
Ch. 78 Skeletal Trauma, p. 1799.

B. False   The scaphoid bone accounts for 75% of carpal fractures.
Ch. 78 Skeletal Trauma, p. 1799.

C. False   Most scaphoid fractures are non-displaced transverse fractures through the middle or waist of the scaphoid.
Ch. 78 Skeletal Trauma, p. 1799.

D. False   By 7–10 days local osteoclasis will have occurred to widen the fracture line and make it perceptible.
Ch. 78 Skeletal Trauma, p. 1799.

E. False   Osteonecrosis occurs in the proximal fragment and is due to damage of the blood supply from the recurrent artery that enters the distal scaphoid and supplies the bone from distal to proximal.
Ch. 78 Skeletal Trauma, p. 1800.

Q **7.20**   Concerning fractures of the carpus

A. Sclerosis of the proximal fragment of a scaphoid fracture suggests ischaemia.

B. Fractures of the triquetrum account for approximately 15% of carpal bone fractures.

C. Trapezium fractures are typically horizontal.

D. Disruption of the scapholunate and lunotriquetral ligaments are the commonest soft-tissue injuries.

E. Wrist arthrography is as accurate as MRI for assessing the integrity of the carpal ligaments.

Q **7.21**   Regarding fractures to the spine

A. The 'swimmers view' is necessary to see the upper 3 thoracic vertebra.

B. Compression fractures are the commonest injury to the thoracic spine.

C. Fracture dislocation most commonly occurs in the upper thoracic spine and lower lumbar spine.

D. The Chance fracture is associated with significant vertebral body compression.

E. Isolated fractures of the posterior elements are common isolated injuries.

(Answers overleaf)

A **7.20** Concerning fractures of the carpus

A. True
Ch. 78 Skeletal Trauma, p. 1800.

B. True The most common pattern of this injury is a small avulsion fragment from the dorsal surface of the bone at the attachment site of the dorsal radiocarpal ligament.
Ch. 78 Skeletal Trauma, p. 1801.

C. False Trapezium fractures occur secondarily to abduction and hyperextension of the thumb and manifest as vertical fractures in the lateral aspect of the bone.
Ch. 78 Skeletal Trauma, p. 1801.

D. True These ligaments are important soft-tissue injuries.
Ch. 78 Skeletal Trauma, p. 1801.

E. True Recent studies have shown that MRI can be as accurate to assess the scapholunate and lunotriquetral ligaments though it should be born in mind that the cost of such procedure versus a simple arthrogram is significantly different. Moreover, the clinical relevance of such disruption is still a subject of much debate.
Ch. 78 Skeletal Trauma, p. 1801.

A **7.21** Regarding fractures to the spine

A. True
Ch. 78 Skeletal Trauma, p. 1828.

B. True
Ch. 78 Skeletal Trauma, p. 1828.

C. False These dislocations occur in the lower thoracic spine and upper lumbar spine.
Ch. 78 Skeletal Trauma, p. 1830.

D. False
Ch. 78 Skeletal Trauma, p. 1832.

E. False Isolated fractures of the posterior elements are unusual with the exception of those involving the transverse processes.
Ch. 78 Skeletal Trauma, p. 1832.

Q **7.22** Concerning the general characteristics of benign bone lesions

A. Histopathology is required in all cases.

B. The histopathological diagnosis must be in accordance with the radiological report.

C. The responsibility for the final diagnosis rests with the histopathologist.

D. Core biopsy is mandatory in benign lesions.

E. Benign lesions may require chemotherapy.

Q **7.23** The following are recognized features of benign bone lesions

A. Less than 10 years old.

B. Solitary lesions.

C. Giant cell tumours and chondroblastomas metastasize.

D. A Lodwick type III pattern.

E. A thick well-defined periosteal reaction.

(Answers overleaf)

A **7.22**   Concerning the general characteristics of benign bone lesions

A. False
> *Ch. 79 Bone Tumours (1): General Characteristics, Benign Lesions, p. 1835.*

B. True
> *Ch. 79 Bone Tumours (1): General Characteristics, Benign Lesions, p. 1835.*

C. True
> *Ch. 79 Bone Tumours (1): General Characteristics, Benign Lesions, p. 1835.*

D. False
> *Ch. 79 Bone Tumours (1): General Characteristics, Benign Lesions, p. 1835.*

E. True
> *Ch. 79 Bone Tumours (1): General Characteristics, Benign Lesions, p. 1836.*

A **7.23**   The following are recognized features of benign bone lesions

A. False
> *Ch. 79 Bone Tumours (1): General Characteristics, Benign Lesions, p. 1836.*

B. False   Benign tumours are generally solitary, though multiple lesions including chondromas and angiomas are also benign.
> *Ch. 79 Bone Tumours (1): General Characteristics, Benign Lesions, p. 1837.*

C. True
> *Ch. 79 Bone Tumours (1): General Characteristics, Benign Lesions, p. 1837.*

D. False   There are three typical patterns that are useful indicators of the rate of growth of bone: The Lodwick Classification (from I-III) takes into account the zone of transition. Typically, a well-demarcated lesion obtains a Lodwick I and suggests it is a relatively benign lesion. The Lodwick III pattern is composed of multiple coalescing small ill-defined lesions with a poor zone of transition and extending over several centimetres of bone. The Lodwick II rests between I-III and gives a moth-eaten type pattern of bony appearances.
> *Ch. 79 Bone Tumours (1): General Characteristics, Benign Lesions, p. 1837.*

E. False
> *Ch. 79 Bone Tumours (1): General Characteristics, Benign Lesions, p. 1838.*

Q 7.24   Regarding the benign bone tumour – chondroma

A. Enchondromas typically affect the hands and feet in 50% of cases.
B. Sixty per cent of chondromas in the hands present as fractures.
C. Men are significantly more affected than women.
D. The carpal bones are affected in approximately 40% of cases.
E. The ratio of chondrosarcomas to chondromas presenting outside the hands and feet is 5.1.

Q 7.25   Concerning benign tumours of chondroid origin

A. Chondromas rarely occur in the soft tissue.
B. Multiple enchondromas associated with soft-tissue angiomas are typical of Ollier's disease.
C. Ollier's disease is typically unilateral.
D. The metaphyses are typically dysplastic in diaphyseal aclasis.
E. Malignant generation in diaphyseal aclasis occurs in approximately 10% of patients.

Q 7.26   Concerning chondroblastoma

A. The lesion typically occurs in the diaphysis.
B. Most tumours affect the immature skeleton.
C. Pain is the predominant presenting feature.
D. The main differential diagnosis is a giant cell tumour.
E. There is a high recurrence rate after curettage.

(Answers overleaf)

A **7.24**   Regarding the benign bone tumour – chondroma

A. True
> *Ch. 79 Bone Tumours (1): General Characteristics, Benign Lesions, p. 1839.*

B. True
> *Ch. 79 Bone Tumours (1): General Characteristics, Benign Lesions, p. 1839.*

C. False
> *Ch. 79 Bone Tumours (1): General Characteristics, Benign Lesions, p. 1839.*

D. False   Carpal bones are rarely affected.
> *Ch. 79 Bone Tumours (1): General Characteristics, Benign Lesions, p. 1839.*

E. True
> *Ch. 79 Bone Tumours (1): General Characteristics, Benign Lesions, p. 1840.*

A **7.25**   Concerning benign tumours of chondroid origin

A. True
> *Ch. 79 Bone Tumours (1): General Characteristics, Benign Lesions, p. 1840.*

B. False   This is a typical finding of Maffucci syndrome.
> *Ch. 79 Bone Tumours (1): General Characteristics, Benign Lesions, p. 1840.*

C. True
> *Ch. 79 Bone Tumours (1): General Characteristics, Benign Lesions, p. 1840.*

D. True
> *Ch. 79 Bone Tumours (1): General Characteristics, Benign Lesions, p. 1842.*

E. True   This is probably an overestimation.
> *Ch. 79 Bone Tumours (1): General Characteristics, Benign Lesions, p. 1842.*

A **7.26**   Concerning chondroblastoma

A. False   This is typically a epiphyseal lesion of a long bone.
> *Ch. 79 Bone Tumours (1): General Characteristics, Benign Lesions, p. 1843.*

B. True
> *Ch. 79 Bone Tumours (1): General Characteristics, Benign Lesions, p. 1843.*

C. True
> *Ch. 79 Bone Tumours (1): General Characteristics, Benign Lesions, p. 1842.*

D. False   The radiological differential diagnosis in a typical age group is relatively straightforward as few other neoplasms are confined to the epiphysis. However, subchrondral cysts may have to be considered. Giant cell tumours are rare in children.
> *Ch. 79 Bone Tumours (1): General Characteristics, Benign Lesions, p. 1844*

E. False
> *Ch. 79 Bone Tumours (1): General Characteristics, Benign Lesions, p. 1845.*

Q **7.27**   Concerning tumours of osteoid origin

A. Bone islands are typically located within the cortex.
B. Ivory osteomas commonly affect the paranasal sinuses.
C. Osteoid osteomas are most common in the 2nd and 3rd decades.
D. The commonest site for osteoid osteoma is in the lower limbs.
E. The commonest spinal site for osteoblastoma is in the vertebral arch.

Q **7.28**   Concerning cysts of bone

A. A simple bone cyst is typically unilocular.
B. Over 90% of simple bone cysts occur under the age of 20 years.
C. The 'falling fragment' sign is virtually pathognomonic for bone cyst.
D. The majority of aneurysmal bone cysts occur below the age of 20 years.
E. The typical site for an aneurysmal bone cyst is the metaphysis.

Q **7.29**   Concerning giant cell tumours

A. Most lesions are locally aggressive.
B. Local recurrence after curretage occurs in 50% of patients.
C. Most patients are under 20 years old.
D. A tumour is highly unlikely in the subcortical region of a fused apophysis.
E. Less than 1% of giant cell tumours produce lung metastasis.

(Answers overleaf)

A **7.27** Concerning tumours of osteoid origin

A. False
> *Ch. 79 Bone Tumours (1): General Characteristics, Benign Lesions, p. 1846.*

B. True
> *Ch. 79 Bone Tumours (1): General Characteristics, Benign Lesions, p. 1846.*

C. True
> *Ch. 79 Bone Tumours (1): General Characteristics, Benign Lesions, p. 1846.*

D. True
> *Ch. 79 Bone Tumours (1): General Characteristics, Benign Lesions, p. 1847.*

E. True
> *Ch. 79 Bone Tumours (1): General Characteristics, Benign Lesions, p. 1850.*

A **7.28** Concerning cysts of bone

A. False
> *Ch. 79 Bone Tumours (1): General Characteristics, Benign Lesions, p. 1852.*

B. True
> *Ch. 79 Bone Tumours (1): General Characteristics, Benign Lesions, p. 1852.*

C. True
> *Ch. 79 Bone Tumours (1): General Characteristics, Benign Lesions, p. 1853.*

D. True
> *Ch. 79 Bone Tumours (1): General Characteristics, Benign Lesions, p. 1853.*

E. True
> *Ch. 79 Bone Tumours (1): General Characteristics, Benign Lesions, p. 1853.*

A **7.29** Concerning giant cell tumours

A. True
> *Ch. 79 Bone Tumours (1): General Characteristics, Benign Lesions, p. 1855.*

B. True
> *Ch. 79 Bone Tumours (1): General Characteristics, Benign Lesions, p. 1855.*

C. False
> *Ch. 79 Bone Tumours (1): General Characteristics, Benign Lesions, p. 1846.*

D. False Giant cell tumours are nearly always found towards the end of the margin of bone, either in the subarticular region or in the subcortical region of a fused apophysis.
> *Ch. 79 Bone Tumours (1): General Characteristics, Benign Lesions, p. 1857.*

E. True
> *Ch. 79 Bone Tumours (1): General Characteristics, Benign Lesions, p. 1857.*

Q **7.30**   Concerning benign bone lesions

A. Size is the only criteria that differentiates a fibrous cortical defect from a non-ossifying fibroma.

B. The typical site for a post traumatic cortical desmoid tumour (Bufkin lesion) is at the insertion of the lateral head of Gastrocnemius.

C. In massive osteolysis (Gorham's disease) there is little or no evidence of callus formation.

D. Fibrous dysplasia is typically painful.

E. Metastases are more common than benign lesions.

Q **7.31**   The following are associated

A. The talus: attaches to abductor digiti minimi.

B. Talar fracture: osteonecrosis of the proximal fragment.

C. Avulsion fractures of the neck of the talus: avascular necrosis of the talus.

D. Osteochrondral fractures of the talar dome: commonly missed on plain radiographs.

E. Boehler's angle: normal range is between 28% and 40%.

(Answers overleaf)

A **7.30**   **Concerning benign bone lesions**

A. True
> *Ch. 79 Bone Tumours (1): General Characteristics, Benign Lesions, p. 1858.*

B. False
> *Ch. 79 Bone Tumours (1): General Characteristics, Benign Lesions, p. 1860.*

C. True
> *Ch. 79 Bone Tumours (1): General Characteristics, Benign Lesions, p. 1863.*

D. False   Unlike many bone tumours fibrous dysplasia is not usually painful unless fracture has occurred. Most lesions are benign and indolent.
> *Ch. 79 Bone Tumours (1): General Characteristics, Benign Lesions, p. 1866.*

E. True
> *Ch. 79 Bone Tumours (1): General Characteristics, Benign Lesions, p. 1837.*

A **7.31**   **The following are associated**

A. False   The talus has no muscular or tendonus attachments.
> *Ch. 78 Skeletal Trauma, p. 1813.*

B. True   Most of the blood supply to the talar dome enters through the more distal talus, a fracture of the talar neck can result in osteonecrosis of the dome.
> *Ch. 78 Skeletal Trauma, p. 1813.*

C. False   Avulsion fractures of the dorsal surface of the head and neck of the talus are not uncommon.
> *Ch. 78 Skeletal Trauma, p. 1813.*

D. True   MRI is the imaging modality of choice.
> *Ch. 78 Skeletal Trauma, p. 1813.*

E. True   Boehler's angle is formed by the intersection of lines drawn on the lateral view form the anterior superior and posterior superior edges of the calcaneus to the highest point of the articular surface.
> *Ch. 78 Skeletal Trauma, p. 1813.*

Q 7.32   Regarding fractures of the midfoot and forefoot

A. Fractures of the dorsal surface of the navicular are rare.
B. The Lisfranc injury is frequently seen in the diabetic foot.
C. The Lisfranc injury may be divergent or homolateral.
D. The march fracture has a seasonal variation.
E. Freiberg's infraction is seen in the 3rd metatarsal head.

Q 7.33   Regarding spinal injuries

A. Image reconstruction is usually required when CT has been performed.
B. There is a direct correlation between the MR signal characteristics and the histopathology of spinal cord trauma.
C. Isolated fractures of the vertebral body or posterior elements are usually stable.
D. Unstable fractures arise from multilevel injury.
E. Lumbar spine haematomas are easily demonstrated on AP radiographs.

(Answers overleaf)

285

A **7.32**   **Regarding fractures of the mid foot and forefoot**

A. False   These are the commonest avulsion injuries of the mid and forefoot.
Ch. 78 Skeletal Trauma, p. 1814.

B. True
Ch. 78 Skeletal Trauma, p. 1814.

C. True   Lisfranc injuries are classified into homolateral (in which all the metatarsals are shifted laterally) or divergent (in which the 1st metatarsal shifts medially and the remainder of the forefoot shifts laterally).
Ch. 78 Skeletal Trauma, p. 1814.

D. False   The March fracture refers to marching rather than the month.
Ch. 78 Skeletal Trauma, p. 1814.

E. False
Ch. 78 Skeletal Trauma, p. 1814.

A **7.33**   **Regarding spinal injuries**

A. True
Ch. 78 Skeletal Trauma, p. 1816.

B. True
Ch. 78 Skeletal Trauma, p. 1816.

C. True
Ch. 78 Skeletal Trauma, p. 1820.

D. False
Ch. 78 Skeletal Trauma, p. 1820.

E. False   The haematomas present have retropharyngeal masses in the cervical spine and paraspinal mass on the frontal projection in the dorsal spine but are difficult to identify in the lumbar spine because they are the same density as the para spinal muscles.
Ch. 78 Skeletal Trauma, p. 1820.

Q **7.34** **The following are common sites for fractures and dislocations of the spine**

    A. C4 to C7.
    B. C1 to C2.
    C. L4 to S1.
    D. T3 to T10.
    E. T10 to L2.

Q **7.35** **The following are associated in spinal injuries**

    A. Flexion: anterior wedge fracture.
    B. Extension injury: Pars fracture.
    C. Flexion distraction fracture: Chance fracture.
    D. Distraction (tension injury): tetter–totter fracture.
    E. Shearing injury: anterior fracture dislocation.

(Answers overleaf)

A **7.34** **The following are common sites for fractures and dislocations of the spine**

A. True

Ch. 78 Skeletal Trauma, p. 1816,

B. True

Ch. 78 Skeletal Trauma, p. 1816.

C. False

Ch. 78 Skeletal Trauma, p. 1816.

D. False

Ch. 78 Skeletal Trauma, p. 1816.

E. True

Ch. 78 Skeletal Trauma, p. 1816.

A **7.35** **The following are associated in spinal injuries**

A. True

Ch. 78 Skeletal Trauma, p. 1819.

B. True

Ch. 78 Skeletal Trauma, p. 1819.

C. False

Ch. 78 Skeletal Trauma, p. 1819.

D. False A flexion distraction injury is a tetter–totter fracture whereas a distraction (tension injury) is a Chance fracture.
Ch. 78 Skeletal Trauma, p. 1819.

E. True

Ch. 78 Skeletal Trauma, p. 1819.

Q 7.36   Regarding fractures of the atlas (C1)

A. A gap in the neural arch of C1 is a typical normal variant.
B. A posterior arch fracture is the commonest injury to C1.
C. The Jefferson fracture is typically produced by hanging.
D. A hyperflexion injury typically produces a fracture of the posterior arch at C1.
E. On an AP radiograph, unilateral offset of the lateral mass of C1 is typically positional.

Q 7.37   Concerning fractures of the axis (C2)

A. Traumatic spondylolysis of the axis results from a hyperflexion fall.
B. The Hangman's fracture is associated with dislocation of C2 on C3.
C. The Hangman's fracture typically produces severe compromise of the spinal canal.
D. A low fracture of the dens is difficult to identify on frontal radiographs.
E. Multidetector CT is the best technique to image dens fractures.

(Answers overleaf)

A 7.36   Regarding fractures of the atlas (C1)

A. True
> *Ch. 78 Skeletal Trauma, p. 1821.*

B. True
> *Ch. 78 Skeletal Trauma, p. 1821.*

C. False   The Jefferson fracture is an uncommon injury characterized by disruption of the anterior and posterior arches of the atlas.
> *Ch. 78 Skeletal Trauma, p. 1822.*

D. False   This is an hyperextension injury.
> *Ch. 78 Skeletal Trauma, p. 1822.*

E. False   A tilting or rotation of the head may produce unilateral offset, but this should be associated with the corresponding inset of the lateral masses on the contralateral side. If this is not demonstrated then a non-tilted view should be undertaken.
> *Ch. 78 Skeletal Trauma, p. 1822.*

A 7.37   Concerning fractures of the axis (C2)

A. False   This is typically from a hyperextension fall – the Hangman's fracture.
> *Ch. 78 Skeletal Trauma, p. 1822.*

B. True
> *Ch. 78 Skeletal Trauma, p. 1823.*

C. False   The neurological consequences of the Hangman's fracture are often less severe than might be anticipated. Firstly, the normal cervical cord occupies only approximately one-third to a half of the AP diameter of the normal spinal canal at this level. Secondly, the bilateral isthmus fracture produces decompression of the canal rather than compromise.
> *Ch. 78 Skeletal Trauma, p. 1823.*

D. True   Type 3 or low fractures of the dens may not be evident on the frontal projection except by noting the dens is tilted by 7° or more off the vertical axis on the body of C2 on the lateral radiograph.
> *Ch. 78 Skeletal Trauma, p. 1823.*

E. True   Plain film tomography is usually superior to CT in the detection of subtle dens fractures because fracture line may lie precisely in the plain of the CT images cut. A low dens fracture has a 35% incidence of non-union. (Many centres do not use tomography, therefore, CT is the best.)
> *Ch. 78 Skeletal Trauma, p. 1823.*

Q **7.38** **The following are associations in fractures of the cervical spine**

    A. The extension teardrop fracture: fracture of the anterior inferior corner of the body of C3.

    B. The extension teardrop fracture: severe neurological deficit.

    C. Torticollis: a unilateral facet dislocation.

    D. Burst fracture: mandatory CT.

    E. Teardrop fracture: spinal cord injury.

Q **7.39** **The following are features of hyperextension fracture dislocation of the cervical spine**

    A. Disruption of the lateral column.

    B. Disorganization of the articular masses.

    C. Flattened facet joints

    D. Interfacetal dislocation.

    E. An anterior teardrop.

(Answers overleaf)

A **7.38** The following are associations in fractures of the cervical spine

A. False The extension teardrop fracture is a fracture of the anterior inferior body of C2 avulsed by the intact anterior longitudinal ligament.
Ch. 78 Skeletal Trauma, p. 1824.

B. False
Ch. 78 Skeletal Trauma, p. 1824.

C. False Torticollis is also known as rotational subluxational physiological dislocation of the atlanto-axial relationship, this results in a very confusing radiographic appearance as neither true subluxation or dislocation occurs at the atlanto-axial articulation.
Ch. 78 Skeletal Trauma, p. 1824.

D. True
Ch. 78 Skeletal Trauma, p. 1824.

E. True The teardrop fracture is a fracture dislocation due to flexion and axial compression. These are usually associated with spinal cord injury.
Ch. 78 Skeletal Trauma, p. 1825.

A **7.39** The following are features of hyperextension fracture dislocation of the cervical spine

A. True
Ch. 78 Skeletal Trauma, p. 1826.

B. True
Ch. 78 Skeletal Trauma, p. 1826.

C. True
Ch. 78 Skeletal Trauma, p. 1826.

D. True
Ch. 78 Skeletal Trauma, p. 1826.

E. False
Ch. 78 Skeletal Trauma, p. 1826.

Q **7.40**   **Regarding fractures of the cervical spine**

  A. Fractures are commonly associated with hyperflexion sprain.
  B. The hyperflexion sprain demonstrates fanning of the posterior elements.
  C. A hyperextension injury in spondylosis may produce cord injury with minimal trauma.
  D. The clayshoveller's fracture demonstrates avulsion of the transverse process of C6, C7, or T1.
  E. The whiplash injury is typically unstable.

Q **7.41**   **Concerning skeletal metastases**

  A. About 10% of metastases are solitary.
  B. A solitary metastasis is more common than a primary neoplasm at any age.
  C. Fifty per cent of metastases to the hands are from bronchial tumours.
  D. Most breast tumours are osteolytic.
  E. Prostate metastases are predominantly osteoblastic or mixed.

(Answers overleaf)

A **7.40**   **Regarding fractures of the cervical spine**

A. False
> *Ch. 78 Skeletal Trauma, p. 1827.*

B. True
> *Ch. 78 Skeletal Trauma, p. 1827.*

C. True
> *Ch. 78 Skeletal Trauma, p. 1827.*

D. False The spinous process.
> *Ch. 78 Skeletal Trauma, p. 1828.*

E. False
> *Ch. 78 Skeletal Trauma, p. 1828.*

A **7.41**   **Concerning skeletal metastases**

A. True
> *Ch. 80 Bone Tumours (2): Malignant Lesions, p. 1869.*

B. True
> *Ch. 80 Bone Tumours (2): Malignant Lesions, p. 1870.*

C. True
> *Ch. 80 Bone Tumours (2): Malignant Lesions, p. 1871.*

D. True
> *Ch. 80 Bone Tumours (2): Malignant Lesions, p. 1873.*

E. True
> *Ch. 80 Bone Tumours (2): Malignant Lesions, p. 1873.*

Q **7.42**   **The following tumours usually cause lytic metastases**

    A. Renal carcinoma.
    B. Thyroid carcinoma.
    C. Stomach carcinoma.
    D. Carcinoma of the uterine body.
    E. Melanoma.

Q **7.43**   **The following favour the diagnosis of metastasis rather than primary tumour of bone**

    A. Diaphyseal location.
    B. Florid periosteal reaction.
    C. Absence of tumour bone formation.
    D. Vertebral body involvement.
    E. Absence of vertebral pedicular involvement.

(Answers overleaf)

A **7.42**   The following tumours usually cause lytic metastases

A. True
   Ch. 80 Bone Tumours (2): Malignant Lesions, p. 1874.

B. True
   Ch. 80 Bone Tumours (2): Malignant Lesions, p. 1874.

C. True
   Ch. 80 Bone Tumours (2): Malignant Lesions, p. 1874.

D. False   Carcinoma of the uterine body is typically adenocarcinoma and like that the
   ovary may produce blastic metastases particularly of the vertebra.
   Ch. 80 Bone Tumours (2): Malignant Lesions, p. 1874.

E. True
   Ch. 80 Bone Tumours (2): Malignant Lesions, p. 1874.

A **7.43**   The following favour the diagnosis of metastasis rather than primary tumour of bone

A. True
   Ch. 80 Bone Tumours (2): Malignant Lesions, p. 1875.

B. False
   Ch. 80 Bone Tumours (2): Malignant Lesions, p. 1875.

C. True
   Ch. 80 Bone Tumours (2): Malignant Lesions, p. 1875.

D. True
   Ch. 80 Bone Tumours (2): Malignant Lesions, p. 1875.

E. False
   Ch. 80 Bone Tumours (2): Malignant Lesions, p. 1875.

Q 7.44 Concerning chondrosarcoma

A. Angiography is helpful for assessing the tumour.
B. A periosteal reaction is identifiable in upto 50% of patients.
C. Cortical thickness is usually decreased.
D. A cartilage cap of greater than 20 mm is likely to be malignant.
E. Chondrosacomas respond well to radiotherapy and cytotoxic drugs

Q 7.45 Concerning osteosarcoma

A. Osteosarcoma is the commonest primary malignant tumour of bone after myeloma.
B. Eighty per cent of patients are older than 25 years.
C. There is a second peak incidence towards middle age.
D. The tumour typically elevates the serum acid phosphatase.
E. Regional lymph nodes are not usually involved early in the disease.

(Answers overleaf)

A **7.44** Concerning chondrosarcoma

A. False Most chondrosarcomas are poorly vascularized. Angiography is usually non-specific and unhelpful.
Ch. 80 Bone Tumours (2): Malignant Lesions, p. 1870.

B. True
Ch. 80 Bone Tumours (2): Malignant Lesions, p. 1879.

C. False Despite cortical scalloping the laying down apositional new bone by the periosteum usually means that the cortical thickness is increased.
Ch. 80 Bone Tumours (2): Malignant Lesions, p. 1879.

D. True Most osteochondromas have cartilage caps no thicker than 5 mm. A cap in excess of 20 mm is likely to be malignant.
Ch. 80 Bone Tumours (2): Malignant Lesions, p. 1879.

E. False
Ch. 80 Bone Tumours (2): Malignant Lesions, p. 1880.

A **7.45** Concerning osteosarcoma

A. True
Ch. 80 Bone Tumours (2): Malignant Lesions, p. 1881.

B. False
Ch. 80 Bone Tumours (2): Malignant Lesions, p. 1881.

C. True
Ch. 80 Bone Tumours (2): Malignant Lesions, p. 1881.

D. False The tumour accounts for more than 75% of osteosarcomas. Elevation of the serum alkaline phosphatase may occur with larger tumours.
Ch. 80 Bone Tumours (2): Malignant Lesions, p. 1881.

E. True
Ch. 80 Bone Tumours (2): Malignant Lesions, p. 1881.

Q **7.46**   Concerning osteogenic tumours

A. Osteosarcoma typically arises in the diaphysis.
B. Sunburst spiculation is characteristic of osteosarcoma.
C. Codman's triangles are specific for primary bone tumours.
D. A CT is mandatory to exclude the presence of lung metastases in patients with osteogenic sarcoma.
E. Parosteal osteosarcoma is more common than periosteal osteosarcoma.

Q **7.47**   Concerning tumours arising in Paget's disease

A. Osteosarcoma is the commonest type.
B. Osteosarcoma in Paget's disease has a better prognosis than in normal bone.
C. Giant cell tumours are well recognized.
D. Malignant fibrous histiocytomas are rare.
E. The fibula is a common site.

Q **7.48**   The following are necessary to establish a diagnosis of radiation induced skeletal sarcoma

A. A previously normal radiograph.
B. A latent period of at least 10 years.
C. Radiological evidence of lytic and blastic changes.
D. Most patients have had in excess of 60 Gy.
E. Malignant fibrous histiocytoma is one of the commonest radiation induced tumours.

(Answers overleaf)

A **7.46**   **Concerning osteogenic tumours**

A. False   This tumour typically arises from the metaphysis.
Ch. 80 Bone Tumours (2): Malignant Lesions, p. 1882.

B. True   Sunburst spiculation is characteristic, but not specific.
Ch. 80 Bone Tumours (2): Malignant Lesions, p. 1882.

C. False
Ch. 80 Bone Tumours (2): Malignant Lesions, p. 1882.

D. True
Ch. 80 Bone Tumours (2): Malignant Lesions, p. 1884.

E. True
Ch. 80 Bone Tumours (2): Malignant Lesions, p. 1886.

A **7.47**   **Concerning tumours arising in Paget's disease**

A. True
Ch. 80 Bone Tumours (2): Malignant Lesions, p. 1887.

B. False
Ch. 80 Bone Tumours (2): Malignant Lesions, p. 1887.

C. False
Ch. 80 Bone Tumours (2): Malignant Lesions, p. 1887.

D. False
Ch. 80 Bone Tumours (2): Malignant Lesions, p. 1887.

E. False
Ch. 80 Bone Tumours (2): Malignant Lesions, p. 1887.

A **7.48**   **The following are necessary to establish a diagnosis of radiation induced skeletal sarcoma**

A. True   Histopathological evidence of the nature of pre-existing benign lesion, or in the case of incidental radiation, a previous normal radiograph.
Ch. 80 Bone Tumours (2): Malignant Lesions, p. 1887.

B. False   A latent period of at least 4 years (range 4–40 years with an average of 11 years).
Ch. 80 Bone Tumours (2): Malignant Lesions, p. 1888.

C. False   Though radiological evidence is highly suggestive, histological evidence is required.
Ch. 80 Bone Tumours (2): Malignant Lesions, p. 1888.

D. False   Although the precise threshold dosage is unknown most patients have received in excess of 30 Gy.
Ch. 80 Bone Tumours (2): Malignant Lesions, p. 1887.

E. True   Osteosarcoma, MFH (malignant fibrous histiocytoma) and fibrosarcoma are the most frequently reported.
Ch. 80 Bone Tumours (2): Malignant Lesions, p. 1888.

Q 7.49   Concerning tumours of marrow origin

    A. Most patients with Ewing's sarcoma are under the age of 20 years old.
    B. Ewing's sarcoma has a greater predilection for the lower skeleton.
    C. Saucerization is a typical radiological finding.
    D. Ewing's sarcoma is readily differentiated from osteomyelitis.
    E. Ewing's sarcoma metastasizes early in the disease to lungs.

Q 7.50   Regarding bone tumours

    A. 5-HIAA (5-hydroxyindoleaceticacid) levels are typically elevated in patients with neuroblastoma.
    B. A chordoma may occur in ribs.
    C. Adamantinoma may occur in the midshaft of the fibula.
    D. Most primary lymphomas of bone are high-grade malignancy.
    E. Primary bone tumours are commoner in the elderly than the young patient.

(Answers overleaf)

A **7.49** Concerning tumours of marrow origin

A. **True** Seventy five per cent are under the age of 20 years old, most between 5–15 years old.
Ch. 80 Bone Tumours (2): Malignant Lesions, p. 1890.

B. **True**
Ch. 80 Bone Tumours (2): Malignant Lesions, p. 1891.

C. **True**
Ch. 80 Bone Tumours (2): Malignant Lesions, p. 1891.

D. **False**
Ch. 80 Bone Tumours (2): Malignant Lesions, p. 1892.

E. **False** The prognosis for Ewing's sarcoma is not improved to the same extent as osteosarcoma. The poor prognosis is probably due to the extent of the marrow spread and the early pulmonary spread.
Ch. 80 Bone Tumours (2): Malignant Lesions, p. 1892.

A **7.50** Regarding bone tumours

A. **False** The levels of vanyl mandellic acid and other urinary catecolamines are usually elevated.
Ch. 80 Bone Tumours (2): Malignant Lesions, p. 1894.

B. **False**
Ch. 80 Bone Tumours (2): Malignant Lesions, p. 1895.

C. **False** This is a rare tumour typically involving the midshaft of the tibia.
Ch. 80 Bone Tumours (2): Malignant Lesions, p. 1895.

D. **True**
Ch. 80 Bone Tumours (2): Malignant Lesions, p. 1893.

E. **True**
Ch. 80 Bone Tumours (2): Malignant Lesions, p. 1895.

Q **7.51** **Concerning thalassaemia**

    A. Thalassaemia major has a good prognosis.
    B. Cardiac enlargement occurs before hepatosplenomegaly.
    C. The anterior ends of the ribs are grossly expanded.
    D. The ethmoid air cells are typically spared.
    E. Diffuse bony sclerosis is typical.

Q **7.52** **The following produce the Erlenmeyer flask deformity**

    A. Gaucher's disease.
    B. Thalassaemia major.
    C. Osteopetrosis.
    D. Morquio's syndrome.
    E. Fallot's pentalogy

(Answers overleaf)

A **7.51** Concerning thalassaemia

A. False Thalassaemia major is severe anaemia in infants and young children with high mortality.
Ch. 81 Myeloproliferative and Similar Disorders, p. 1901

B. False The typical changes are rodent-like facies and hepatosplenomegaly. In later childhood cardiac enlargement tends to mirror the degree of anaemia.
Ch. 81 Myeloproliferative and Similar Disorders, p. 1902.

C. False Posterior ends.
Ch. 81 Myeloproliferative and Similar Disorders, p. 1901.

D. True The ethmoid air cells contain no red bone marrow.
Ch. 81 Myeloproliferative and Similar Disorders, p. 1902.

E. False The bony features are typically osteopenia.
Ch. 81 Myeloproliferative and Similar Disorders, p. 1902.

A **7.52** The following produce the Erlenmeyer flask deformity

A. True
Ch. 81 Myeloproliferative and Similar Disorders, p. 1902.

B. True
Ch. 81 Myeloproliferative and Similar Disorders, p. 1902.

C. True
Ch. 81 Myeloproliferative and Similar Disorders, p. 1902.

D. False
Ch. 81 Myeloproliferative and Similar Disorders, p. 1902.

E. False
Ch. 81 Myeloproliferative and Similar Disorders, p. 1902.

Q **7.53** **Concerning sickle cell disease**

A. Congenital malaria affords protection against sickle cell disease.
B. Cardiomegaly is a typical feature of the homozygous sickle cell subject.
C. Hepatosplenomegaly is typically in adults.
D. Bony crisis are typical in the hands and feet during infancy and childhood.
E. Muscle infarction is a typical finding in Hb S-S disease.

Q **7.54** **The radiological changes of sickle cell disease are**

A. Early skeletal maturation.
B. Marrow hyperplasia.
C. Bone infarction.
D. Soft-tissue calcification.
E. Secondary osteomyelitis.

(Answers overleaf)

305

A **7.53** Concerning sickle cell disease

A. False Invasion of affected erythrocytes by the malarial parasite causes them to sickle. They are removed from the circulation by the spleen. The merozoites are not, therefore, released into the systemic circulation affording some protection against malaria.
Ch. 81 Myeloproliferative and Similar Disorders, p. 1904.

B. True Cardiomegaly is present in 80% of homozygous sickle cell patients.
Ch. 81 Myeloproliferative and Similar Disorders, p. 1904.

C. False Splenomegaly is found up to the age of 10 years old in S-S disease, but infrequently thereafter, as a result of repeated splenic infarction.
Ch. 81 Myeloproliferative and Similar Disorders, p. 1904.

D. True
Ch. 81 Myeloproliferative and Similar Disorders, p. 1904.

E. True
Ch. 81 Myeloproliferative and Similar Disorders, p. 1904.

A **7.54** The radiological changes of sickle cell disease are

A. False
Ch. 81 Myeloproliferative and Similar Disorders, p. 1905.

B. True
Ch. 81 Myeloproliferative and Similar Disorders, p. 1905.

C. True
Ch. 81 Myeloproliferative and Similar Disorders, p. 1905.

D. False
Ch. 81 Myeloproliferative and Similar Disorders, p. 1905.

E. True
Ch. 81 Myeloproliferative and Similar Disorders, p. 1905.

Q 7.55   The typical leukaemic bone changes in children include

A. Metaphyseal lucencies.
B. Diffuse bone destruction.
C. Osteoblastic lesions
D. Periosteal reaction.
E. Osteolytic lesions.

Q 7.56   Regarding lymphoma

A. Bony changes are indicative of late disease.
B. Approximately 2% of patients with Hodgkin's disease present with a skeletal lesion.
C. Approximately 5% of lesions are solitary.
D. Hodgkin's disease typically preserves the bony cortex and endplates within the vertebral body.
E. Bony involvement is more common in non-Hodgkin's lymphoma.

Q 7.57   Regarding plasma cell disorders

A. Plasmacytoma typically presents below the age of 30 years.
B. The serum electrophoresis is usually normal in patients with plasmacytoma.
C. Most plasmacytoma lesions are typically destructive.
D. Involvement of the vertebral body is a typical finding in plasmacytoma.
E. Extension across the disc space is a common finding for plasmacytoma.

(Answers overleaf)

307

A **7.55**   **The typical leukaemic bone changes in children include**

A. True
> *Ch. 81 Myeloproliferative and Similar Disorders, p. 1909.*

B. True
> *Ch. 81 Myeloproliferative and Similar Disorders, p. 1909.*

C. True
> *Ch. 81 Myeloproliferative and Similar Disorders, p. 1909.*

D. True
> *Ch. 81 Myeloproliferative and Similar Disorders, p. 1909.*

E. True
> *Ch. 81 Myeloproliferative and Similar Disorders, p. 1909.*

A **7.56**   **Regarding lymphoma**

A. True   Involvement of bone, by any criteria, usually indicates extensive or late disease (stage IV). Primary non-Hodgkin's lymphoma of the bone is very unusual. Primary Hodgkin's lymphoma of bone is even rarer.
> *Ch. 81 Myeloproliferative and Similar Disorders, p. 1910.*

B. True   Unlike carcinoma, approximately 2% of patients with Hodgkin's disease present initially with a skeletal lesion.
> *Ch. 81 Myeloproliferative and Similar Disorders, p. 1910.*

C. False   About 30% of skeletal lesions are solitary.
> *Ch. 81 Myeloproliferative and Similar Disorders, p. 1911.*

D. True
> *Ch. 81 Myeloproliferative and Similar Disorders, p. 1911.*

E. True   Bony involvement occurs in 15–25% of all patients.
> *Ch. 81 Myeloproliferative and Similar Disorders, p. 1912.*

A **7.57**   **Regarding plasma cell disorders**

A. False   Few patients present below the age of 40 years, the overall age presentation tends to be earlier than the age range of generalized myelomatosis.
> *Ch. 81 Myeloproliferative and Similar Disorders, p. 1913.*

B. True
> *Ch. 81 Myeloproliferative and Similar Disorders, p. 1913.*

C. True   Sclerosis is very unusual.
> *Ch. 81 Myeloproliferative and Similar Disorders, p. 1913.*

D. True
> *Ch. 81 Myeloproliferative and Similar Disorders, p. 1913.*

E. False
> *Ch. 81 Myeloproliferative and Similar Disorders, p. 1913.*

Q **7.58** **Concerning multiple myeloma**

A. This is the commonest primary malignancy of bone.
B. Widespread skeletal involvement is demonstrated in 40% of patients at presentation.
C. Bence Jones protein is present in the urine in over half the patients presenting with myeloma.
D. Bony lesions appear typically well defined.
E. A typical radiological finding includes generalized osteopenia.

Q **7.59** **The following are associated in patients with Langerhans cell histiocytosis**

A. Letterer-Siwe syndrome: children under 2 years.
B. Letterer-Siwe syndrome: acute visceral involvement.
C. Hand-Schüller-Christian syndrome: exomphalos.
D. Eosinophilic granuloma: vertebra plana.
E. Eosinophilic granuloma: benign self-limiting disease.

(Answers overleaf)

A **7.58**   **Concerning multiple myeloma**

A. True

    Ch. 81 Myeloproliferative and Similar Disorders, p. 1913.

B. False

    Ch. 81 Myeloproliferative and Similar Disorders, p. 1914.

C. True

    Ch. 81 Myeloproliferative and Similar Disorders, p. 1914.

D. True   The classical appearance of myelomatosis consists of well defined 'punched out' lesions throughout the skeleton most characteristic in the skull.
    Ch. 81 Myeloproliferative and Similar Disorders, p. 1914.

E. True

    Ch. 81 Myeloproliferative and Similar Disorders, p. 1915.

A **7.59**   **The following are associated in patients with Langerhans cell histiocytosis**

A. True

    Ch. 81 Myeloproliferative and Similar Disorders, p. 1916.

B. True

    Ch. 81 Myeloproliferative and Similar Disorders, p. 1916.

C. False   The triad of calvarial lesions, *exophthalmos* and diabetes insipidus are not constant, being found in only 10% of cases.
    Ch. 81 Myeloproliferative and Similar Disorders, p. 1916.

D. True

    Ch. 81 Myeloproliferative and Similar Disorders, p. 1917.

E. True

    Ch. 81 Myeloproliferative and Similar Disorders, p. 1918.

Q **7.60** The following are associated as part of the growth plate

A. The reserve zone: non-calcified cartilaginous matrix.
B. The hypertrophic zone: no calcification.
C. The subzone of provisional calcification: the beginning of the radiographically calcified metaphysis.
D. The growth plate: the physis.
E. The zone of primary spongiosa: chondrocyte meiosis.

Q **7.61** Concerning the physiology and anatomy of normal bone

A. The Haversian system is demonstrated throughout the bony medulla.
B. Bone turnover is in the order of 50% per year.
C. 1 alpha, 25 dihydroxy vitamin D is converted in the kidney to its active metabolite.
D. Vitamin D inhibits calcium mobilization from mature bone.
E. Parathyroid hormone requires the presence of vitamin D in order to function.

(Answers overleaf)

311

A **7.60** The following are associated as part of the growth plate

A. True

Ch. 82 Metabolic and Endocrine Disease of the Skeleton, p. 1925.

B. False Hypertrophic zone includes subzones at maturation, degeneration and provisional calcification.

Ch. 82 Metabolic and Endocrine Disease of the Skeleton, p. 1925.

C. True

Ch. 82 Metabolic and Endocrine Disease of the Skeleton, p. 1925.

D. True

Ch. 82 Metabolic and Endocrine Disease of the Skeleton, p. 1925.

E. False In the zone of primary and secondary spongiosa the calcified cartilaginous columns are surrounded by osteoblasts, which produce bone via endochondral bone formation. Furthermore, meiosis is the incorrect term.

Ch. 82 Metabolic and Endocrine Disease of the Skeleton, p. 1925.

A **7.61** Concerning the physiology and anatomy of normal bone

A. False Cortical bone (compact bone) is more dense and has fewer spaces. It is composed of a number of semi cylindrical canals termed the Haversian system. This Haversian system is only present within the cortex not within the medulla.

Ch. 82 Metabolic and Endocrine Disease of the Skeleton, p. 1926.

B. False Bone turnover is 5–10%.

Ch. 82 Metabolic and Endocrine Disease of the Skeleton, p. 1927.

C. False 25 hydroxy cholecalciferol is converted in the kidney to 1 alpha 25-dihydroxy cholecalciferol (1 alpha 25-dihydroxy vitamin D). This step is influenced by the serum phosphate level.

Ch. 82 Metabolic and Endocrine Disease of the Skeleton, p. 1927.

D. False

Ch. 82 Metabolic and Endocrine Disease of the Skeleton, p. 1927.

E. True The converse is also true.

Ch. 82 Metabolic and Endocrine Disease of the Skeleton, p. 1925.

Q 7.62   The following are associated with a general loss of bone density

A. Osteogenesis imperfecta.
B. Addison's disease.
C. Hyperpituitarism.
D. Sickle cell anaemia.
E. Hyperphosphatasia.

Q 7.63   The following influence the loss of skeletal mass

A. The size of skeleton achieved during growth and development.
B. Exercise.
C. Progesterone.
D. Smoking.
E. Weightlessness.

(Answers overleaf)

313

A **7.62** The following are associated with a general loss of bone density

A. True

Ch. 82 Metabolic and Endocrine Disease of the Skeleton, p. 1928.

B. True

Ch. 82 Metabolic and Endocrine Disease of the Skeleton, p. 1928.

C. True

Ch. 82 Metabolic and Endocrine Disease of the Skeleton, p. 1928.

D. False

Ch. 82 Metabolic and Endocrine Disease of the Skeleton, p. 1928.

E. False Hyperphosphatasia gives a radiological finding similar to that of Paget's disease, whereas, hypophosphatasia affects the metabolic pathways of vitamin D producing generalized loss of bone density.
Ch. 82 Metabolic and Endocrine Disease of the Skeleton, p. 1928.

A **7.63** The following influence the loss of skeletal mass

A. True

Ch. 82 Metabolic and Endocrine Disease of the Skeleton, p. 1929.

B. True

Ch. 82 Metabolic and Endocrine Disease of the Skeleton, p. 1929.

C. True Though the dominant hormone is oestrogen in women.
Ch. 82 Metabolic and Endocrine Disease of the Skeleton, p. 1929.

D. False There is no direct link.
Ch. 82 Metabolic and Endocrine Disease of the Skeleton, p. 1929.

E. True

Ch. 82 Metabolic and Endocrine Disease of the Skeleton, p. 1929.

Q **7.64** **The following are typical features of osteoporosis**

    A. Osteopenia.
    B. Loss of cortical definition in the vertebra.
    C. Accentuation of the primary trabeculae.
    D. Biconcave vertebra.
    E. Fractured neck of humerus

Q **7.65** **The following are typical of Cushing's disease**

    A. Normal bone density.
    B. Poor callus formation.
    C. Avascular necrosis in the humeral head.
    D. Delayed skeletal maturation.
    E. Excess soft tissue around the knee joint.

Q **7.66** **The following are recognized features of osteomalacia**

    A. Pseudo fractures.
    B. Scoliosis.
    C. Basilar invagination.
    D. Avascular necrosis of the femoral heads.
    E. High serum calcium.

(Answers overleaf)

A 7.64   The following are typical features of osteoporosis

A. True
> *Ch. 82 Metabolic and Endocrine Disease of the Skeleton, p. 1929.*

B. False   The typical findings are thinning and accentuation of the cortices.
> *Ch. 82 Metabolic and Endocrine Disease of the Skeleton, p. 1929.*

C. True   This is associated with thinning of the secondary trabeculae.
> *Ch. 82 Metabolic and Endocrine Disease of the Skeleton, p. 1929.*

D. True
> *Ch. 82 Metabolic and Endocrine Disease of the Skeleton, p. 1929.*

E. False
> *Ch. 82 Metabolic and Endocrine Disease of the Skeleton, p. 1929.*

A 7.65   The following are typical of Cushing's disease

A. False   Typically the patients are osteoporotic.
> *Ch. 82 Metabolic and Endocrine Disease of the Skeleton, p. 1930.*

B. False   Typically patients with Cushing's disease have exuberant callus formation, which forms increased density around the endplates in vertebral crush fractures.
> *Ch. 82 Metabolic and Endocrine Disease of the Skeleton, p. 1930.*

C. True   Avascular necrosis (osteonecrosis) typically occurs in the femoral head, although it can be demonstrated in many bones throughout the body.
> *Ch. 82 Metabolic and Endocrine Disease of the Skeleton, p. 1930.*

D. True
> *Ch. 82 Metabolic and Endocrine Disease of the Skeleton, p. 1930.*

E. False
> *Ch. 82 Metabolic and Endocrine Disease of the Skeleton, p. 1930.*

A 7.66   The following are recognized features of osteomalacia

A. True
> *Ch. 82 Metabolic and Endocrine Disease of the Skeleton, p. 1933.*

B. True   Scoliosis occasionally develops and the vertebral bodies may assume a bi-concave appearance.
> *Ch. 82 Metabolic and Endocrine Disease of the Skeleton, p. 1933.*

C. True
> *Ch. 82 Metabolic and Endocrine Disease of the Skeleton, p. 1933.*

D. False
> *Ch. 82 Metabolic and Endocrine Disease of the Skeleton, p. 1933.*

E. False
> *Ch. 82 Metabolic and Endocrine Disease of the Skeleton, p. 1933.*

Q 7.67 Concerning rickets

A. The bone changes of neonatal rickets occur around the age of 2 months after birth.
B. Tumour associated rickets is primarily due to calcium loss.
C. Narrowing of the growth plate is a recognized feature.
D. Cupping of the metaphases is a recognized feature.
E. Osteopenia is common.

Q 7.68 The following are causes of rickets in patients under 6 months

A. Biliary atresia.
B. Vitamin-D-dependent rickets.
C. Multiple epiphyseal dysplasia.
D. Mucopolysaccharidoses.
E. Holt-Oram syndrome.

Q 7.69 The following are radiological features of renal osteodystrophy

A. Osteosclerosis.
B. Osteoporosis.
C. Osteopenia.
D. Osteomalacia.
E. Osteopetrosis

(Answers overleaf)

317

A **7.67** Concerning rickets

A. True

Ch. 82 Metabolic and Endocrine Disease of the Skeleton, p. 1933.

D. False Tumour associated rickets is probably related phosphate loss. The typical tumour associated with rickets is a haemangiopericytoma.

Ch. 82 Metabolic and Endocrine Disease of the Skeleton, p. 1933.

C. False A typical imaging finding is widening of the growth plate.

Ch. 82 Metabolic and Endocrine Disease of the Skeleton, p. 1933.

D. True Splaying and cupping of the metaphases and costochondral junctions is a typical finding

Ch. 82 Metabolic and Endocrine Disease of the Skeleton, p. 1934.

E. True

Ch. 82 Metabolic and Endocrine Disease of the Skeleton, p. 1934.

A **7.68** The following are causes of rickets in patients under 6 months

A. True

Ch. 82 Metabolic and Endocrine Disease of the Skeleton, p. 1933.

B. True

Ch. 82 Metabolic and Endocrine Disease of the Skeleton, p. 1933.

C. False

Ch. 82 Metabolic and Endocrine Disease of the Skeleton, p. 1933.

D. False

Ch. 82 Metabolic and Endocrine Disease of the Skeleton, p. 1933.

E. False

Ch. 82 Metabolic and Endocrine Disease of the Skeleton, p. 1933.

A **7.69** The following are radiological features of renal osteodystrophy

A. True

Ch. 82 Metabolic and Endocrine Disease of the Skeleton, p. 1935.

B. True

Ch. 82 Metabolic and Endocrine Disease of the Skeleton, p. 1935.

C. True

Ch. 82 Metabolic and Endocrine Disease of the Skeleton, p. 1935.

D. True

Ch. 82 Metabolic and Endocrine Disease of the Skeleton, p. 1935.

E. False

Ch. 82 Metabolic and Endocrine Disease of the Skeleton, p. 1935.

Q 7.70   Regarding osteodystrophy

A. Brown tumours are a common presentation in patients with primary hyperparathyroidism.
B. Brown tumours have well-defined margins.
C. Fifty per cent of patients develop osteosclerosis.
D. Aluminium toxicity typically produces dense bones.
E. Periarticular calcification is a recognized feature.

Q 7.71   In primary hyperparathyroidism

A. Subperiosteal bone resorption is demonstrated in most patients.
B. Subperiosteal bone resorption typically occurs in the radial aspect of the middle phalanges of the 2nd and 3rd digits.
C. Cortical striations are seen in more than 50% of patients.
D. A giant cell tumour is a recognized feature.
E. Chondrocalcinosis is present in 70% of patients.

Q 7.72   Regarding metabolic bone disease

A. Scurvy results from lack of vitamin A.
B. Radiological changes in scurvy may develop within weeks.
C. Excessive periosteal elevation occurs in patients with scurvy.
D. Acromegaly is associated with scalloped vertebral bodies.
E. Increased height of vertebra in patients with acromegaly.

(Answers overleaf)

319

A **7.70**   **Regarding osteodystrophy**

A. **False**   Brown tumours nowadays are a manifestation of secondary hyperparathyroidism.
Ch. 82 Metabolic and Endocrine Disease of the Skeleton, p. 1936.

B. **True**
Ch. 82 Metabolic and Endocrine Disease of the Skeleton, p. 1936.

C. **False**   From 10 to 20% of patients with renal osteodystrophy develop osteosclerosis.
Ch. 82 Metabolic and Endocrine Disease of the Skeleton, p. 1936.

D. **False**   Aluminium toxicity produces osteopenia, multiple rib fractures and looser's zones.
Ch. 82 Metabolic and Endocrine Disease of the Skeleton, p. 1937.

E. **True**
Ch. 82 Metabolic and Endocrine Disease of the Skeleton, p. 1938.

A **7.71**   **In primary hyperparathyroidism**

A. **False**   Typically this is only seen in 10% of patients.
Ch. 82 Metabolic and Endocrine Disease of the Skeleton, p. 1939.

B. **True**
Ch. 82 Metabolic and Endocrine Disease of the Skeleton, p. 1939.

C. **True**
Ch. 82 Metabolic and Endocrine Disease of the Skeleton, p. 1939.

D. **False**   Typically, the patients develop brown tumours (osteoclastomas). Unfortunately, these look similar to giant cell tumours at microscopy and, therefore, it is important to know the serum calcium in patients with suspected bone tumours.
Ch. 82 Metabolic and Endocrine Disease of the Skeleton, p. 1941.

E. **False**   Chondrocalcinosis occurs in approximately 10–20% of patients.
Ch. 82 Metabolic and Endocrine Disease of the Skeleton, p. 1941.

A **7.72**   **Regarding metabolic bone disease**

A. **False**   This disorder results from long-term deficiency of vitamin C.
Ch. 82 Metabolic and Endocrine Disease of the Skeleton, p. 1941.

B. **False**   Typically it takes 4–6 months.
Ch. 82 Metabolic and Endocrine Disease of the Skeleton, p. 1941.

C. **True**
Ch. 82 Metabolic and Endocrine Disease of the Skeleton, p. 1942.

D. **True**
Ch. 82 Metabolic and Endocrine Disease of the Skeleton, p. 1942.

E. **False**   The vertebral bodies show an increase in the AP dimension, not the height.
Ch. 82 Metabolic and Endocrine Disease of the Skeleton, p. 1948.

Q 7.73 Regarding osteogenesis imperfecta

    A. Most forms are autosomal dominant.
    B. There is diffuse loss in bone density.
    C. Bowed bones are atypical.
    D. Early fusion of the occipitoparietal suture is a radiological feature.
    E. Exuberant callus formation is a radiological feature.

Q 7.74 The following are associated with a generalized decrease in bone density and delayed skeletal maturation

    A. Hypopituitrism.
    B. Hypothyroidism.
    C. Hypogonadism.
    D. Diabetes insipidus.
    E. Multiple epiphyseal dysplasia.

Q 7.75 The following are typical findings in Turner's syndrome

    A. Normal bone density.
    B. Normal skeletal maturation.
    C. Short 5th metacarpal.
    D. Depression of the lateral tibial plateau.
    E. Coarctation of the aorta.

(Answers overleaf)

321

A 7.73   Regarding osteogenesis imperfecta

A. **True**
   Ch. 82 Metabolic and Endocrine Disease of the Skeleton, p. 1945.

B. **True**
   Ch. 82 Metabolic and Endocrine Disease of the Skeleton, p. 1946.

C. **False**   Multiple fractures and bowing of the bones is a typical finding.
   Ch. 82 Metabolic and Endocrine Disease of the Skeleton, p. 1946.

D. **False**   There is normal fusion with wormian bones.
   Ch. 82 Metabolic and Endocrine Disease of the Skeleton, p. 1946.

E. **True**
   Ch. 82 Metabolic and Endocrine Disease of the Skeleton, p. 1946.

A 7.74   The following are associated with a generalized decrease in bone density and delayed skeletal maturation

A. **True**
   Ch. 82 Metabolic and Endocrine Disease of the Skeleton, p. 1949.

B. **True**
   Ch. 82 Metabolic and Endocrine Disease of the Skeleton, p. 1949.

C. **True**
   Ch. 82 Metabolic and Endocrine Disease of the Skeleton, p. 1949.

D. **False**   Diabetes mellitus.
   Ch. 82 Metabolic and Endocrine Disease of the Skeleton, p. 1949.

E. **False**

A 7.75   The following are typical findings in Turner's syndrome

A. **False**   Osteoporosis.
   Ch. 82 Metabolic and Endocrine Disease of the Skeleton, p. 1951.

B. **False**   Delayed skeletal maturation with delayed fusion in the epiphysis.
   Ch. 82 Metabolic and Endocrine Disease of the Skeleton, p. 1951.

C. **False**   Typically short 4th metacarpal.
   Ch. 82 Metabolic and Endocrine Disease of the Skeleton, p. 1951.

D. **False**   Depression of the medial tibial plateau and associated overgrowth in medial femoral condyle.
   Ch. 82 Metabolic and Endocrine Disease of the Skeleton, p. 1951.

E. **True**
   Ch. 82 Metabolic and Endocrine Disease of the Skeleton, p. 1951.

Q **7.76** **The following are typical features of reflex sympathetic dystrophy syndrome**

    A. Patchy osteoporosis.
    B. Soft-tissue swelling.
    C. Bone marrow oedema on MRI.
    D. Endosteal scalloping.
    E. Cortical tunnelling.

Q **7.77** **The following are associated**

    A. Gorham's disease: disappearing bone.
    B. Carpotarsal osteolysis syndrome: nephropathy.
    C. Transient regional osteoporosis: the femoral head and acetabulum are typically involved.
    D. Dense bones: pyknodysostosis.
    E. Fluorosis: enthesopathy

Q **7.78** **The following are associated with dense metaphyseal bands**

    A. Normal variant.
    B. Untreated rickets.
    C. Scurvy.
    D. Hyperthyroidism.
    E. Hypervitaminosis D.

(Answers overleaf)

323

A **7.76** **The following are typical features of reflex sympathetic dystrophy syndrome**

A. True

Ch. 82 Metabolic and Endocrine Disease of the Skeleton, p. 1953.

B. True

Ch. 82 Metabolic and Endocrine Disease of the Skeleton, p. 1953.

C. True

Ch. 82 Metabolic and Endocrine Disease of the Skeleton, p. 1953.

D. True

Ch. 82 Metabolic and Endocrine Disease of the Skeleton, p. 1953.

E. True

Ch. 82 Metabolic and Endocrine Disease of the Skeleton, p. 1953.

A **7.77** **The following are associated**

A. True

Ch. 82 Metabolic and Endocrine Disease of the Skeleton, p. 1956.

B. True

Ch. 82 Metabolic and Endocrine Disease of the Skeleton, p. 1956.

C. False Typically it is the femoral head not the acetabulum.
Ch. 82 Metabolic and Endocrine Disease of the Skeleton, p. 1957.

D. True

Ch. 82 Metabolic and Endocrine Disease of the Skeleton, p. 1958.

E. True

Ch. 82 Metabolic and Endocrine Disease of the Skeleton, p. 1959.

A **7.78** **The following are associated with dense metaphyseal bands**

A. True

Ch. 82 Metabolic and Endocrine Disease of the Skeleton, p. 1963.

B. False Treated rickets.
Ch. 82 Metabolic and Endocrine Disease of the Skeleton, p. 1963.

C. True

Ch. 82 Metabolic and Endocrine Disease of the Skeleton, p. 1963.

D. False Hypothyroidism.
Ch. 82 Metabolic and Endocrine Disease of the Skeleton, p. 1963.

E. True

Ch. 82 Metabolic and Endocrine Disease of the Skeleton, p. 1963.

Q 7.79 The following are associated with hyperostosis of cortical bone

- **A.** Pachydermoperiostosis.
- **B.** Thyroid acropachy.
- **C.** Paget's disease.
- **D.** Infantile cortical hyperostosis.
- **E.** Fibrous dysplasia.

Q 7.80 Regarding abnormalities of the skeleton

- **A.** Skeletal dysplasias are usually a generalized abnormality of bone growth and development.
- **B.** A malformation syndrome has no skeletal involvement.
- **C.** One per cent of live births have a skeletal abnormality.
- **D.** One per cent of skeletal abnormalities are unclassifiable.
- **E.** A precise diagnosis of a skeletal dysplasia can be obtained by antenatal ultrasound.

(Answers overleaf)

A **7.79** The following are associated with hyperostosis of cortical bone

A. True

Ch. 82 Metabolic and Endocrine Disease of the Skeleton, p. 1963.

B. True

Ch. 82 Metabolic and Endocrine Disease of the Skeleton, p. 1963.

C. True

Ch. 82 Metabolic and Endocrine Disease of the Skeleton, p. 1963.

D. True

Ch. 82 Metabolic and Endocrine Disease of the Skeleton, p. 1963.

E. False

Ch. 82 Metabolic and Endocrine Disease of the Skeleton, p. 1963.

A **7.80** Regarding abnormalities of the skeleton

A. True

Ch. 83 Skeletal Dysplasias and Malformation Syndromes, p. 1967.

B. False Malformation syndromes are conditions in which the structural abnormalities are present in several systems, which may include the skeletal system.
Ch. 83 Skeletal Dysplasias and Malformation Syndromes, p, 1967.

C. True

Ch. 83 Skeletal Dysplasias and Malformation Syndromes, p. 1967.

D. False A significant proportion of cases (approximately 30%) are unclassifiable because the combination of findings does not conform to any recognized condition.
Ch. 83 Skeletal Dysplasias and Malformation Syndromes, p. 1967.

E. False Skeletal ultrasounds are highly significant but not very specific and in general it is unwise to offer a precise diagnosis.
Ch. 83 Skeletal Dysplasias and Malformation Syndromes, p. 1968.

Q **7.81** **Concerning skeletal dysplasias and malformation syndromes, the following are associated**

A. Thanatophoric dysplasia: the most common lethal neonatal dysplasia.
B. Achondroplasia : a severe platyspondyly.
C. Achondrogenesis: lethal skeletal dysplasia.
D. Pierre Robin abnormality: Stickler syndrome.
E. Morquio disease: absent odontoid peg.

Q **7.82** **The following are typical features of the syndromes**

A. Dyschondrosteosis (Leri-Weill syndrome): Madelung deformity.
B. Osteogenesis imperfecta: blue sclera.
C. Osteopetrosis: cranial nerve palsies.
D. Osteopoikilosis: the bone resembles running wax.
E. Enchondromatosis (Ollier's disease): Madelung deformity.

(Answers overleaf)

A **7.81**   Concerning skeletal dysplasias and malformation syndromes, the following are associated

A. True

   Ch. 83 Skeletal Dysplasias and Malformation Syndromes, p. 1972.

B. False   Achondroplasia results in a decrease in a decrease in the interpodicular distance in the lumbar spine cordally, short vertebral pedicles and posterior vertebral scallopings.
   Ch. 83 Skeletal Dysplasias and Malformation Syndromes, p. 1973.

C. True

   Ch. 83 Skeletal Dysplasias and Malformation Syndromes, p. 1974.

D. True

   Ch. 83 Skeletal Dysplasias and Malformation Syndromes, p. 1976.

E. True

   Ch. 83 Skeletal Dysplasias and Malformation Syndromes, p. 1979.

A **7.82**   The following are typical features of the syndromes

A. True

   Ch. 83 Skeletal Dysplasias and Malformation Syndromes, p. 1985.

B. True

   Ch. 83 Skeletal Dysplasias and Malformation Syndromes, p. 1985.

C. True

   Ch. 83 Skeletal Dysplasias and Malformation Syndromes, p. 1985.

D. False   This refers to melorheostosis.
   Ch. 83 Skeletal Dysplasias and Malformation Syndromes, p. 1986.

E. True   This gives rise typically to the reverse Madelung deformity.
   Ch. 83 Skeletal Dysplasias and Malformation Syndromes, p. 1990.

Q 7.83   Concerning rheumatoid arthritis

A. Symmetrical soft-tissue swelling is typical.
B. Marginal erosions occurring in the 'bare area' of bones.
C. Subchondral cysts and bone erosions are typical.
D. Joint malalignment without evidence of bony erosions.
E. Generalized osteopenia

Q 7.84   Regarding rheumatoid arthritis

A. Elbow involvement occurs in approximately 10% of patients.
B. Resorption of the proximal clavicle.
C. Focal loss of cartilage around the fovea of the hip joint.
D. Rheumatoid arthritis in the hand is three times as common as rheumatoid arthritis in the foot.
E. Fusion of the sacroiliac joints is occasionally seen.

Q 7.85   Concerning connective-tissue disorders

A. In patients with systemic lupus erythematosus the joint radiographs are frequently normal.
B. Soft-tissue calcification is a common finding in patients with scleroderma.
C. Bone erosions occur in approximately 50% of patients with dermatomyositis.
D. Malalignment is an early feature of multicentric reticulohistiocytosis.
E. Enthesitis is an atypical finding in patients with ankylosing spondylitis.

(Answers overleaf)

329

A **7.83**   Concerning rheumatoid arthritis

A. True
> *Ch. 84A Joint Disease, p. 1995.*

B. True   Marginal erosions are due to inflamed synovium destroying the white cortical line and underlying bone, and they occur firstly at the joint where the synovium is applied to bone that is not covered by cartilage – the so-called bare area.
> *Ch. 84A Joint Disease, p. 1995.*

C. True   Subchondral cysts and bone erosions are typical manifestations of rheumatoid joint destruction.
> *Ch. 84A Joint Disease, p. 1996.*

D. False
> *Ch. 84A Joint Disease, p. 1996.*

E. True   Generalized osteopenia reflects a more chronic stage of the disease. It is accentuated in an older person, women, reduced activity and steroid therapy.
> *Ch. 84A Joint Disease, p. 1996.*

A **7.84**   Regarding rheumatoid arthritis

A. False   Elbow involvement occurs in 50% of patients.
> *Ch. 84A Joint Disease, p. 1998.*

B. False   Typical findings are resorption of the distal clavicle.
> *Ch. 84A Joint Disease, p. 1999.*

C. False   In the hip the early changes are focal loss of cartilage superiorly.
> *Ch. 84A Joint Disease, p. 1999.*

D. False   They are both equally common.
> *Ch. 84A Joint Disease, p. 1999.*

E. True
> *Ch. 84A Joint Disease, p. 2000.*

A **7.85**   Concerning connective-tissue disorders

A. True
> *Ch. 84A Joint Disease, p. 2004.*

B. True
> *Ch. 84A Joint Disease, p. 2005.*

C. False   Joint changes are extremely rare in this disorder.
> *Ch. 84A Joint Disease, p. 2005.*

D. False   Malalignment is not a feature of the disease until late.
> *Ch. 84A Joint Disease, p. 2005.*

E. False
> *Ch. 84A Joint Disease, p. 2006.*

Q **7.86**   Concerning psoriatic arthropathy

A. Forty per cent of patients with psoriasis develop psoriatic arthropathy.
B. The arthritis rarely presents before psoriatic skin changes.
C. A rheumatoid arthritis pattern of disease distribution is the rarest presentation.
D. A sacroiliitis occurs in about 1% of patients with psoriatic arthropathy
E. Bone mineralization is rarely affected.

Q **7.87**   The following are correct associations in patients with joint disease

A. Reiter's syndrome: urethritis.
B. Lyme arthritis: spirochete infection.
C. Chronic tophaceous gout: intraosseous tophi.
D. Chondrocalcinosis: pseudogout.
E. Dialysis arthropathy: amyloid deposition.

(Answers overleaf)

A **7.86** Concerning psoriatic arthropathy

A. False Psoriasis affects about 1% of the population and about 7% of these individuals have psoriatic arthropathy.
Ch. 84A Joint Disease, p. 2009.

B. True
Ch. 84A Joint Disease, p. 2009.

C. False The most common pattern (about 70%) is at a single joint or a few random joints whilst the second pattern is indistinguishable from rheumatoid arthritis (15%). The third, or classic, presentation (5%) is in the distal interphalangeal joints, almost invariably accompanied by no abnormalities. The fourth presentation is a primary spondylisis with or without peripheral joint involvement. The fifth type is with aggressive arthritis mutilans.
Ch. 84A Joint Disease, p. 2009.

D. False Sacroiliitis occurs in approximately 25%.
Ch. 84A Joint Disease, p. 2009.

E. True
Ch. 84A Joint Disease, p. 2010.

A **7.87** The following are correct associations in patients with joint disease

A. True
Ch. 84A Joint Disease, p. 2010.

B. True
Ch. 84A Joint Disease, p. 2010.

C. True
Ch. 84A Joint Disease, p. 2013.

D. True Most people with chondrocalcinosis never have a single acute episode of pseudo gout.
Ch. 84A Joint Disease, p. 2014.

E. True
Ch. 84A Joint Disease, p. 2016.

Q **7.88** **The following are typical causes of neuropathic arthropathy**

    A. Diabetes mellitus.
    B. Yaws.
    C. Syringomyelia.
    D. Herpes zoster infection.
    E. Poliomyelitis.

Q **7.89** **The following are associated with hypertrophic osteoarthropathy**

    A. Bronchogenic carcinoma.
    B. Cystic fibrosis.
    C. Infected aortic grafts.
    D. Mesothelioma.
    E. Graves' disease.

(Answers overleaf)

A **7.88** The following are typical causes of neuropathic arthropathy

A. True

Ch. 84A Joint Disease, p. 2019.

B. False

C. True

Ch. 84A Joint Disease, p. 2019.

D. False

E. False

A **7.89** The following are associated with hypertrophic osteoarthropathy

A. True

Ch. 84A Joint Disease, p. 2024.

B. True

Ch. 84A Joint Disease, p. 2024.

C. True

Ch. 84A Joint Disease, p. 2024.

D. True

Ch. 84A Joint Disease, p. 2024.

E. False

Ch. 84A Joint Disease, p. 2024.

Q **7.90**   Concerning MRI and joint disease

A. A 'double line' sign is an MRI feature of avascular necrosis of the hip.
B. The MRI findings of transient osteoporosis of the hip are specific.
C. The rim of an iliopsoas bursa typically enhances after intravenous gadolinium DTPA .
D. A discoid meniscus typically occurs in the medial joint space
E. Joint fluid is easily missed on T1 weighted MRI images of the knee.

Q **7.91**   Concerning anterior cruciate ligament disruption

A. Posterior tibial translation may be seen.
B. An over-straightened patella ligament.
C. A 'bunched up' posterior cruciate ligament.
D. The accuracy of MRI is approximately 70%.
E. The Segond fracture is present in over 95% of patients with ACL disruption.

(Answers overleaf)

A 7.90 Concerning MRI and joint disease

A. True In 80% of cases the line of demarcation between normal and abnormal bone is characterized by a 'double line', which is thought to be related to granulation tissue in the adjacent viable reactive bone. However, it has been shown more recently to be related to a chemical shift artefact.
Ch. 84B Joint Disease: MRI Aspects, p. 2029.

B. False The MRI appearances are non-specific and consist of bone-marrow oedema. The differential diagnosis includes early avascular necrosis, malignancy, infection or trauma.
Ch. 84B Joint Disease: MRI Aspects, p. 2029.

C. True The rim of an iliopsoas bursa typically enhances after intravenous gadolinium DTPA.
Ch. 84B Joint Disease: MRI Aspects, p. 2032.

D. False A discoid meniscus typically occurs in the medial joint space.
Ch. 84B Joint Disease: MRI Aspects, p. 2034.

E. True Joint fluid is easily missed on T1 weighted MRI images of the knee.
Ch. 84B Joint Disease: MRI Aspects, p. 2034.

A 7.91 Concerning anterior cruciate ligament disruption

A. False This typically anterior tibial translation.
Ch. 84B Joint Disease: MRI Aspects, p. 2035.

B. False Typically a wavy patella ligament is demonstrated.
Ch. 84B Joint Disease: MRI Aspects, p. 2035.

C. True
Ch. 84B Joint Disease: MRI Aspects, p. 2035.

D. False The accuracy of MRI for detecting anterior cruciate ligament ruptures is in excess of 95%.
Ch. 84B Joint Disease: MRI Aspects, p. 2035.

E. False A fracture or bone bruising involving the posterior lateral tibial plateau (Segond's fracture) and lateral femoral condyle have been shown to be a relatively specific sign for an acute complete anterior cruciate ligament, present in more than 95% of such injuries. The converse is not true.
Ch. 84B Joint Disease: MRI Aspects, p. 2036.

Q 7.92 Concerning musculo skeletal radiology

A. Patella tendonitis typically occurs in the mid portion of the patella tendon.
B. A bursa of the pes anserinus is demonstrated on the lateral aspect of the tibia.
C. Fifty per cent of meniscal cysts are associated with tears of the meniscus.
D. Tenosynovitis may occur in the Achilles tendon.
E. The anterior talofibular ligament is the most frequent lateral ankle ligament injury.

Q 7.93 Concerning musculoskeletal disorders of the upper limb

A. The supraspinatus tendon may demonstrate the magic angle phenomenon on MRI.
B. Subscapularis tendon tears frequently occur in isolation.
C. Kienböck's disease is an avascular necrosis of the triquetral bone.
D. MRI imaging of the temporomandibular joint should be obtained in the open and closed position.
E. MRI is the test of choice for scaphoid fractures cash not withstanding.

Q 7.94 The following are associated

A. Soft-tissue calcification: hypoparathyroidism.
B. Cysticercosis: oval calcifications within muscle.
C. Fibrodysplasia ossificans progressiva: bone tumours.
D. Calcium hydroxyapatite deposition disease: supraspinatus tendonosis.
E. Pigmented villonodular synovitis: high signal intensity lesions on T1 weighted images.

(Answers overleaf)

A **7.92** Concerning musculo skeletal radiology

A. False

    Ch. 84B Joint Disease: MRI Aspects, p. 2037.

B. False The pes anserinus is a medial structure.

C. False A meniscal cyst is an accumulation of fluid in association with an adjacent meniscal tear extending from the joint surface to its outer border.
    Ch. 84B Joint Disease: MRI Aspects, p. 2038.

D. False The Achilles tendon does not have a tendon sheath and thus inflammation around the outside of the Achilles tendon is termed peritendonitis.
    Ch. 84B Joint Disease: MRI Aspects, p. 2040.

E. True

    Ch. 84B Joint Disease: MRI Aspects, p. 2042.

A **7.93** Concerning musculoskeletal disorders of the upper limb

A. True When using a T1-weighted imaging sequence an area of intermediate signal intensity or signal inhomogeneity may be demonstrated in the distal supraspinatus tendon. This relates to the tendon fibrila orientation and is at 55% to the main magnetic field.
    Ch. 84B Joint Disease: MRI Aspects, p. 2044.

B. False They typically occur with other tears of the rotator cuff.
    Ch. 84B Joint Disease: MRI Aspects, p. 2044.

C. False This eponymous disease refers to avascular necrosis of the lunate.
    Ch. 84B Joint Disease: MRI Aspects, p. 2050.

D. True

    Ch. 84B Joint Disease: MRI Aspects, p. 2052.

E. True

A **7.94** The following are associated

A. True

    Ch. 86 Imaging of Soft Tissues, p. 2080.

B. True

    Ch. 86 Imaging of Soft Tissues, p. 2082.

C. False This disorder, previously known as miositis ossificans progressiva, is an inherited autosomal dominant disorder of the variable penetrance.
    Ch. 86 Imaging of Soft Tissues, p. 2083.

D. True

    Ch. 86 Imaging of Soft Tissues, p. 2084.

E. False

    Ch. 86 Imaging of Soft Tissues, p. 2090.

Q 7.95   Concerning non-accidental injury in children

A.   Non-accidental injury most commonly occurs in the first 6 months of life.
B.   Metaphyseal fractures are highly specific for abuse.
C.   Linear skull fractures of the parietal bone have a high specificity for non-accidental injury.
D.   The spleen is the most frequently involved visceral organ.
E.   Radiology may provide the only documentation of abuse.

Q 7.96   Concerning paediatric musculoskeletal disease

A.   A supracondylar fracture of the humerus may damage the brachial artery.
B.   Perthes' disease is bilateral in approximately 5–20% of cases.
C.   Sternocleidomastoid tumour (fibromatosis colli) is usually self limiting.
D.   Acute osteomyelitis in children is monostotic in only 50% of patients.
E.   Ultrasound reliably demonstrates hip-joint effusion.

(Answers overleaf)

339

A **7.95** Concerning non-accidental injury in children

A. False The frequency of skeletal trauma in non-accidental injury has been variously reported between 11 and 55%. It is common in children under 3 years, although others have quoted 1 year.
Ch. 88 The Radiology of Nonaccidental Injury p. 2113.

B. True
Ch. 88 The Radiology of Nonaccidental Injury p. 2113.

C. False
Ch. 88 The Radiology of Nonaccidental Injury p. 2114.

D. False In abuse the liver is injured more frequently than the spleen or the kidneys, but in accidental trauma the reverse is true.
Ch. 88 The Radiology of Nonaccidental Injury p. 2119.

E. True
Ch. 88 The Radiology of Nonaccidental Injury p. 2123.

A **7.96** Concerning paediatric musculoskeletal disease

A. True
Ch. 89 Paediatric Musculoskeletal Trauma, p. 2130.

B. True
Ch. 89 Paediatric Musculoskeletal Trauma, p. 2135.

C. True
Ch. 91 Radiology of Soft Tissues in Children, p. 2159.

D. False Acute osteomyelitis is more common in boys. It is monostotic in 95% and typically affects long tubular bones such as the tibia and femur.
Ch. 92 Bone and Soft-tissue Infection in Children, p. 2163.

E. True
Ch. 92 Bone and Soft-tissue Infection in Children, p. 2171.

Q **7.97** **Concerning injuries to the hand**

A. Scapholunate dislocation is best demonstrated in ulnar deviation of the carpus on the PA radiograph.

B. Disruption of the scapholunate, lunocapitate and lunotriquitral ligaments is necessary for a perilunate dislocation to occur.

C. On the PA radiograph of the wrist the normal triangular configuration of the lunate bone becomes trapezoidal in shape when this bone is dislocated (lunate dislocation).

D. The fracture of the midshaft of the second metacarpal is termed a boxer's fracture.

E. It is rare for a dislocation to occur without the presence of significant carpal instability.

Q **7.98** **The following associations are correct**

A. The Bennett's fracture: an oblique fracture through the base of the 5th metacarpal.

B. A Ronaldo's fracture: a comminuted fracture of the base of the 1st metacarpal.

C. Skier's thumb: ulnar collateral ligament disruption.

D. The Stenner lesion: disruption of the ulnar collateral ligament and interposition of the abductor pollicis longus muscle.

E. Hitch-hiker's thumb: distal phalangeal fracture.

(Answers overleaf)

A **7.97** Concerning injuries to the hand

A. True In scapholunate dislocation widening of the scapholunate space is demonstrated on the PA film. Normal intercarpol distance is approximately 2 mm. A space wider than 4 mm is abnormal, the so-called 'Terry Thomas' sign, after the famous English comedian, or the 'David Letterman' sign.
Ch. 78 Skeletal Trauma, p. 1802.

B. True
Ch. 78 Skeletal Trauma, p. 1802.

C. False The lunate appears trapezoidal in the non-dislocated state.
Ch. 78 Skeletal Trauma, p. 1802.

D. False A boxer's fracture is associated with oblique fractures of the 4th and 5th metacarpals.
Ch. 78 Skeletal Trauma, p. 1802.

E. True
Ch. 78 Skeletal Trauma, p. 1802.

A **7.98** The following associations are correct

A. False This is an oblique fracture through the base of the 1st metacarpal Bennett's fractures are usually unstable as the distal fragment is distracted by the unopposed abductor pollicis longus muscle, which may require surgical intervention.
Ch. 78 Skeletal Trauma, p. 1803.

B. False Ronaldo is a footballer. The fracture described is a Rolando's fracture.
Ch. 78 Skeletal Trauma, p. 1803.

C. True
Ch. 78 Skeletal Trauma, p. 1803.

D. False The Stenner lesion describes the disruption of the ulnar collateral ligament with interposition of the adductor pollicis brevis muscle aponeurosis.
Ch. 78 Skeletal Trauma, p. 1803.

E. False
Ch. 78 Skeletal Trauma, p. 1803.

Q 7.99   Concerning fractures of the hip

A. The risk of avascular necrosis is directly related to the proximity of the femoral neck fracture to the femoral head.

B. The majority of femoral neck fractures, in the elderly, occur in the subcapital region.

C Intertrochanteric fractures do not disrupt the blood supply to the femoral head.

D. Isolated fractures of the greater trochanter are uncommon.

E. Isolated fractures of the lesser trochanter are common in the elderly.

Q 7.100   Concerning fractures of the lower limb

A. Subtrochanteric fractures are frequently pathological.

B. Skeletal scintigraphy is more sensitive than MRI for occult hip fractures.

C. Skeletal scintigraphy for the dissection of occult fractures may yield false-negative results under 24 hours.

D. MRI may demonstrate false-positive findings for occult fractures within 2–6 hours on presentation.

E. Most hip dislocations occur posteriorly.

(Answers overleaf)

A **7.99** Concerning fractures of the hip

A. True It is because the blood supply to the adult femoral head is principally via recurrent arteries entering the hip joint from the lateral aspect of the femoral neck, fractures proximal to this site may disrupt the blood flow to the femoral head resulting in avascular necrosis.
Ch. 78 Skeletal Trauma, p. 1805.

B. True
Ch. 78 Skeletal Trauma, p. 1805.

C. True
Ch. 78 Skeletal Trauma, p. 1805.

D. False These injuries commonly occur in the elderly.
Ch. 78 Skeletal Trauma, p. 1806.

E. False These are uncommon and when they are seen a pathological cause should be sought.
Ch. 78 Skeletal Trauma, p. 1806.

A **7.100** Concerning fractures of the lower limb

A. True Subtrochanteric fractures are frequently pathological and they are usually transverse in orientation and are often seen in the setting of metastatic disease, myeloma and Paget's disease.
Ch. 78 Skeletal Trauma, p. 1806.

B. False Skeletal scintigraphy and MRI have been shown to be highly sensitive for undisplaced fractures and should be suspected if a hip fracture cannot be demonstrated on routine radiography.
Ch. 78 Skeletal Trauma, p. 1806.

C. True
Ch. 78 Skeletal Trauma, p. 1806.

D. True
Ch. 78 Skeletal Trauma, p. 1806.

E. True A dislocation of the hip is usually related to motor vehicle accidents and is the result of the femur being driven posteriorly by the dashboard.
Ch. 78 Skeletal Trauma, p. 1807.

Q 7.101 Concerning injuries to the knee

A. Lateral tibial plateau fractures are more common than medial tibial plateau fractures.

B. The Segond fracture is associated with damage to the posterior cruciate ligament.

C. The bipartite patella can usually be distinguished from a fracture.

D. A typical site for an osteochondral fracture is on the articular surfaces of the tibial plateau.

E. A lipohaemarthrosis is typically present in the suprapatella recess of the knee joint on a cross table view.

Q 7.102 Concerning internal derangements of the knee joint

A. An anterior cruciate ligament injury is unlikely without the presence of joint effusion.

B. The typical site for ACL rupture is at its tibial insertion.

C. Posterior cruciate ligament injury is usually caused by a hyperflexion manoeuvre.

D. Lateral collateral ligament injury is more frequent than medial collateral ligament injury.

E. The medial collateral ligament injury is most often associated with varus stress of the knee joint.

(Answers overleaf)

A **7.101** Concerning injuries to the knee

A. True They are generally due to valgus impaction injuries.
Ch. 78 Skeletal Trauma, p. 1808.

B. False A small fracture of the lateral margin of the tibial plateau may represent avulsion of the lateral collateral ligamentous complex of the knee. There is a high association with disruption of the anterior cruciate ligament – this is the Segond injury.
Ch. 78 Skeletal Trauma, p. 1808.

C. True The bipartite patella has a separate ossification centre in the superior lateral aspect of the patella. The fragment of the bipartite patella is well corticated edge unlike the acute fracture fragment.
Ch. 78 Skeletal Trauma, p. 1809.

D. False Osteochondral fractures of the knee usually occur in the articular surface of the femoral condyle. MRI can demonstrate the size and location with considerable ease.
Ch. 78 Skeletal Trauma, p. 1809.

E. True
Ch. 78 Skeletal Trauma, p. 1809.

A **7.102** Concerning internal derangements of the knee joint

A. False This may occur in the chronically injured ACL.
Ch. 78 Skeletal Trauma, p. 1810.

B. False This is a rare injury of the anterior cruciate ligament and is often associated with an avulsion fracture.
Ch. 78 Skeletal Trauma, p. 1810.

C. False This injury typically occurs in hyperextension though it can be produced in complex mechanisms of injury.
Ch. 78 Skeletal Trauma, p. 1810.

D. False The medial collateral ligament is more frequently disrupted than the lateral collateral ligament.
Ch. 78 Skeletal Trauma, p. 1810.

E. False This is typically produced by a valgus stress and other complex rotational knee injuries.
Ch. 78 Skeletal Trauma, p. 1810.

Q 7.103   Concerning the menisci of the knee

A. MRI has a high sensitivity and low specificity for meniscal tears.
B. Tears are of high signal on all sequences.
C. Extension of linear high signal within a meniscus to the capsular surface does not represent a tear.
D. Bucket handle tears are best demonstrated in the coronal image plane.
E. The anterior third of the medial meniscus is smaller than the posterior third.

Q 7.104   There is an association between the following injuries

A. Fibula head fracture: peroneal nerve injury.
B. Anterior middle third tibial cortical fracture: stress fracture.
C. Posterior fibula dislocation: equestrian injury.
D. Anterior fibula head dislocation: parachuting injury.
E. Impaction fracture of the fibula neck: weight lifters.

(Answers overleaf)

A 7.103   Concerning the menisci of the knee

A. False   Both the sensitivity and the specificity are high (and are greater than 90%).
Ch. 78 Skeletal Trauma, p. 1810.

B. True   Undoubtedly certain image sequences may suppress the high signal created from the menisci when a tear is present, though these are unusal and this question should be taken at its face value.
Ch. 78 Skeletal Trauma, p. 1810.

C. True
Ch. 78 Skeletal Trauma, p. 1810.

D. True
Ch. 78 Skeletal Trauma, p. 1811.

E. True   Remember normal anatomy!
Ch. 78 Skeletal Trauma, p. 1811.

A 7.104   There is an association between the following injuries

A. False   This injury typically occurs with fractures of the fibula neck.
Ch. 78 Skeletal Trauma, p. 1811.

B. True   This is the typical stress fracture that is often seen in long-distance runners.
Ch. 78 Skeletal Trauma, p. 1811.

C. True
Ch. 78 Skeletal Trauma, p. 1811.

D. True
Ch. 78 Skeletal Trauma, p. 1811.

E. False   This ought to be true but it is not.
Ch. 78 Skeletal Trauma, p. 1811.

Q **7.105** Concerning ankle injuries

   A. Standard radiographic evaluation includes an AP view, lateral view and an internally rotated oblique view (mortis view).
   B. Stress views may be necessary to demonstrate ligamentous laxity.
   C. MRI is poor at assessing the ankle ligament.
   D. The Maisonneuve fracture occurs in an eversion injury.
   E. The trimalleolar fracture and the pylon fracture are synonymous.

Q **7.106** The following are associated with achilles tendon rupture

   A. Diabetes mellitus.
   B. Gout.
   C. Ehlers Danlos syndrome.
   D. Smoking.
   E. Hyperparathyroidism.

(Answers overleaf)

A **7.105** Concerning ankle injuries

A. True
Ch. 78 Skeletal Trauma, p. 1812.

B. True
Ch. 78 Skeletal Trauma, p. 1812.

C. False
Ch. 78 Skeletal Trauma, p. 1812.

D. True Rarely, an eversion injury may result in an avulsion of the medial malleolus without the visible lateral malleolar fracture. The force may be dissipated superiorly causing disruption of the interosseous ligaments joining the shafts of the fibula and tibia, with a fracture of the proximal fibula.
Ch. 78 Skeletal Trauma, p. 1813.

E. False The posterior lip of the distal tibia may be fractured, even in combination with the medial and lateral malleoli, due to massive force (trimalleolar fracture) or due to a vertical compressive force in the dorsiflex foot driving the Talar dome superiorly into the distal tibia (pylon fracture).
Ch. 78 Skeletal Trauma, p. 1813.

A **7.106** The following are associated with achilles tendon rupture

A. True
Ch. 78 Skeletal Trauma, p. 1813.

B. True
Ch. 78 Skeletal Trauma, p. 1813.

C. False
Ch. 78 Skeletal Trauma, p. 1813.

D. False
Ch. 78 Skeletal Trauma, p. 1813.

E. True
Ch. 78 Skeletal Trauma, p. 1813.

8 Obstetrics and gynaecology

Q 8.1 Regarding ultrasound in obstetrics and gynaecology

A. Continuous wave Doppler uses greater wave intensity than pulsed Doppler imaging.

B. Pulsed Doppler transducers emit sound waves with intensity in the range 10–100 mW per centimetre^2.

C. A yolk sac is visible on transabdominal ultrasound when the β-hCG is 500 mIU per ml.

D. Transvaginal ultrasound can detect a gestational sac at 4–5 weeks post last menstrual period.

E. Free intraperitoneal fluid is found in tubal abortion.

Q 8.2 Concerning gestational age on ultrasound

A. An embryo is not detected on transvaginal ultrasound until 8 weeks post last menstrual period (LMP).

B. Foetal heart is not detected on transvaginal ultrasound until 8 weeks post LMP.

C. Biparietal diameter is not an accurate means of establishing gestational age until 10 weeks post LMP.

D. The rhombencephalon is a precursor of the ventricular system.

E. Molar pregnancy can be reliably exclude before 10 weeks.

(Answers overleaf)

A **8.1** Regarding ultrasound in obstetrics and gynaecology

A. False Pulsed imaging requires greater intensity than continuous wave Doppler.
Ch. 93 Ultrasound in Obstetrics and Gynaecology, p. 2179.

B. False Pulsed Doppler transducers may emit relatively high intensity waves approximately 1000 mW per centimetre^2 and are currently under restriction by the Federal Drugs Administration in the USA.
Ch. 93 Ultrasound in Obstetrics and Gynaecology, p. 2178.

C. False Gestational sac can be seen when the β-hCG is between 500 and 1500 mIU per ml whereas with transabdominal sonography it is first detectable between 1500 and 2000 mIU per ml.
Ch. 93 Ultrasound in Obstetrics and Gynaecology, p. 2178.

D. True
Ch. 93 Ultrasound in Obstetrics and Gynaecology, p. 2178.

E. True It is also seen in ruptured ectopic pregnancy.
Ch. 93 Ultrasound in Obstetrics and Gynaecology, p. 2178.

A **8.2** Concerning gestational age on ultrasound

A. False An embryo can be detected at 5 weeks.
Ch. 93 Ultrasound in Obstetrics and Gynaecology, p. 2178.

B. False It can be seen at 6 weeks.
Ch. 93 Ultrasound in Obstetrics and Gynaecology, p. 2178.

C. True Biparietal diameter is useful between weeks 10 and 33.
Ch. 93 Ultrasound in Obstetrics and Gynaecology, p. 2178.

D. True
Ch. 93 Ultrasound in Obstetrics and Gynaecology, p. 2179.

E. False Before 10 weeks the molar tissue may not demonstrate the hydropic villi that are diagnostic of this abnormality.
Ch. 93 Ultrasound in Obstetrics and Gynaecology, p. 2180.

Q **8.3** **Signs of complicated pregnancy on ultrasound include**

A. Deflated yolk sac.
B. A hypo echoic band deep to the choriodecidua.
C. Septated fluid collection behind the foetal neck.
D. An echogenic ring in the maternal adnexa.
E. Herniation of mid gut into the base of the umbilical cord at 10 weeks.

Q **8.4** **Causes of abnormally elevated amniotic fluid a-fetoprotein in pregnancy include**

A. Incorrect dates.
B. Multiple pregnancy.
C. Down's syndrome.
D. Meningomyelocoele.
E. Maternal diabetes.

Q **8.5** **Regarding gynaecological ultrasound**

A. Normal post menopausal endometrial thickness is 10 mm or less.
B. Endometrial polyps are detected more readily when fluid is instilled into the uterine cavity.
C. Low velocity high impedance flow on Doppler ultrasound in an ovarian mass indicates malignancy.
D. Endometrial polyps appear as echogenic masses between the two endometrial layers.
E. Myometrial cysts in patient taking tamoxifen are likely to represent metastatic disease from primary breast carcinoma.

(Answers overleaf)

353

A 8.3 Signs of complicated pregnancy on ultrasound include

A. True Deflated yolk sac within an enlarged gestational sac indicates the demise of an embryo.
Ch. 93 Ultrasound in Obstetrics and Gynaecology, p. 2190.

B. True This indicates a retrochorionic bleed.
Ch. 93 Ultrasound in Obstetrics and Gynaecology, p. 2181.

C. True This is a sign of cystic hygroma.
Ch. 93 Ultrasound in Obstetrics and Gynaecology, p. 2181.

D. True This is a sign of ectopic pregnancy.
Ch. 93 Ultrasound in Obstetrics and Gynaecology, p. 2181.

E. False This is a normal finding from 8–11 weeks.
Ch. 93 Ultrasound in Obstetrics and Gynaecology, p. 2181.

A 8.4 Causes of abnormally elevated amniotic fluid a fetoprotein in pregnancy include

A. True
Ch. 93 Ultrasound in Obstetrics and Gynaecology, p. 2181.

B. True
Ch. 93 Ultrasound in Obstetrics and Gynaecology, p. 2181.

C. True
Ch. 93 Ultrasound in Obstetrics and Gynaecology, p. 2181.

D. True
Ch. 93 Ultrasound in Obstetrics and Gynaecology, p. 2181.

E. False
Ch. 93 Ultrasound in Obstetrics and Gynaecology, p. 2181.

A 8.5 Regarding gynaecological ultrasound

A. False It is less than 5 mm.
Ch. 93 Ultrasound in Obstetrics and Gynaecology, p. 2189.

B. True Installation of sterile saline and subsequent insonation is called sonohysterography and is a useful technique for demonstrating endometrial polyps.
Ch. 93 Ultrasound in Obstetrics and Gynaecology, p. 2189.

C. False A vascular bed of low impedance, high-velocity flow is a sign of malignancy.
Ch. 93 Ultrasound in Obstetrics and Gynaecology, p. 2191.

D. True
Ch. 93 Ultrasound in Obstetrics and Gynaecology, p. 2192.

E. False They are likely to represent benign cysts that are reactivated adenomyomas.
Ch. 93 Ultrasound in Obstetrics and Gynaecology, p. 2192.

Q **8.6** Regarding normal imaging findings in gynaecological imaging

A. Secretory endometrium is hyper-reflective on ultrasound.
B. The internal iliac artery lies anterior to the ipsilateral ovary.
C. The endometrial canal has low attenuation compared to enhancing myometrium on CT.
D. Endometrium has high signal on T2-weighted MRI.
E. The low signal junctional zone on MRI represents serosa.

Q **8.7** Concerning hysterosalpinography

A. The optimal time for this examination is day 18–22 of the menstrual cycle.
B. Pregnancy is a contraindication.
C. Ionic contrast medium is more irritant to the peritoneum than non-ionic.
D. Non-filling of the lateral half of the tube is caused by cornual spasm.
E. Antibiotics are routinely administered for 3 days post procedure.

Q **8.8** Causes of pelvic pain in women include

A. Adenomyosis.
B. Pelvic varices.
C. Uterus didelphys.
D. Transverse vaginal septum.
E. Leiomyoma.

(Answers overleaf)

A **8.6** Regarding normal imaging findings in gynaecological imaging

A. True
> *Ch. 94A Imaging in Gynaecology, p. 2202.*

B. False It lies immediately posterior.
> *Ch. 94A Imaging in Gynaecology, p. 2202.*

C. True This is not to be confused with fluid.
> *Ch. 94A Imaging in Gynaecology, p. 2203.*

D. True
> *Ch. 94A Imaging in Gynaecology, p. 2203.*

E. False This layer identifies the inner myometrium.
> *Ch. 94A Imaging in Gynaecology, p. 2203.*

A **8.7** Concerning hysterosalpinography

A. False Towards the end of the first week is the best time when the isthmus is most distensible and the fallopian tubes are most readily filled by contrast media.
> *Ch. 94A Imaging in Gynaecology, p. 2204.*

B. True
> *Ch. 94A Imaging in Gynaecology, p. 2204.*

C. True
> *Ch. 94A Imaging in Gynaecology, p. 2204.*

D. False
> *Ch. 94A Imaging in Gynaecology, p. 2204.*

E. False This is still somewhat controversial but most workers reserve antibiotic administration for cases where infection is suspected or discovered at the time of the examination.
> *Ch. 94A Imaging in Gynaecology, p. 2204.*

A **8.8** Causes of pelvic pain in women include

A. True
> *Ch. 94A Imaging in Gynaecology, p. 2208.*

B. True
> *Ch. 94A Imaging in Gynaecology, p. 2208.*

C. False
> *Ch. 94A Imaging in Gynaecology, p. 2206.*

D. True This may cause cyclical abdominal pain in teenagers and a hematocolpos may be palpable within the pelvis.
> *Ch. 94A Imaging in Gynaecology, p. 2207.*

E. True
> *Ch. 94A Imaging in Gynaecology, p. 2208.*

Q 8.9 Features of uterine adenomyosis include

A. The presence of endometrial tissue within myometrium.
B. High signal foci on T1-weighted images.
C. On ultrasound focal adenomyosis can be readily distinguished from leiomyoma.
D. Hysterosalpingography demonstrates associated pseudopolyps.
E. Calcification is seen in 5–10% of cases on computed tomography.

Q 8.10 Regarding imaging findings in endometrial carcinoma

A. Polycystic ovaries are a risk factor for the development of malignancy.
B. Normal post menopausal endometrial thickness is 10 mm or less.
C. An intracavitary polyp is a recognized finding.
D. Unenhanced T1-weighted MRI shows the majority of endometrial tumours.
E. Ultrasound is used to evaluate stage I disease.

(Answers overleaf)

A **8.9**   **Features of uterine adenomyosis include**

A. True
> *Ch. 94A Imaging in Gynaecology, p. 2210.*

B. True   These foci are felt to represent endometrial rests and/or small punctate haemorrhages.
> *Ch. 94A Imaging in Gynaecology, p. 2210.*

C. False   These two conditions are difficult to differentiate on ultrasound.
> *Ch. 94A Imaging in Gynaecology, p. 2210.*

D. False   HSG may demonstrate pseudodiverticula (i.e. invading endometrial glands).
> *Ch. 94A Imaging in Gynaecology, p. 2210.*

E. False
> *Ch. 94A Imaging in Gynaecology, p. 2210.*

A **8.10**   **Regarding imaging findings in endometrial carcinoma**

A. True
> *Ch. 94A Imaging in Gynaecology, p. 2211.*

B. False   It is 5 mm thick or less.
> *Ch. 94A Imaging in Gynaecology, p. 2211.*

C. True   Asymmetrical thickening is an alternative presentation.
> *Ch. 94A Imaging in Gynaecology, p. 2211.*

D. False   Routine use of dynamic IV contrast enhancement is necessary for adequate MRI evaluation of endometrial carcinoma because endometrial carcinoma is isointense with normal endometrium on T1-weighted images.
> *Ch. 94A Imaging in Gynaecology, p. 2211.*

E. True   It can identify the degree of myometrial invasion.
> *Ch. 94A Imaging in Gynaecology, p. 2212.*

Q **8.11** Regarding ovarian cystic disease

A. Persistent corpus luteum cyst simulates ectopic pregnancy.
B. Theca lutein cysts are usually bilateral.
C. Endometriomas appear hyperintense on T1- and T2-weighted images.
D. The majority of patients with polycystic ovarian disease are hirsute and obese.
E. Polycystic ovary syndrome causes dysmenorrhoea, bleeding and infertility.

Q **8.12** Theca lutein cysts are found in association with

A. Polycystic ovary syndrome.
B. Hydatid disease.
C. Cholangiocarcinoma.
D. Mucinous ovarian carcinoma.
E. Clomiphene therapy.

Q **8.13** Regarding pelvic inflammatory disease

A. There is good correlation between the extent of tubal damage and the presence of symptoms.
B. The endometrium is thickened with hyporeflective margins on ultrasound.
C. MRI allows an adnexal abscess to be reliably differentiated from necrotic tumour.
D. Crohn's disease presents as acute salpingitis.
E. Antibiotic therapy reverses the changes of salpingitis isthmica nodosa.

(Answers overleaf)

A **8.11**   Regarding ovarian cystic disease

A. True   Local pain, tenderness and delayed menstruation or amenorrhoea are features.
Ch. 94A Imaging in Gynaecology, p. 2215.

B. True   They are usually large and bilateral.
Ch. 94A Imaging in Gynaecology, p. 2215.

C. True   Owing to blood products.
Ch. 94A Imaging in Gynaecology, p. 2216.

D. False
Ch. 94A Imaging in Gynaecology, p. 2216.

E. False   This condition is characterized by secondary amenorrhoea or oligomenorrhoea and infertility. The combination of dysmenorrhoea, bleeding and infertility is usually found in endometriosis.
Ch. 94A Imaging in Gynaecology, p. 2216.

A **8.12**   Theca lutein cysts are found in association with

A. True
Ch. 94A Imaging in Gynaecology, p. 2215.

B. False
Ch. 94A Imaging in Gynaecology, p. 2215.

C. False   They are, however, associated with choriocarcinoma.
Ch. 94A Imaging in Gynaecology, p. 2215.

D. False
Ch. 94A Imaging in Gynaecology, p. 2215.

E. False
Ch. 94A Imaging in Gynaecology, p. 2215.

A **8.13**   Regarding pelvic inflammatory disease

A. False   No such correlation exists.
Ch. 94A Imaging in Gynaecology, p. 2217.

B. True   Due to endometrial oedema.
Ch. 94A Imaging in Gynaecology, p. 2217.

C. False
Ch. 94A Imaging in Gynaecology, p. 2217.

D. True
Ch. 94A Imaging in Gynaecology, p. 2217.

E. False   Antibiotic therapy has no effect on this condition, which is probably due to a non-inflammatory process similar to adenomyosis or related to diverticulosis in other organs.
Ch. 94A Imaging in Gynaecology, p. 2217.

Q **8.14** Regarding imaging of gynaecological malignancy

 A. Malignant neovascularity in the ovary has a high resistivity index.
 B. Amorphous calcification in an ovarian cyst makes it more likely to be benign.
 C. The presence of a pleural effusion on CT implies stage IV disease.
 D. Ovarian cyst wall thickness of 4 mm is associated with malignancy.
 E. Ureteric stricture after radiotherapy for carcinoma of the cervix is almost always caused by recurrent tumour.

Q **8.15** Concerning hystersalpingography technique

 A. Twenty millilitres of contrast is injected under fluoroscopic control.
 B. Gentle cephalad pressure on the cervix allows better visualization of the entire uterus.
 C. Rapid injection of contrast medium is recommended as it allows better tubal distension.
 D. Inadvertent hysterosalpingography during pregnancy is likely to result in an abortion.
 E. Venous intravasation of non-ionic contrast medium is an indication to terminate the procedure immediately.

(Answers overleaf)

A **8.14** Regarding imaging of gynaecological malignancy

A. False The thin walls which contains little smooth muscle allow for high velocity low resisitivity flow.
Ch. 94A Imaging in Gynaecology, p. 2219.

B. False Organized calcification may be seen in dermoids containing teeth. Amorphous coarse calcification is a sign of malignancy.
Ch. 94A Imaging in Gynaecology, p. 2219.

C. False There are many causes of pleural effusion. Positive cytology is required to demonstrate stage IV disease.
Ch. 94A Imaging in Gynaecology, p. 2219.

D. True
Ch. 94A Imaging in Gynaecology, p. 2220.

E. True Less than 1% is secondary to irradiation fibrosis.
Ch. 94A Imaging in Gynaecology, p. 2222.

A **8.15** Concerning hystersalpingography technique

A. False From 5 to 10 ml is adequate to demonstrate uterine and tubal anatomy.
Ch. 94B Hysterosalpingography, p. 2227.

B. True Forward pressure allows full visualization of the uterus when imaged with both obliques. It is an alternative to cervical traction.
Ch. 94B Hysterosalpingography, p. 2227.

C. False The pain of this procedure is reduced by injecting contrast medium gently. Uterine and tubal distension caused by rapid or forced injection can be associated with severe pain.
Ch. 94B Hysterosalpingography, p. 2230.

D. False There is little evidence in those cases reported in the literature to suggest harm to the foetus as the result of an inadvertent HSG.
Ch. 94B Hysterosalpingography, p. 2230.

E. False When this occurs (as it does in up to 7% of examinations) it is usually of no clinical significance. However, the rapid flow of contrast into the venous system usually precludes further useful imaging.
Ch. 94B Hysterosalpingography, p. 2230.

Q **8.16**   Regarding mammographic technique

A.   Compression allows a lower kVp to be used.

B.   Carcinomas are rendered more conspicuous by compression.

C.   A beam of 24–28 kVp is optimal.

D.   Dose is lower with higher kVp settings.

E.   A molybdenum target with aluminium filtration is optimal

Q **8.17**   Regarding mammographic technique

A.   A rhodium tube with rhodium filtration is used for examining larger breasts.

B.   Focal spot size should be between 0.2 and 0.5 mm.

C.   High mA output is desirable.

D.   Grids are not used as they cause an excessive increase in dose.

E.   A magnification factor of ×3 is optimal for magnification mammography.

(Answers overleaf)

A **8.16** **Regarding mammographic technique** .

A. **True** This improves contrast by reducing scatter.
Ch. 95 The Breast, p. 2241.

B. **True** Cysts and normal glandular tissue are more easily compressed allowing the more rigid carcinomas to be highlighted.
Ch. 95 The Breast, p. 2241.

C. **True**
Ch. 95 The Breast, p. 2241.

D. **True** But contrast is reduced.
Ch. 95 The Breast, p. 2241.

E. **False** A molybdenum target is used with molybdenum filtration. Aluminium filters cause excessive beam hardening.
Ch. 95 The Breast, p. 2241.

A **8.17** **Regarding mammographic technique**

A. **True**
Ch. 95 The Breast, p. 2242.

B. **True**
Ch. 95 The Breast, p. 2242.

C. **True** This allows short exposure times thereby reducing motion unsharpness.
Ch. 95 The Breast, p. 2242.

D. **False** They are mandatory to increase contrast.
Ch. 95 The Breast, p. 2243.

E. **False** Magnification ×1.5–×2 is the optimal factor. Higher magnification results in an unacceptably high dose.
Ch. 95 The Breast, p. 2243.

9 The skull and brain: methods of examination and the anatomy

Q **9.1** **Regarding radiography of the skull**

A. The anthropological base line is drawn from the lower margin of the orbit to the superior border of the external auditory meatus.
B. The orbito-meatal line is drawn from the outer canthus to the superior border of the external auditory meatus.
C. The interpupillary line is perpendicular to the median sagittal plane.
D. The median sagittal plane is the anatomical line.
E. The frontal biauricular plane is in the coronal plane.

Q **9.2** **Concerning an occipito-frontal radiographic projection**

A. The midsagittal and orbito-meatal planes are perpendicular to the film.
B. The tube is angled 40° caudally.
C. The beam is centred on the nasion.
D. An antero-posterior projection should not be used as it causes magnification and blurring of the more important anterior structures.
E. The petrous ridges should be projected at or near the inferior orbital margins.

Q **9.3** **Regarding the Towne's projection**

A. This is a half axial postero-anterior projection.
B. The dorsum sellae is obscured by the upper cervical vertebrae.
C. The temporo-mandibular joints are projected over the petrous ridge.
D. The lambdoid and coronal sutures are visualized.
D. The groove for the transverse sinus is projected superior to the foramen magnum.

(Answers overleaf)

A **9.1** Regarding radiography of the skull

A. True This line is also known as Reid's or the Frankfurt line.
Ch. 97 The Skull and Brain: Methods of Examination and Anatomy, p. 2300.

B. False It extends from the outer canthus to the centre of the meatus.
Ch. 97 The Skull and Brain: Methods of Examination and Anatomy, p. 2300.

C. True
Ch. 97 The Skull and Brain: Methods of Examination and Anatomy, p. 2300.

D. True
Ch. 97 The Skull and Brain: Methods of Examination and Anatomy, p. 2300.

E. True
Ch. 97 The Skull and Brain: Methods of Examination and Anatomy, p. 2300.

A **9.2** Concerning an occipito-frontal radiographic projection

A. True This is achieved by resting the nose and forehead on the cassette.
Ch. 97 The Skull and Brain: Methods of Examination and Anatomy, p. 2300.

B. False The angulation should be 20° caudally.
Ch. 97 The Skull and Brain: Methods of Examination and Anatomy, p. 2300.

C. True
Ch. 97 The Skull and Brain: Methods of Examination and Anatomy, p. 2300.

D. True
Ch. 97 The Skull and Brain: Methods of Examination and Anatomy, p. 2300.

E. True
Ch. 97 The Skull and Brain: Methods of Examination and Anatomy, p. 2300.

A **9.3** Regarding the Towne's projection

A. False It is taken AP.
Ch. 97 The Skull and Brain: Methods of Examination and Anatomy, p. 2300.

B. False It should be seen through the foramen magnum.
Ch. 97 The Skull and Brain: Methods of Examination and Anatomy, p. 2300.

C. False
Ch. 97 The Skull and Brain: Methods of Examination and Anatomy, p. 2300.

D. True
Ch. 97 The Skull and Brain: Methods of Examination and Anatomy, p. 2300

E. True
Ch. 97 The Skull and Brain: Methods of Examination and Anatomy, p. 2302

Q **9.4** Regarding the submentovertical projection

A. The patient is prone.
B. The neck is fully hyperextended.
C. The anthropological baseline is parallel with the film.
D. A thick pillow or bolster may be placed between the face and the table.
E. On a satisfactory radiograph the angles of the mandible lie just anterior to the middle ear cavities.

Q **9.5** Concerning CT of the brain

A. Slice thickness in the posterior fossa should be increased to reduce beam hardening artefact.
B. Imaging of the pituitary is performed with the patient prone and the head maximally extended.
C. An intravenous injection of iodinated contrast medium containing a dose equivalent of 15–30 g of iodine is appropriate.
D. The electron density of grey matter is slightly greater than white.
E. The decussation of the superior cerebellar peduncles can be differentiated in the brain stem.

Q **9.6** In a good-quality submentovertical radiograph

A. The odontoid peg is projected over the centre of the foramen magnum.
B. The internal occipital protuberance is not visualized.
C. The hyoid bone cannot be identified.
D. The Eustachian tube is lateral to the carotid canal.
E. The zygomatic arches are projected anterior to the external auditory meatus.

(Answers overleaf)

A **9.4** Regarding the submentovertical projection

A. False The patient should be supine.
Ch. 97 The Skull and Brain: Methods of Examination and Anatomy, p. 2300.

B. True
Ch. 97 The Skull and Brain: Methods of Examination and Anatomy, p. 2300.

C. True
Ch. 97 The Skull and Brain: Methods of Examination and Anatomy, p. 2300.

D. False Inadvisable. It may help to place a thick pillow under the shoulders of the supine patient.
Ch. 97 The Skull and Brain: Methods of Examination and Anatomy, p. 2300.

E. True
Ch. 97 The Skull and Brain: Methods of Examination and Anatomy, p. 2300.

A **9.5** Concerning computed tomography of the brain

A. False Slice thickness of 5 mm or less is advised for the posterior fossa in attempt to reduce beam hardening artefact.
Ch. 97 The Skull and Brain: Methods of Examination and Anatomy, p. 2302.

B. True This technique involves imaging in the direct coronal plane. An alternative is to image it in the axial plane with multi-planar reformatting to generate views in the coronal plane as appropriate.
Ch. 97 The Skull and Brain: Methods of Examination and Anatomy, p. 2302.

C. True Some centres use twice or even three times this dose.
Ch. 97 The Skull and Brain: Methods of Examination and Anatomy, p. 2303.

D. True
Ch. 97 The Skull and Brain: Methods of Examination and Anatomy, p. 2305.

E. True
Ch. 97 The Skull and Brain: Methods of Examination and Anatomy, p. 2305.

A **9.6** In a good-quality submentovertical radiograph

A. False
Ch. 97 The Skull and Brain: Methods of Examination and Anatomy, p. 2303.

B. False
Ch. 97 The Skull and Brain: Methods of Examination and Anatomy, p. 2303.

C. False
Ch. 97 The Skull and Brain: Methods of Examination and Anatomy, p. 2303.

D. True
Ch. 97 The Skull and Brain: Methods of Examination and Anatomy, p. 2303.

E. True
Ch. 97 The Skull and Brain: Methods of Examination and Anatomy, p. 2303.

Q **9.7** Concerning the anatomy of the sellar region

A. The tuberculum sellae is superior to the anterior clinoid process.
B. Cortical bone can be seen lining the sella turcica.
C. The anterior clinoid process is lateral to the ipsilateral posterior clinoid process.
D. The optic canal is lateral to the tuberculum sellae.
E. The middle clinoid process is a constant feature.

Q **9.8** Regarding cranial foramina and canals

A. The optic canal extends from the orbital apex to the middle cranial fossa.
B. The superior orbital fissure contains the superior ophthalmic vein.
C. The foramen rotundum extends from middle cranial fossa to pterygopalatine fossa.
D. The pterygoid (vidian) canal is best seen on the occipito-frontal view.
E. The foramen spinosum penetrates the greater wing of sphenoid postero-lateral to the foramen ovale.

(Answers overleaf)

369

A **9.7**   **Concerning the anatomy of the sellar region**

A.   **False**
> *Ch. 97 The Skull and Brain: Methods of Examination and Anatomy, p. 2303.*

B.   **True**
> *Ch. 97 The Skull and Brain: Methods of Examination and Anatomy, p. 2303.*

C.   **True**
> *Ch. 97 The Skull and Brain: Methods of Examination and Anatomy, p. 2303.*

D.   **True**
> *Ch. 97 The Skull and Brain: Methods of Examination and Anatomy, p. 2303.*

E.   **False**
> *Ch. 97 The Skull and Brain: Methods of Examination and Anatomy, p. 2303.*

A **9.8**   **Regarding cranio-foramina and canals**

A.   **True**   It contains the optic nerve and sheath and ophthalmic artery.
> *Ch. 97 The Skull and Brain: Methods of Examination and Anatomy, p. 2304.*

B.   **True**   This extends from orbital apex and middle cranial fossa lying between the greater and lesser wings of sphenoid. Is also transmits the middle meningeal artery branch and also cranial nerves III, IV and VI, as well as the first branch of the trigeminal nerve.
> *Ch. 97 The Skull and Brain: Methods of Examination and Anatomy, p. 2304.*

C.   **True**   It may be surrounded by extensive sphenoid sinus and it contains the second division of the second trigeminal nerve as well as the artery of the foramen rotundum.
> *Ch. 97 The Skull and Brain: Methods of Examination and Anatomy, p. 2304.*

D.   **True**
> *Ch. 97 The Skull and Brain: Methods of Examination and Anatomy, p. 2304.*

E.   **True**   This extends from the middle cranial fossa to the infratemporal fossa and transmits the middle meningeal artery.
> *Ch. 97 The Skull and Brain: Methods of Examination and Anatomy, p. 2304.*

Q 9.9 Regarding the jugular foramen

A. It extends between the petrous temporal bone and the basiocciput.
B. It contains the inferior petrosal sinus.
C. It transmits the ascending pharyngeal and occipital arteries.
D. It is best seen on an under-tilted submentovertical projection.
E. It transmits the glossopharyngeal nerve.

Q 9.10 During CT cisternography

A. It is best to start imaging in the axial plane.
B. Carotid arterial compression is applied.
C. Intrathecal contrast extends into the optic nerve sheaths.
D. Iohexol 350 mg per ml x 20 ml is required in most cases.
E. It is important that the patient is actually leaking at the time of the examination.

Q 9.11 Physiological intracranial calcification is seen in

A. Glial rests.
B. Diaphragm sellae.
C. Habenular commissure.
D. Petroclinoid ligaments.
E. Arachnoid villi.

(Answers overleaf)

A **9.9** Regarding the jugular foramen

A. True
> Ch. 97 *The Skull and Brain: Methods of Examination and Anatomy, p. 2304.*

B. True
> Ch. 97 *The Skull and Brain: Methods of Examination and Anatomy, p. 2304.*

C. True
> Ch. 97 *The Skull and Brain: Methods of Examination and Anatomy, p. 2304.*

D. True
> Ch. 97 *The Skull and Brain: Methods of Examination and Anatomy, p. 2304.*

E. True
> Ch. 97 *The Skull and Brain: Methods of Examination and Anatomy, p. 2304.*

A **9.10** During CT cisternography

A. False Generally, it is best to start imaging in the direct coronal plane with the patient prone, as the desired leaking is likely to be maximal in this position.
> Ch. 97 *The Skull and Brain: Methods of Examination and Anatomy, p. 2305.*

B. False Jugular vein compression is applied for 5 minutes to try and encourage leaking if there is any clinical doubt whether this is occurring.
> Ch. 97 *The Skull and Brain: Methods of Examination and Anatomy, p. 2305.*

C. True
> Ch. 97 *The Skull and Brain: Methods of Examination and Anatomy, p. 2307.*

D. False A concentration of 240 mg per ml by 10 ml is usually more than adequate.
> Ch. 97 *The Skull and Brain: Methods of Examination and Anatomy, p. 2305.*

E. True
> Ch. 97 *The Skull and Brain: Methods of Examination and Anatomy, p. 2305.*

A **9.11** Physiological intracranial calcification is seen in

A. False
> Ch. 97 *The Skull and Brain: Methods of Examination and Anatomy, p. 2305.*

B. True
> Ch. 97 *The Skull and Brain: Methods of Examination and Anatomy, p. 2305.*

C. True Seen in 30%.
> Ch. 97 *The Skull and Brain: Methods of Examination and Anatomy, p. 2305.*

D. True Seen in 12% of skull X-rays.
> Ch. 97 *The Skull and Brain: Methods of Examination and Anatomy, p. 2305.*

E. False
> Ch. 97 *The Skull and Brain: Methods of Examination and Anatomy, p. 2305.*

Q 9.12 Concerning diffusion MRI

A. This exploits Brownian motion of water molecules to produce image contrast.

B. Images are acquired by applying a pair of diffusion gradients to a T1-weighted MRI sequence.

C. Regions of relatively stationary water molecules appear dark.

D. The degree of phased shift and signal loss depends on the strength and duration of the diffusion sensitizing gradient.

E. Diffusion in the brain is direction dependent.

Q 9.13 Regarding single photon emission CT (SPECT)

A. SPECT images are formed from detection of gamma rays emitted during radio-nuclide decay.

B. Regional cerebral blood flow can be imaged using ^{133}Xe – HMPAO.

C. Because of lead collimation, SPECT has inherently better resolution than positron emission tomography (PET).

D. Compared to PET SPECT is relatively inexpensive and more readily available.

E. T2*-weighted sequences can identify a tiny increase in signal intensity during neural activation.

(Answers overleaf)

A **9.12** Concerning diffusion MRI

A. True

Ch. 97 The Skull and Brain: Methods of Examination and Anatomy, p. 2309.

B. False A pair of diffusion gradients are applied symmetrically around a 180°
refocusing RF pulse of a T2-weighted MR sequence.
Ch. 97 The Skull and Brain: Methods of Examination and Anatomy, p. 2309.

C. False Relatively stationary water molecules appear much brighter than areas with
higher molecular diffusion.
Ch. 97 The Skull and Brain: Methods of Examination and Anatomy, p. 2309.

D. True

Ch. 97 The Skull and Brain: Methods of Examination and Anatomy, p. 2309.

E. True This is called anisotropy and is particularly prominent in compacted white
matter tracts and least evident in grey matter.
Ch. 97 The Skull and Brain: Methods of Examination and Anatomy, p. 2309.

A **9.13** Regarding single photon emission CT (SPECT)

A. True

Ch. 97 The Skull and Brain: Methods of Examination and Anatomy, p. 2310.

B. False ^{99m}Tc hexamethylpropylene amine oxide (HMPAO) is used for this application.
^{133}Xe can be used on its own as a method of measuring regional cerebral blood
flow.
Ch. 97 The Skull and Brain: Methods of Examination and Anatomy, p. 2310.

C. False The resolution of PET is better than SPECT.
Ch. 97 The Skull and Brain: Methods of Examination and Anatomy, p. 2310.

D. True

Ch. 97 The Skull and Brain: Methods of Examination and Anatomy, p. 2310.

E. True This occurs as a result of the magnetic susceptibility effects of
oxyhaemaglobin. Oxyhaemaglobin is diamagnetic and during cortical
activation there is an increase in cerebral blood flow, which results in a net
increase in oxyhaemaglobin in the vicinity of activated brain. This results in a
tiny increase in MRI signal.
Ch. 97 The Skull and Brain: Methods of Examination and Anatomy, p. 2310.

Q **9.14** **Regarding cranial angiography**

    A. The origin of the external carotid artery lies anterior and medial to that of the internal carotid artery.

    B. Selective vertebral arterial injection causes patients to experience flashing lights in their eyes.

    C. The anterior choroidal artery supplies posterior limb of internal capsule and optic tract.

    D. Vertebral artery enters the foramen transversarium of the 7th cervical vertebra in the majority of cases.

    E. The left vertebral artery is larger than the right in 80% of cases.

Q **9.15** **Typical technical parameters used for spiral CT angiography of the extra cranial and intra cranial vessels are**

    A. Slice collimation of 5 mm.

    B. Table speed of 6 mm/s.

    C. Reconstruction interval of 5 mm.

    D. Gantry rotation time of 3 s.

    E. Injection of 120 ml of contrast medium at a rate of 10ml/s.

(Answers overleaf)

375

A **9.14** Regarding cranial angiography

A. True This is the case in the majority of cases.
Ch. 97 The Skull and Brain: Methods of Examination and Anatomy, p. 2311.

B. True Patients should be warned of this prior to the injection.
Ch. 97 The Skull and Brain: Methods of Examination and Anatomy, p. 2311.

C. True It also supplies the cerebral peduncle, medial temporal lobe and choroid plexus.
Ch. 97 The Skull and Brain: Methods of Examination and Anatomy, p. 2315.

D. False The vertebral artery arises as the first branch of the corresponding subclavian artery and enters the foramen transversarium at C6, subsequently running cranially in the bony vertebral canal formed by these foramina.
Ch. 97 The Skull and Brain: Methods of Examination and Anatomy, p. 2316.

E. True When one of the arteries is very small it is frequently supplied by the ipsilateral posterior inferior cerebellar artery territory. This is called a PICA termination of the vertebral artery.
Ch. 97 The Skull and Brain: Methods of Examination and Anatomy, p. 2316.

A **9.15** Typical technical parameters used for spiral CT angiography of the extra cranial and intra cranial vessels are

A. False The slice collimation of 2 mm per second or less is appropriate.
Ch. 97 The Skull and Brain: Methods of Examination and Anatomy, p. 2312.

B. False Table speed of 3 mm/s is required for optimal resolution.
Ch. 97 The Skull and Brain: Methods of Examination and Anatomy, p. 2312.

C. False A reconstruction interval of 1 mm is required to optimize image detail.
Ch. 97 The Skull and Brain: Methods of Examination and Anatomy, p. 2312.

D. False Gantry rotation time of 0.75 s is a typical rate.
Ch. 97 The Skull and Brain: Methods of Examination and Anatomy, p. 2312.

E. False An injection of 120 ml at a rate of 3 ml/s allows for a 40-s injection that accommodates variations in circulation time in most patients.
Ch. 97 The Skull and Brain: Methods of Examination and Anatomy, p. 2312.

Q **9.16** **Principal anastomotic pathways of collateral arterial supply to brain occur via**

    A. Facial arteries.
    B. Superficial temporal artery.
    C. Superior thyroid artery.
    D. Artery of foramen rotundum.
    E. Occipital artery.

Q **9.17** **Persistent caroticovertebral anastomoses include**

    A. Retroaxial intersegmental artery.
    B. Hypoglossal artery.
    C. The optic artery.
    D. Trigeminal artery.
    E. The ambient artery of Labbé.

(Answers overleaf)

A **9.16** **Principal anastomotic pathways of collateral arterial supply to brain occur via**

A. True This anastomoses with the ophthalmic artery.
Ch. 97 The Skull and Brain: Methods of Examination and Anatomy, p. 2318.

B. True This anastomoses with the ophthalmic artery.
Ch. 97 The Skull and Brain: Methods of Examination and Anatomy, p. 2318.

C. False This does not contribute to an anastomotic pathway to any major extent.
Ch. 97 The Skull and Brain: Methods of Examination and Anatomy, p. 2318.

D. True This anastomoses with the carotid siphon.
Ch. 97 The Skull and Brain: Methods of Examination and Anatomy, p. 2319.

E. True This anastomoses with the vertebral artery.
Ch. 97 The Skull and Brain: Methods of Examination and Anatomy, p. 2319.

A **9.17** **Persistent caroticovertebral anastomoses include**

A. False The pro-atlanto intersegmental artery is a branch of the cervical internal carotid artery that joins the vertebral artery via the foramen magnum.
Ch. 97 The Skull and Brain: Methods of Examination and Anatomy, p. 2319.

B. True This internal carotid arterial branch anastomoses with the vertebral artery via the hypoglossal canal.
Ch. 97 The Skull and Brain: Methods of Examination and Anatomy, p. 2319.

C. False The otic (not optic) artery is a very rare branch of the petrous internal carotid artery that enters the basilar artery via the internal auditory meatus.
Ch. 97 The Skull and Brain: Methods of Examination and Anatomy, p. 2319.

D. True This is a branch of the precavernous internal carotid artery that terminates in the basilar artery.
Ch. 97 The Skull and Brain: Methods of Examination and Anatomy, p. 2319.

E. False Remember when there is negative marking of MCQs *never* make a wild guess.
Ch. 97 The Skull and Brain: Methods of Examination and Anatomy, p. 2319.

Q 9.18   Concerning intracranial venous anatomy

A.   The straight sinus is formed by the confluence of the vein of Galen and the inferior sagittal sinus.

B.   The superior petrosal sinus drains into the jugular bulb.

C.   The great vein of Galen is formed by the confluence of the internal cerebral and both basal veins of Rosenthal.

D.   The internal cerebral vein is formed by the junction of the septal veins and the thalamostriate veins.

E.   The cerebellar hemispheres are drained by veins that usually enter the transverse sinuses.

Q 9.19   Haemorrhagic cerebral lesions are commonly caused by

A.   Metastases from prostatic carcinoma.

B.   Metastases from bronchogenic carcinoma.

C.   Glioblastoma multiforme.

D.   Oligodendroglioma.

E.   Teratoma.

(Answers overleaf)

379

A **9.18**   **Concerning intracranial venous anatomy**

A. True

> *Ch. 97 The Skull and Brain: Methods of Examination and Anatomy, p. 2319.*

B. False   The inferior petrosal sinus drains into the jugular bulb. The superior petrosal sinus extends from the cavernous sinus to the sigmoid sinus.

> *Ch. 97 The Skull and Brain: Methods of Examination and Anatomy, p. 2319.*

C. True

> *Ch. 97 The Skull and Brain: Methods of Examination and Anatomy, p. 2320.*

D. True

> *Ch. 97 The Skull and Brain: Methods of Examination and Anatomy, p. 2320.*

E. True

> *Ch. 97 The Skull and Brain: Methods of Examination and Anatomy, p. 2321.*

A **9.19**   **Haemorrhagic cerebral lesions are commonly caused by**

A. False

> *Ch. 98 Cranial and Intracranial Pathology (1): Intracranial Tumours in Adults, p. 2327.*

B. True

> *Ch. 98 Cranial and Intracranial Pathology (1): Intracranial Tumours in Adults, p. 2327.*

C. True

> *Ch. 98 Cranial and Intracranial Pathology (1): Intracranial Tumours in Adults, p. 2327.*

D. True

> *Ch. 98 Cranial and Intracranial Pathology (1): Intracranial Tumours in Adults, p. 2327.*

E. False   Teratoma often calcifies but haemorrhage is very uncommon.

> *Ch. 98 Cranial and Intracranial Pathology (1): Intracranial Tumours in Adults, p. 2327.*

Q **9.20** Regarding the imaging of brain tumours

A. Perfusion-weighted MRI measuring relative cerebral blood volume discriminates radiation necrosis from active tumour.

B. Overall metastases are commoner than primary brain tumours.

C. Glioblastoma multiforme is the commonest primary intracranial neoplasm in adults.

D. Signal loss on T2-weighted MRI in an oligodendroglioma is caused by calcification or haemorrhage.

E. On unenhanced CT, primary cerebral lymphoma appears hyperdense.

Q **9.21** Regarding brain tumours

A. Pineal region tumours are commoner in adults.

B. Ependymoma appears as a partially calcified tumour with heterogeneous enhancement on CT.

C. The majority of haemangioblastomas occur in associated with von Hippel-Lindau disease.

D. Enlargement of the internal auditory meatus is more common in acoustic schwannoma than meningioma.

E. Vestibular schwannomas almost always show marked enhancement with intravenous contrast medium.

(Answers overleaf)

A **9.20**   Regarding the imaging of brain tumours

A. True   This is emerging as a useful technique in brain tumours that shows that high-grade tumours have a more marked increase in relative cerebral blood volume that low-grade tumours and radiation necrosis shows a degree of cerebral blood volume compared to active tumours.
Ch. 98 Cranial and Intracranial Pathology (1): Intracranial Tumours in Adults, p. 2327.

B. False   Approximately two-thirds of all brain tumours are primary cerebral neoplasms and one-third are metastases.
Ch. 98 Cranial and Intracranial Pathology (1): Intracranial Tumours in Adults, p. 2328.

C. True
Ch. 98 Cranial and Intracranial Pathology (1): Intracranial Tumours in Adults, p. 2329.

D. True
Ch. 98 Cranial and Intracranial Pathology (1): Intracranial Tumours in Adults, p. 2331.

E. True
Ch. 98 Cranial and Intracranial Pathology (1): Intracranial Tumours in Adults, p. 2333.

A **9.21**   Regarding brain tumours

A. False   They account for 1% of adult intracranial tumours and 10% of paediatric brain tumours.
Ch. 98 Cranial and Intracranial Pathology (1): Intracranial Tumours in Adults, p. 2333.

B. True
Ch. 98 Cranial and Intracranial Pathology (1): Intracranial Tumours in Adults, p. 2335.

C. False   About 20% of these tumours are associated with this phakomatosis in which the lesions are often multiple.
Ch. 98 Cranial and Intracranial Pathology (1): Intracranial Tumours in Adults, p. 2336.

D. True
Ch. 98 Cranial and Intracranial Pathology (1): Intracranial Tumours in Adults, p. 2337.

E. True
Ch. 98 Cranial and Intracranial Pathology (1): Intracranial Tumours in Adults, p. 2339.

Q **9.22** Concerning primary tumours in the sellar and parasellar region

A. Pituitary macroadenoma rarely enhances strongly.

B. Trigeminal Schwannoma is usually hyperintense on both T1- and T2-weighted images.

C. Nodular enhancement, calcification and cysts are features of crangiopharyngioma.

D. The Rathke's cleft cyst is hyper intense on T1-weighted MRI.

E. Germ cell tumours are often located in the midline.

Q **9.23** Regarding stroke imaging

A. Haemorrhagic transformation appears hypo intense on T1- and hyper intense on T2-weighted imaging.

B. Serial MR perfusion scans show an increase of relative cerebral blood volume in the infarcted region in the subacute stage.

C. Evanescent high signal in the cortical spinal tract on T2-weighting occurs in Wallerian degeneration.

D. Infarction in the middle cerebral artery territory involves the superior temporal lobe.

E. Haemorrhagic and multi-focal lesions are suggestive of venous infarction.

(Answers overleaf)

A **9.22** Concerning primary tumours in the sellar and parasellar region

A. False Strong enhancement is a typical feature.
Ch. 98 Cranial and Intracranial Pathology (1): Intracranial Tumours in Adults, p. 2342.

B. False It is usually hypo intense on T1 and hyper intense on T2, and exhibits strong enhancement with gadolinium.
Ch. 98 Cranial and Intracranial Pathology (1): Intracranial Tumours in Adults, p. 2342.

C. True
Ch. 98 Cranial and Intracranial Pathology (1): Intracranial Tumours in Adults, p. 2342.

D. True
Ch. 98 Cranial and Intracranial Pathology (1): Intracranial Tumours in Adults, p. 2342.

E. True
Ch. 98 Cranial and Intracranial Pathology (1): Intracranial Tumours in Adults, p. 2342.

A **9.23** Regarding stroke imaging

A. False This indicates secondary bleeding into an ischaemic zone that occurs during the first 2 weeks and is probably due to reperfusion of the infarcted area. Haemorrhagic transformation appears hyper intense on T1 and hypo intense on T2-weighted images
Ch. 99A Cranial and Intracranial Pathology (2): Cerebrovascular Disease and Nontraumatic Intracranial Haemorrhage, p. 2355.

B. True This is often associated with recanalization of the occluded vessel on MRA, which is subsequently followed by a decrease in the relative cerebral blood volume in the chronic phase.
Ch. 99A Cranial and Intracranial Pathology (2): Cerebrovascular Disease and Nontraumatic Intracranial Haemorrhage, p. 2355.

C. True
Ch. 99A Cranial and Intracranial Pathology (2): Cerebrovascular Disease and Nontraumatic Intracranial Haemorrhage, p. 2356.

D. True
Ch. 99A Cranial and Intracranial Pathology (2): Cerebrovascular Disease and Nontraumatic Intracranial Haemorrhage, p. 2358.

E. True
Ch. 99A Cranial and Intracranial Pathology (2): Cerebrovascular Disease and Nontraumatic Intracranial Haemorrhage, p. 2358.

Q 9.24 **Lesions commonly simulating cerebral infarcts on axial CT and MRI include**

- **A.** Mineralizing angiopathy.
- **B.** Glioma.
- **C.** Dysembryoblastic neuroepithelial tumour.
- **D.** Gangliocytoma.
- **E.** Progressive multifocal leucoencephalopathy.

Q 9.25 **Regarding subarachnoid haemorrhage**

- **A.** If subarachnoid blood is confined to the perimesencephalic area, cerebral angiography is likely to be positive.
- **B.** A patient with subarachnoid haemorrhage whose angiogram does not show an aneurysm has a worse long-term prognosis than if the angiogram was positive.
- **C.** Presence of high signal FLAIR images in the pontine cistern and around the ventricular foramina indicates subarachnoid haemorrhage.
- **D.** High signal on T1-weighted images caused by methaemoglobin persists longer than hyper density of acute subarachnoid haemorrhage on CT.
- **E.** Fusiform cerebral aneurysms become clinically manifest through mass effect rather than rupture.

(Answers overleaf)

A 9.24 Lesions commonly simulating cerebral infarcts on axial CT and MRI imaging include

A. False Tramline calcification in this entity has quite a characteristic appearance.
Ch. 99A Cranial and Intracranial Pathology (2): Cerebrovascular Disease and Nontraumatic Intracranial Haemorrhage, p. 2360.

B. True
Ch. 99A Cranial and Intracranial Pathology (2): Cerebrovascular Disease and Nontraumatic Intracranial Haemorrhage, p. 2360.

C. True
Ch. 99A Cranial and Intracranial Pathology (2): Cerebrovascular Disease and Nontraumatic Intracranial Haemorrhage, p. 2360.

D. True
Ch. 99A Cranial and Intracranial Pathology (2): Cerebrovascular Disease and Nontraumatic Intracranial Haemorrhage, p. 2360.

E. True An early presentation of this condition can simulate infarction.
Ch. 99A Cranial and Intracranial Pathology (2): Cerebrovascular Disease and Nontraumatic Intracranial Haemorrhage, p. 2360.

A 9.25 Regarding subarachnoid haemorrhage

A. False This may be caused by bleeding from a perimesencephalic vein and is often the cause of an angiogram-negative subarachnoid haemorrhage.
Ch. 99A Cranial and Intracranial Pathology (2): Cerebrovascular Disease and Nontraumatic Intracranial Haemorrhage, p. 2365.

B. False The prognosis is better and there is a low risk of further bleeding.
Ch. 99A Cranial and Intracranial Pathology (2): Cerebrovascular Disease and Nontraumatic Intracranial Haemorrhage, p. 2365.

C. False Flow artefacts cause these changes and need to be interpreted with caution.
Ch. 99A Cranial and Intracranial Pathology (2): Cerebrovascular Disease and Nontraumatic Intracranial Haemorrhage, p. 2366.

D. True
Ch. 99A Cranial and Intracranial Pathology (2): Cerebrovascular Disease and Nontraumatic Intracranial Haemorrhage, p. 2366.

E. True
Ch. 99A Cranial and Intracranial Pathology (2): Cerebrovascular Disease and Nontraumatic Intracranial Haemorrhage, p. 2366.

Q **9.26**   Regarding saccular cerebral aneurysms

A. Clot in the septum pellucidum is virtually diagnostic of anterior cerebral arterial haemorrhage.

B. Basilar artery tip aneurysms frequently present with mass effect.

C. Areas of increased signal intensity on MRI indicate turbulent slow flow or thrombus.

D. Oncotic aneurysms occur more peripherally than Berry aneurysms.

E. Mycotic aneurysms rarely present with haemorrhage.

Q **9.27**   Regarding intracerebral haemorrhage

A. Peripheral or lobal haemorrhages in the elderly, particularly if they are multi-focal, are suggestive of amyloidosis.

B. Preferential site of hypertensive haemorrhage is basal ganglia, thalamus and pons.

C. Acute haemorrhage reaches around 100 HU on CT.

D. In severely anaemic patients, haematoma are isodense with surrounding brain.

E. In early subacute haemorrhage intrasellar methaemoglobin is hyper intense on T2-weighted on MRI.

(Answers overleaf)

A **9.26** Regarding saccular cerebral aneurysms

A. False Bleeding from an aneurysm arising in the anterior communicating artery causes this sign.
Ch. 99A Cranial and Intracranial Pathology (2): Cerebrovascular Disease and Nontraumatic Intracranial Haemorrhage, p. 2367.

B. True
Ch. 99A Cranial and Intracranial Pathology (2): Cerebrovascular Disease and Nontraumatic Intracranial Haemorrhage, p. 2367.

C. True
Ch. 99A Cranial and Intracranial Pathology (2): Cerebrovascular Disease and Nontraumatic Intracranial Haemorrhage, p. 2368.

D. True Both mycotic and oncotic aneurysms are caused by septic or malignant emboli tend to occur more peripherally than Berry aneurysms, particularly on the MCA branches.
Ch. 99A Cranial and Intracranial Pathology (2): Cerebrovascular Disease and Nontraumatic Intracranial Haemorrhage, p. 2368.

E. False This is their commonest mode of presentation. A peripheral intraparencymal clot, while not specific, is highly suggestive of such a lesion in a patient with known septicaemia or bacterial endocarditis.
Ch. 99A Cranial and Intracranial Pathology (2): Cerebrovascular Disease and Nontraumatic Intracranial Haemorrhage, p. 2368.

A **9.27** Regarding intracerebral haemorrhage

A. False This is suggestive of amyloid angiopathy.
Ch. 99A Cranial and Intracranial Pathology (2): Cerebrovascular Disease and Nontraumatic Intracranial Haemorrhage, p. 2369.

B. True
Ch. 99A Cranial and Intracranial Pathology (2): Cerebrovascular Disease and Nontraumatic Intracranial Haemorrhage, p. 2369.

C. True
Ch. 99A Cranial and Intracranial Pathology (2): Cerebrovascular Disease and Nontraumatic Intracranial Haemorrhage, p. 2369.

D. True
Ch. 99A Cranial and Intracranial Pathology (2): Cerebrovascular Disease and Nontraumatic Intracranial Haemorrhage, p. 2369.

E. False It is hyper intense on T1-weighted images but hypo intense on T2-weighted images.
Ch. 99A Cranial and Intracranial Pathology (2): Cerebrovascular Disease and Nontraumatic Intracranial Haemorrhage, p. 2369.

Q **9.28** Concerning MRI signal characteristics of intracerebral haemorrhage

A. In the first few hours deoxyhaemoglobin is the predominant form of haem iron.

B. Late subacute extra cellular methaemaglobin is hyper intense on T1- and T2-weighted images.

C. Deoxyhaemaglobin is hypointense on T2-weighted images.

D. Intracellular methaemaglobin is hypo intense on T2-weighted images.

E. $T2^*$-weighted images are more sensitive to deoxyhaemaglobin and haemosiderin.

Q **9.29** Regarding brain infection

A. Brain abscesses are most often staphylococcal.

B. High-density contents on unenhanced CT favours abscess over tumour.

C. Flecks of calcification in the basal cisterns are a sign of infection with tuberculosis.

D. Tuberculous arteritis causes cerebral infarction most frequently in the basal ganglia.

E. Continued contrast enhancement of an abscess capsule indicates active infection.

(Answers overleaf)

A **9.28** Concerning MRI signal characteristics of intracerebral haemorrhage

A. False Oxyhaemaglobin is the predominant form in the hyperacute phase.
Ch. 99A Cranial and Intracranial Pathology (2): Cerebrovascular Disease and Nontraumatic Intracranial Haemorrhage, p. 2370.

B. True This is because of methaemaglobin content.
Ch. 99A Cranial and Intracranial Pathology (2): Cerebrovascular Disease and Nontraumatic Intracranial Haemorrhage, p. 2370.

C. True
Ch. 99A Cranial and Intracranial Pathology (2): Cerebrovascular Disease and Nontraumatic Intracranial Haemorrhage, p. 2370.

D. True It is hyper intense on T1-weighted images.
Ch. 99A Cranial and Intracranial Pathology (2): Cerebrovascular Disease and NontraumaticIntracranial Haemorrhage, p. 2370.

E. True
Ch. 99A Cranial and Intracranial Pathology (2): Cerebrovascular Disease and Nontraumatic Intracranial Haemorrhage, p. 2370.

A **9.29** Regarding brain infection

A. False Streptococcus is the usual organism.
Ch. 99A Cranial and Intracranial Pathology (2): Cerebrovascular Disease and Nontraumatic Intracranial Haemorrhage, p. 2377.

B. False Abscesses do not usually contain material of high density before injecting contrast media.
Ch. 99A Cranial and Intracranial Pathology (2): Cerebrovascular Disease and Nontraumatic Intracranial Haemorrhage, p. 2378.

C. True A chronic granulomatous reaction in the basal cistern tracks along the major arteries with a consequent arteritis.
Ch. 99A Cranial and Intracranial Pathology (2): Cerebrovascular Disease and Nontraumatic Intracranial Haemorrhage, p. 2379.

D. True
Ch. 99A Cranial and Intracranial Pathology (2): Cerebrovascular Disease and Nontraumatic Intracranial Haemorrhage, p. 2379.

E. False Prolonged enhancement of an abscess rim occurs even though the contents are sterile.
Ch. 99A Cranial and Intracranial Pathology (2): Cerebrovascular Disease and Nontraumatic Intracranial Haemorrhage, p. 2379.

Q **9.30** Regarding viral infection of the central nervous system

A. Focal haemorrhage in the anterior temporal lobe is a sign of herpes simplex encephalitis.

B. Severe regional cerebral atrophy is a sign of previous herpes encephalitis.

C. Cerebellum and brain stem are spared the atrophic changes of HIV encephalopathy.

D. Cytomegalovirus causes a necrotizing ventriculitis.

E. Moderate enhancement and mass effect are the earliest changes of HIV encephalopathy on MRI.

Q **9.31** The differential diagnosis of 'target' lesions on MRI include

A. Systemic lupus erythematosus.

B. Anti-phospholipid syndrome.

C. Sardoidosis.

D. Multiple sclerosis.

E. Behçet's syndrome.

(Answers overleaf)

A **9.30** **Regarding viral infection of the central nervous system**

A. True

Ch. 99A Cranial and Intracranial Pathology (2): Cerebrovascular Disease and Nontraumatic Intracranial Haemorrhage, p. 2380.

B. True

Ch. 99A Cranial and Intracranial Pathology (2): Cerebrovascular Disease and Nontraumatic Intracranial Haemorrhage, p. 2380.

C. False Cerebral atrophy is its commonest radiological manifestation but the cerebellum and brain stem are also involved.

Ch. 99A Cranial and Intracranial Pathology (2): Cerebrovascular Disease and Nontraumatic Intracranial Haemorrhage, p. 2382.

D. True

Ch. 99A Cranial and Intracranial Pathology (2): Cerebrovascular Disease and Nontraumatic Intracranial Haemorrhage, p. 2382.

E. False This is the slowly progressive white matter disease that is characterized by poorly defined hyper intense lesions on T2-weighted images unaccompanied by enhancement or mass effect.

Ch. 99A Cranial and Intracranial Pathology (2): Cerebrovascular Disease and Nontraumatic Intracranial Haemorrhage, p. 2382.

A **9.31** **The differential diagnosis of 'target' lesions on MRI include**

A. True

Ch. 99A Cranial and Intracranial Pathology (2): Cerebrovascular Disease and Nontraumatic Intracranial Haemorrhage, p. 2389.

B. True

Ch. 99A Cranial and Intracranial Pathology (2): Cerebrovascular Disease and Nontraumatic Intracranial Haemorrhage, p. 2389.

C. True

Ch. 99A Cranial and Intracranial Pathology (2): Cerebrovascular Disease and Nontraumatic Intracranial Haemorrhage, p. 2389.

D. True

Ch. 99A Cranial and Intracranial Pathology (2): Cerebrovascular Disease and Nontraumatic Intracranial Haemorrhage, p. 2389.

E. True

Ch. 99A Cranial and Intracranial Pathology (2): Cerebrovascular Disease and Nontraumatic Intracranial Haemorrhage, p. 2389.

Q **9.32** Regarding cranial trauma

  A. Bubbles of air outlining the brain are likely to lie in the subarachnoid space.
  B. Diffuse axonal injury predominantly involves the grey matter initially.
  C. Traumatic caroticocavernous fistula most commonly drains to the inferior orbital vein.
  D. A hyperdense comma shape on the tentorium is a sign of interhemispheric subdural haematoma on CT.
  E. All isodense haematomas are subacute.

Q **9.33** Regarding spinal anatomy and imaging techniques

  A. Intervertebral foramina contain epidural fat.
  B. The anterior epidural space lies between the posterior longitudinal ligament and the posterior surface of the vertebral body.
  C. The dura matter is separated from the anterior cortex of the spinous processes by the anterior internal vertebral veins.
  D. Lumbar puncture should be performed through a laminectomy scar because of the technical ease and improved patient comfort.
  E. Epilepsy is a contra-indication for myelography with non-ionic contrast media.

(Answers overleaf)

A **9.32** **Regarding cranial trauma**

A. True This indicates that the leptomeninges have been torn.
Ch. 100 Cranial and Intracranial Pathology (3): Trauma, Bone Pathology, CSF Disturbances, Degenerative Disorders, Epilepsy, p. 2395.

B. False It affects the white matter including the corpus callosum.
Ch. 100 Cranial and Intracranial Pathology (3): Trauma, Bone Pathology, CSF Disturbances, Degenerative Disorders, Epilepsy, p. 2398.

C. False The commonest draining vein is the superior ophthalmic vein that is associated with enlargement of one or both superior orbital fissures.
Ch. 100 Cranial and Intracranial Pathology (3): Trauma, Bone Pathology, CSF Disturbances, Degenerative Disorders, Epilepsy, p. 2400.

D. True
Ch. 100 Cranial and Intracranial Pathology (3): Trauma, Bone Pathology, CSF Disturbances, Degenerative Disorders, Epilepsy, p. 2396.

E. False New bleeds can be isodense in a very anaemic patient, and continual leakage of blood into a chronic haematoma can make it isodense.
Ch. 100 Cranial and Intracranial Pathology (3): Trauma, Bone Pathology, CSF Disturbances, Degenerative Disorders, Epilepsy, p. 2396.

A **9.33** **Regarding spinal anatomy and imaging techniques**

A. True
Ch. 101 The Spine: Methods of Examination, p. 2418.

B. True
Ch. 101 The Spine: Methods of Examination, p. 2419.

C. False The dura matter is usually loosely attached to the anterior cortex of the spinous processes. The anterior epidural space contains the anterior internal vertebral vein as well as the basivertebral veins.
Ch. 101 The Spine: Methods of Examination, p. 2419.

D. False A laminectomy scar should be avoided wherever possible because of the risk of chronic and occult postoperative infection. Furthermore, adhesion of neural structures and arachnoiditis at such a site is sufficiently common for attempts at puncture to be an excruciatingly painful experience for the patient.
Ch. 101 The Spine: Methods of Examination, p. 2421.

E. False
Ch. 101 The Spine: Methods of Examination, p. 2423.

Q **9.34** Concerning the vascular supply to the spinal cord

A. Paired postero-medial arteries supply the posterior cord.
B. In the lower cervical region the major contribution to the anterior spinal artery is from common carotid arterial branches.
C. The sulcocommisural artery is usually formed by penetrating branches of the postero-lateral spinal arteries.
D. The deep cervical artery is usually a branch of the innominate artery.
E. Arteria radicularis magna of Adamkiewicz is usually right sided between T8 and L1/2 level.

Q **9.35** Concerning developmental abnormalities of the spine

A. Intramedullary lipoma is most oftenly found in the lumbo-sacral area.
B. Intraspinal neurenteric cysts may contain intrathecal contrast medium on delayed CT cisternography.
C. In diastematomyelia a separate anterior spinal artery supplies each hemicord.
D. The Chiari I malformation is an acquired lesion.
E. Most cases of diastematomyelia occur in the thoracic cord.

Q **9.36** Features of neurofibromatosis type I on plain film include

A. Absence of spinal pedicles.
B. C1/2 subluxation.
C. Anterior scalloping of a vertebral body.
D. Absent superior orbital fissure.
E. Scoliosis concave to the side of the neurofibroma.

(Answers overleaf)

A **9.34** Concerning the vascular supply to the spinal cord

A. False The two posterior spinal arteries are postero-lateral in position.
Ch. 101 The Spine: Methods of Examination, p. 2424.

B. False Deep cervical and vertebral arterial branches supply the cord in the lower cervical region.
Ch. 101 The Spine: Methods of Examination, p. 2424.

C. False These arteries arise from the anterior spinal artery.
Ch. 101 The Spine: Methods of Examination, p. 2424.

D. False It usually arises from the subclavian artery.
Ch. 101 The Spine: Methods of Examination, p. 2424.

E. False The level of origin is variable but it is usually on the left side between T8 and L1/2.
Ch. 101 The Spine: Methods of Examination, p. 2424.

A **9.35** Concerning developmental abnormalities of the spine

A. False These lesions occur most often in the thoraco-cervical or cranio-vertebral junctions.
Ch. 102 The Imaging of Spinal Pathology, p. 2430.

B. True
Ch. 102 The Imaging of Spinal Pathology, p. 2430.

C. True
Ch. 102 The Imaging of Spinal Pathology, p. 2430.

D. True
Ch. 102 The Imaging of Spinal Pathology, p. 2430.

E. True
Ch. 102 The Imaging of Spinal Pathology, p. 2430.

A **9.36** Features of neurofibromatosis type I on plain film include

A. True
Ch. 102 The Imaging of Spinal Pathology, p. 2434.

B. True
Ch. 102 The Imaging of Spinal Pathology, p. 2434.

C. False
Ch. 102 The Imaging of Spinal Pathology, p. 2434.

D. True
Ch. 98 Cranial and Intracranial Pathology (1): Intracranial Tumours in Adults, p. 2347.

E. False The scoliosis is caused by dysplasia not neurofibroma.
Ch. 102 The Imaging of Spinal Pathology, p. 2434.

Q **9.37**   In syringomyelia

A. The spinal cord is usually smaller than normal.
B. Clinical disability is proportional to the size of the syrnix relative to remaining cord substance.
C. Involvement of the thoracic cord only is a feature.
D. Most syrinxes extend above C2.
E. Most cases are associated with cerebellar ectopia.

Q **9.38**   Regarding degenerative spinal disease

A. Posterior disc bulging greater than 4 mm is associated with annulus fibrosis fissures.
B. Disc protrusions usually breach the posterior longitudinal ligament.
C. Osteophytes narrow the spinal canal more frequently in the cervical than the lumbar region.
D. Ossification of the posterior longitudinal ligament occurs most commonly in the lumbar spine.
E. Synovial cysts occur most commonly in the thoracic spine.

Q **9.39**   Regarding intervertebral disc disease

A. On T2-weighting migratory fragments are rarely brighter than the nucleus of the disc of origin.
B. Myelography is more sensitive than CT at detecting far lateral disc protrusions.
C. Myelomalacia is not depicted by myelography.
D. Post-operative pseudomeningoceles imply breach of the dura during surgery.
E. Recurrent disc material is often enclosed in enhancing fibrous tissue.

(Answers overleaf)

A **9.37** **In syringomyelia**

A. False
> *Ch. 102 The Imaging of Spinal Pathology, p. 2435.*

B. False
> *Ch. 102 The Imaging of Spinal Pathology, p. 2435.*

C. True
> *Ch. 102 The Imaging of Spinal Pathology, p. 2435.*

D. False
> *Ch. 102 The Imaging of Spinal Pathology, p. 2435.*

E. True Between 70 and 90% of cases the cerebellar tonsils are low-lying usually at the level of C1 or between C1 and C2.
> *Ch. 102 The Imaging of Spinal Pathology, p. 2436.*

A **9.38** **Regarding degenerative spinal disease**

A. True
> *Ch. 102 The Imaging of Spinal Pathology, p. 2437.*

B. False
> *Ch. 102 The Imaging of Spinal Pathology, p. 2438.*

C. True
> *Ch. 102 The Imaging of Spinal Pathology, p. 2438.*

D. False It involves the mid and lower cervical regions in over 90% of cases.
> *Ch. 102 The Imaging of Spinal Pathology, p. 2438.*

E. False They usually occur in the lower lumbar or mid and lower cervical region.
> *Ch. 102 The Imaging of Spinal Pathology, p. 2439.*

A **9.39** **Regarding intervertebral disc disease**

A. False It is common for fragments to be conspicuously brighter than their nucleus of origin.
> *Ch. 102 The Imaging of Spinal Pathology, p. 2442*

B. False Most far lateral posterior disc protrusions will not be shown by myelography.
> *Ch. 102 The Imaging of Spinal Pathology, p. 2443.*

C. False Intramedullary contrast penetration and retention can be seen on myelography and even more sensitively on delayed post-myelography CT.
> *Ch. 102 The Imaging of Spinal Pathology, p. 2443.*

D. True
> *Ch. 102 The Imaging of Spinal Pathology, p. 2444.*

E. True
> *Ch. 102 The Imaging of Spinal Pathology, p. 2444.*

Q **9.40** **Common causes of metastases spreading via cerebral spinal fluid include**

    A. Neuroblastoma.
    B. Melanoma.
    C. Choriocarcinoma.
    D. Optic glioma
    E. Chordoma.

Q **9.41** **Regarding spinal tumours**

    A. Meningiomas are common in the lumbar spine.
    B. Heavily calcified intradural extra medullary mass is usually caused by a meningioma.
    C. Most intramedullary tumours are gliomas.
    D. Ependymoma metastasizes to the lung.
    E. Most intramedullary tumours have an associated cyst.

(Answers overleaf)

A **9.40** Common causes of metastases spreading via cerebral spinal fluid include

A. False

 Ch. 102 The Imaging of Spinal Pathology, p. 2445.

B. True

 Ch. 102 The Imaging of Spinal Pathology, p. 2446.

C. False

 Ch. 102 The Imaging of Spinal Pathology, p. 2447.

D. False

 Ch. 102 The Imaging of Spinal Pathology, p. 2446.

E. False

 Ch. 102 The Imaging of Spinal Pathology, p. 2446.

A **9.41** Regarding spinal tumours

A. False They are very rare in this location.
 Ch. 102 The Imaging of Spinal Pathology, p. 2448.

B. False Marked calcification is uncommon in meningiomas and hyperostosis is uncommon with spinal meningiomas because bone is rarely infiltrated.
 Ch. 102 The Imaging of Spinal Pathology, p. 2448.

C. True Ependymomas and astrocytomas occur with approximately equal frequency in the spinal cord.
 Ch. 102 The Imaging of Spinal Pathology, p. 2449.

D. True Rarely ependymomas arise from the extra dural part of the filum terminalae and present as a focus of sacral destruction which is prone to metastasize to the lung.
 Ch. 102 The Imaging of Spinal Pathology, p. 2449.

E. True

 Ch. 102 The Imaging of Spinal Pathology, p. 2450.

Q 9.42 Regarding inflammatory disorders of the spine

A. A pyogenic vertebral osteomyelitis is more likely to result in neurological involvement than tuberculous osteomyelitis.

B. Retropharyngeal sepsis is a cause of atlanto-axial subluxation.

C. Arachnoidits follows spinal subarachnoid haemorrhage.

D. Diffuse enhancement of the outer surface of the cord and spinal roof is a feature of Lyme's disease.

E. Acute myelitis is caused by infection with enterovirus.

Q 9.43 Regarding scoliosis

A. It is commoner in females.

B. It is defined as a Cobb angle of greater than 5%.

C. Plain radiographs should be taken AP.

D. MRI should be avoided as movement of stainless steel implants is hazardous.

E. Scoliosis is associated with oesophageal atresia.

(Answers overleaf)

A 9.42   Regarding inflammatory disorders of the spine

A. False   Neurological involvement results from intraspinal extension of infection or more rarely instability in only 1% of cases caused by pyogenic organisms but is much more common in tuberculous infection.
Ch. 102 The Imaging of Spinal Pathology, p. 2454.

B. True
Ch. 102 The Imaging of Spinal Pathology, p. 2454.

C. True
Ch. 102 The Imaging of Spinal Pathology, p. 2454.

D. True   There is an intense spinal meningitis that exhibits this appearance.
Ch. 102 The Imaging of Spinal Pathology, p. 2455.

E. True
Ch. 102 The Imaging of Spinal Pathology, p. 2456.

A 9.43   Regarding scoliosis

A. True
Ch. 103 Scoliosis, p. 2464.

B. False   A simple lateral curvature of the spine of 5% is classed as spinal asymmetry that is not unusual.
Ch. 103 Scoliosis, p. 2464.

C. False   The PA projection is used to reduce the radiation dose to breast tissue.
Ch. 103 Scoliosis, p. 2467.

D. False   Presence of stainless steel implants is not an absolute contraindication to MRI. Very poor images will be obtained, however, and the ferromagnetic quality of the implant may cause uncomfortable heat sensation.
Ch. 103 Scoliosis, p. 2467.

E. True   A group of anomalies grouped under the acronym VACTERLS (vertebral bars and blocks, Anus, Cardiac, Tracheal, oEsophageal atresia, Renal, Limb, Single umbilical artery).
Ch. 103 Scoliosis, p. 2467.

Q 9.44 Concerning neonatal ultrasound

A. On pulsed Doppler increased intracranial pressure is correlated with increased resistivity index.

B. Intraventricular haemorrhage has a similar appearance to choroid plexus.

C. Fusion of the two hemicords in diastematomyelia into a single distal cord is readily visible on ultrasound.

D. A low conus position below L1 is a characteristic finding of tethered cord on ultrasound.

E. Radial arrangement of medial cerebral sulci on ultrasound is a feature of agenesis of the corpus callosum.

Q 9.45 Common causes of obstructive hydrocephalus in children

A. Subarachnoid haemorrhage.

B. Tumour.

C. Aqueduct stenosis.

D. Arachnoid cyst.

E. Chiari malformation.

Q 9.46 Regarding congenital cerebral malformations

A. Anencephaly is an extreme form of hydrocephalus.

B. Anencephaly is the most common severe cerebral malformation in the foetus.

C. In Chiari II malformation interdigitation of gyri is a feature.

D. Holoprosencephaly is associated with maternal warfarin ingestion.

E. Megalencephaly is caused by on overproduction of neurones.

(Answers overleaf)

A **9.44**   **Concerning neonatal ultrasound**

A. True
        Ch. 104 Neonatal Head and Spine Ultrasound, p. 2470.

B. True   Both are strongly echogenic.
        Ch. 104 Neonatal Head and Spine Ultrasound, p. 2471.

C. True
        Ch. 104 Neonatal Head and Spine Ultrasound, p. 2474.

D. False   Conus position below L3 is associated with tethered cord.
        Ch. 104 Neonatal Head and Spine Ultrasound, p. 2474.

E. True
        Ch. 104 Neonatal Head and Spine Ultrasound, p. 2472.

A **9.45**   **Common causes of obstructive hydrocephalus in children**

A. False
        Ch. 105 Paediatric Neurology, p. 2484.

B. True
        Ch. 105 Paediatric Neurology, p. 2484.

C. True
        Ch. 105 Paediatric Neurology, p. 2484.

D. True
        Ch. 105 Paediatric Neurology, p. 2484.

E. False
        Ch. 105 Paediatric Neurology, p. 2484.

A **9.46**   **Regarding congenital cerebral malformations**

A. False   There is no cerebral mantle in anencephaly whereas one is usually visible even in extreme hydrocephalus
        Ch. 105 Paediatric Neurology, p. 2484.

B. True   It is incompatible with life. Most anencephalics are stillborn but some live for a few days.
        Ch. 105 Paediatric Neurology, p. 2484.

C. True   The falx is partially absent or fenestrated with consequent interdigitation of gyri across the midline.
        Ch. 105 Paediatric Neurology, p. 2487.

D. False   No such association exists.
        Ch. 105 Paediatric Neurology, p. 2487.

E. True
        Ch. 105 Paediatric Neurology, p 2489.

Q 9.47   Regarding the phakomatoses

A. The most frequent brain abnormality of neurofibromatosis type I is subependymal hamartoma.

B. Angiomyolipoma of the thyroid are seen in tuberous sclerosis.

C. Giant cell astrocytomas occur most commonly at the foramen of luschka.

D. Cortical hamartomas are pre-malignant.

E. Subependymal hamartomas have their long axis parallel to the ventricular wall.

Q 9.48   Concerning paediatric neuroimaging

A. If an intradural extramedullary tumour is found, brain examination is mandatory.

B. Gelastic seizures suggest the presence of underlying hypothalamic inflammatory demyelination.

C. Precocious puberty in boys always requires imaging.

D. Craniopharyngiomas cause growth retardation.

E. Medulloblastoma is a primitive neuroectodermal tumour.

(Answers overleaf)

405

A **9.47** Regarding the phakomatoses

A. False The most frequent abnormality is a Glial tumour of the optic pathways.
Ch. 105 Paediatric Neurology, p. 2489.

B. True Angiomyolipomas occur in the kidneys, liver, lungs, thyroid and testes.
Ch. 105 Paediatric Neurology, p. 2489.

C. False They are usually located at the foramen of monro where they cause obstructive hydrocephalus.
Ch. 105 Paediatric Neurology, p. 2489.

D. True
Ch. 105 Paediatric Neurology, p. 2490.

E. False In contrast to subependymal heterotpia of grey matter, subependymal hamartomas have their long axis perpendicular to the ventricular wall.
Ch. 105 Paediatric Neurology, p. 2489.

A **9.48** Concerning paediatric neuroimaging

A. True This is because of the possibility of metastases from haemangioblastoma.
Ch. 105 Paediatric Neuroradiology, p. 2495.

B. False Such seizures (e.g. inappropriate laughter at a funeral) are a sign of an underlying hypothalamic hamartoma.
Ch. 105 Paediatric Neurology, p. 2489.

C. True
Ch. 105 Paediatric Neurology, p. 2497.

D. True Even though they are non-secreting tumours the mass effect can impair the function of the pituitary – hypothalamic axis.
Ch. 105 Paediatric Neurology, p. 2497.

E. True
Ch. 105 Paediatric Neurology, p. 2497.

10 The orbit; ear, nose and throat; face and teeth

Q 10.1 Regarding the anatomy of the orbit

A. The arterial connection between middle meningeal and ophthalmic arteries passes through the superior orbital fissure.
B. The inferior orbital fissure contains the annulus of Zinn.
C. The periorbita is continuous with intracranial dura matter.
D. The lacrimal sac occupies an anterior depression in the lamina papyracea.
E. The four rectus muscles originate from the greater wing of sphenoid.

Q 10.2 Regarding orbital ultrasound

A. It may be useful to instil local anaesthetic into the eye before the examination.
B. The probe can be placed on the closed lid.
C. Colour Doppler flow imaging detects central retinal arterial occlusion.
D. Fifty megahertz is a suitable frequency for examination of the anterior segment.
E. Ultrasound is not useful for evaluation of the orbit outside the globe.

(Answers overleaf)

A **10.1** **Regarding the anatomy of the orbit**

A. **True**

> *Ch. 106 The Orbit; Ear, Nose and Throat; Face; Teeth. p. 2519*

B. **False** The annulus of Zinn describes the four rectus muscles (superior, inferior, medial and lateral), which form the muscle cone separating extra and intraconal spaces. These muscles originate on the inferior root of the lesser wing of sphenoid and are not contained within the inferior orbital fissure.
> *Ch. 106 The Orbit; Ear, Nose and Throat; Face; Teeth, p. 2520.*

C. **True**
> *Ch. 106 The Orbit; Ear, Nose and Throat; Face; Teeth, p. 2520.*

D. **True**
> *Ch. 106 The Orbit; Ear, Nose and Throat; Face; Teeth, p. 2519.*

E. **False** They originate from the lesser wing.
> *Ch. 106 The Orbit; Ear, Nose and Throat; Face; Teeth, p. 2520.*

A **10.2** **Regarding orbital ultrasound**

A. **True** Although ultrasound evaluation of the eye and orbit is a painless examination it is advisable to instil local anaesthetic into the eye first.
> *Ch. 106 The Orbit; Ear, Nose and Throat; Face; Teeth, p. 2521.*

B. **True** It can be placed directly on the conjunctiva or on the closed lid which is covered with some methyl cellulose gel.
> *Ch. 106 The Orbit; Ear, Nose and Throat; Face; Teeth, p. 2521.*

C. **True**
> *Ch. 106 The Orbit; Ear, Nose and Throat; Face; Teeth, p. 2521.*

D. **True** The use of very high-frequency probes and an immersion technique is mandatory to analyze anterior segment structures (cornea, iris, iridocorneal, ciliary body).
> *Ch. 106 The Orbit; Ear, Nose and Throat; Face; Teeth, p. 2523.*

E. **False**
> *Ch. 106 The Orbit; Ear, Nose and Throat; Face; Teeth, p. 2521.*

Q **10.3** **Regarding orbital pathology**

A. The modality of choice for diagnosing retinal detachment.
B. Diabetic retinopathy causes increased retinal thickness and hypo reflectivity on ultrasound.
C. Malignancy melanoma usually arises from the sclera.
D. Melanoma returns high signal relative to vitreous on T1-weighted MRI.
E. Metastases to the orbit most frequently involve the retina.

Q **10.4** **Regarding proptosis**

A. The commonest cause is Graves' ophthalmopathy.
B. Exophthalmos is caused by acromegaly.
C. It is usually unilateral.
D. Inferior and superior oblique muscles are most commonly involved.
E. Exophthalmos is caused by primary hyperadrenalism.

(Answers overleaf)

A **10.3** **Regarding orbital pathology**

A. True

Ch. 106 The Orbit; Ear, Nose and Throat; Face; Teeth, p. 2524.

B. True

Ch. 106 The Orbit; Ear, Nose and Throat; Face; Teeth, p. 2524.

C. False This highly malignant neoplasm arises in the choroid and its commonest symptomatic uveal tract tumour.
Ch. 106 The Orbit; Ear, Nose and Throat; Face; Teeth, p. 2524.

D. True The paramagnetic properties of melanin lead to a characteristic high signal on T1 weighted images an exception is amelanotic melanoma.
Ch. 106 The Orbit; Ear, Nose and Throat; Face; Teeth, p. 2525.

E. False Metastatic tumour is usually to the choroid. It is frequently found at autopsy but is often clinically silent. Carcinoma of the breast, lung and gastrointestinal tract are the usual primary site.
Ch. 106 The Orbit; Ear, Nose and Throat; Face; Teeth, p. 2525.

A **10.4** **Regarding proptosis**

A. True This is the most frequent cause of endocrine exophthalmos and the commonest cause of proptosis.
Ch. 106 The Orbit; Ear, Nose and Throat; Face; Teeth, p. 2529.

B. True

Ch. 106 The Orbit; Ear, Nose and Throat; Face; Teeth, p. 2529.

C. False Proptosis is bilateral in 70% of cases of Graves' ophthalmopathy and most commonly bilateral due to all causes.
Ch. 106 The Orbit; Ear, Nose and Throat; Face; Teeth, p. 2529.

D. False The four rectus muscles especially inferior rectus and superior rectus are most commonly enlarged.
Ch. 106 The Orbit; Ear, Nose and Throat; Face; Teeth, p. 2530.

E. True

Ch. 106 The Orbit; Ear, Nose and Throat; Face; Teeth, p. 2529.

Q **10.5**   Concerning orbital inflammation

A. The extra ocular muscles are the orbital structures most frequently involved by idiopathic pseudotumour.

B. Intense enhancement of sclera and optic nerve by IV gadolinium occurs in MRI of orbital tumour.

C. Ultrasound guided biopsy is usually required to differentiate orbital pseudotumour from lymphoma.

D. Orbital hydatid cysts are usually subconjuntival.

E. Involvement of the orbit by Wegener's granulomatosis occurs when disease spreads from the adjacent paranasal sinus.

Q **10.6**   Concerning the radiology of ENT disorders

A. The size of an acoustic neuroma is related to the degree of deafness.

B. The middle meatus receives mucosal drainage from all of the paranasal sinuses except the posterior ethmoid.

C. Nasal polyposis in children is associated with underlying cystic fibrosis.

D. Proptosis is caused by anterior ethmoid mucocele.

E. The presence of a nasal mass and widened pterygopalatine fissure in an adolescent male with epistaxis is pathognomonic of juvenile angiofibroma.

(Answers overleaf)

A **10.5** **Concerning orbital inflammation**

A. False The lacrimal gland is the orbital structure most frequently affected by this process.
Ch. 106 The Orbit; Ear, Nose and Throat; Face; Teeth, p. 2531.

B. True
Ch. 106 The Orbit; Ear, Nose and Throat; Face; Teeth, p. 2531.

C. False In practice the proof of the diagnosis is rapid sustained improvement with systemic steroid therapy when this fails biopsy may be used to differentiate orbital pseudotumour from lymphoma.
Ch. 106 The Orbit; Ear, Nose and Throat; Face; Teeth, p. 2530.

D. False Hydatid cysts are most often shown as a spherical or ovoid mass of low reflectivity on ultrasound and low density on CT, with or without calcification. These are retrobulbar in the vast majority of cases.
Ch. 106 The Orbit; Ear, Nose and Throat; Face; Teeth, p. 2530.

E. True Unilateral or bilateral retrobulbar masses may be seen in this condition.
Ch. 106 The Orbit; Ear, Nose and Throat; Face; Teeth, p. 2531.

A **10.6** **Concerning the radiology of ENT disorders**

A. False It bears no relationship.
Ch. 107 Ear, Nose and Throat Radiology, p. 2546.

B. False The sphenoid sinus drains into the sphenoethmoid recess.
Ch. 107 Ear, Nose and Throat Radiology, p. 2551.

C. True
Ch. 107 Ear, Nose and Throat Radiology, p. 2553.

D. True Posterior ethmoid mucocele may involve optic nerve and cause visual failure.
Ch. 107 Ear, Nose and Throat Radiology, p. 2554.

E. True
Ch. 107 Ear, Nose and Throat Radiology, p. 2556.

Q **10.7** Concerning imaging of head and neck pathology

A. Vagal neuromas can spread to infiltrate the carotid artery and internal jugular vein.
B. Lymphatic drainage from the infraglottis is to the upper deep cervical nodes.
C. Fractures of the zygoma involve the lateral wall of orbit, lateral wall of maxillary antrum, inferior wall of orbit and zygomatic arch.
D. In a 'blow-out' fracture of the orbit, the orbital rim remains intact.
E. Air outlining the eyeball is a sign of fracture involving the nasal cavity.

Q **10.8** Arthritides involving the TMJ include

A. Systemic lupus erythematosus.
B. Pigmented villonodular synovitis.
C. Psoriasis.
D. Enteropathic arthritis.
E. Reiter's syndrome.

Q **10.9** Regarding arthritis of the TMJ

A. In rheumatoid disease erosions usually affect the glenoid fossa.
B. In osteoarthritis sclerosis usually affects both sides of the joint.
C. In osteoarthritis, osteophytes arise only from the anterior aspect of the mandibular condyle.
D. Septic arthritis destroys the articular surface of the glenoid fossa.
E. Condylar erosions precede the development of osteoarthritis.

(Answers overleaf)

A **10.7** Concerning imaging of head and neck pathology

A. True   This is because of their site of origin within the carotid sheath. They have high T2-weighted signal and enhance avidly with IV contrast medium
Ch. 107 Ear, Nose and Throat Radiology, p. 2561.

B. False   The infraglottis drains to the inferior jugular, peritracheal and media nodes.
Ch. 108 Maxillofacial Radiology, p. 2575.

C. True   It is usually not possible to see all four on one film but if one is seen the others need to be looked for.
Ch. 108 Maxillofacial Radiology, p. 2575

D. True
Ch. 108 Maxillofacial Radiology, p. 2576

E. True   It is also seen when a fracture involves a paranasal sinus.
Ch. 108 Maxillofacial Radiology, p. 2577

A **10.8** Arthritides involving the TMJ include

A. True
Ch. 108 Maxillofacial Radiology p. 2580.

B. True
Ch. 108 Maxillofacial Radiology, p. 2580.

C. True
Ch. 108 Maxillofacial Radiology, p. 2580.

D. True
Ch. 108 Maxillofacial Radiology, p. 2580.

E. True
Ch. 108 Maxillofacial Radiology, p. 2580.

A **10.9** Regarding arthritis of the TMJ

A. False
Ch. 108 Maxillofacial Radiology, p. 2580.

B. False
Ch. 108 Maxillofacial Radiology, p. 2580.

C. True
Ch. 108 Maxillofacial Radiology, p. 2580.

D. True
Ch. 108 Maxillofacial Radiology, p. 2580.

E. True
Ch. 108 Maxillofacial Radiology, p. 2580.

Q **10.10** **Concerning radiology of the salivary glands**

A. Sialography should be routinely used to investigate mass lesions in the parotid gland.

B. Childhood parotid sialectasis is caused by calculus obstruction in over 50% of cases.

C. Sarcoidosis causes glandular enlargement with multiple areas of high attenuation on CT.

D. Multiple intraparotid cysts and enlarged neck nodes seen on ultrasound suggest underlying infection with mumps virus.

E. Perineural spread is a feature of adenoid cystic carcinoma.

(Answers overleaf)

A **10.10** Concerning radiology of the salivary glands

A. **False**

Ch. 108 Maxillofacial Radiology, p. 2582.

B. **False**

Ch. 108 Maxillofacial Radiology, p. 2584.

C. **True**

Ch. 108 Maxillofacial Radiology, p. 2584.

D. **False**

Ch. 108 Maxillofacial Radiology, p. 2585.

E. **True**

Ch. 108 Maxillofacial Radiology, p. 2585.